Agricultural Products Processing and Postharvest Storage

Agricultural Products Processing and Postharvest Storage

Editor

Bengang Wu

MDPI • Basel • Beijing • Wuhan • Barcelona • Belgrade • Manchester • Tokyo • Cluj • Tianjin

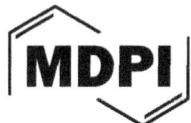

Editor
Bengang Wu
School of Food & Biological
Engineering, Jiangsu University,
Zhenjiang, China

Editorial Office
MDPI
St. Alban-Anlage 66
4052 Basel, Switzerland

This is a reprint of articles from the Special Issue published online in the open access journal *Agriculture* (ISSN 2077-0472) (available at: https://www.mdpi.com/journal/agriculture/special_issues/Agricultural_Products_Postharvest_Storage).

For citation purposes, cite each article independently as indicated on the article page online and as indicated below:

LastName, A.A.; LastName, B.B.; LastName, C.C. Article Title. *Journal Name* **Year**, *Volume Number*, Page Range.

ISBN 978-3-0365-7416-5 (Hbk)
ISBN 978-3-0365-7417-2 (PDF)

© 2023 by the authors. Articles in this book are Open Access and distributed under the Creative Commons Attribution (CC BY) license, which allows users to download, copy and build upon published articles, as long as the author and publisher are properly credited, which ensures maximum dissemination and a wider impact of our publications.

The book as a whole is distributed by MDPI under the terms and conditions of the Creative Commons license CC BY-NC-ND.

Contents

About the Editor vii

Preface to "Agricultural Products Processing and Postharvest Storage" ix

Goretti L. Díaz-Delgado, Elena M. Rodríguez-Rodríguez, Eva Dorta and M. Gloria Lobo
Effects of Peeling, Film Packaging, and Cold Storage on the Quality of Minimally Processed Prickly Pears (*Opuntia ficus-indica* L. Mill.)
Reprinted from: *Agriculture* 2022, 12, 281, doi:10.3390/agriculture12020281 1

Hao Hu, Shipeng Li, Danjie Pan, Kaijun Wang, Mingming Qiu, Zhuzhu Qiu, et al.
The Variation of Rice Quality and Relevant Starch Structure during Long-Term Storage
Reprinted from: *Agriculture* 2022, 12, 1211, doi:10.3390/agriculture12081211 19

Francileni Pompeu Gomes, Osvaldo Resende, Elisabete Piancó de Sousa, Juliana Aparecida Célia and Kênia Borges de Oliveira
Application of Mathematical Models and Thermodynamic Properties in the Drying of Jambu Leaves
Reprinted from: *Agriculture* 2022, 12, 1252, doi:10.3390/agriculture12081252 31

Kun Luo, Zhengmin Wu, Chengmao Cao, Kuan Qin, Xuechen Zhang and Minhui An
Biomechanical Characterization of Bionic Mechanical Harvesting of Tea Buds
Reprinted from: *Agriculture* 2022, 12, 1361, doi:10.3390/agriculture12091361 43

Xiulan Bao, Biyu Chen, Peng Dai, Yishu Li and Jincheng Mao
Construction and Verification of Spherical Thin Shell Model for Revealing Walnut Shell Crack Initiation and Expansion Mechanism
Reprinted from: *Agriculture* 2022, 12, 1446, doi:10.3390/agriculture12091446 57

Hong Zhang, Hualong Liu, Yong Zeng, Yurong Tang, Zhaoguo Zhang and Ji Che
Design and Performance Evaluation of a Multi-Point Extrusion Walnut Cracking Device
Reprinted from: *Agriculture* 2022, 12, 1494, doi:10.3390/agriculture12091494 71

Bengang Wu, Chengcheng Qiu, Yiting Guo, Chunhong Zhang, Dan Li, Kun Gao, et al.
Comparative Evaluation of Physicochemical Properties, Microstructure, and Antioxidant Activity of Jujube Polysaccharides Subjected to Hot Air, Infrared, Radio Frequency, and Freeze Drying
Reprinted from: *Agriculture* 2022, 12, 1606, doi:10.3390/agriculture12101606 89

Jun-Wen Bai, Yi Dai, Yu-Chi Wang, Jian-Rong Cai, Lu Zhang and Xiao-Yu Tian
Potato Slices Drying: Pretreatment Affects the Three-Dimensional Appearance and Quality Attributes
Reprinted from: *Agriculture* 2022, 12, 1841, doi:10.3390/agriculture12111841 103

Mattia Rapa, Vanessa Giannetti and Maurizio Boccacci Mariani
Characterization of Polyphenols in a Sicilian Autochthonous White Grape Variety (PDO) for Monitoring Production Process and Shelf-Life of Wines
Reprinted from: *Agriculture* 2022, 12, 1888, doi:10.3390/agriculture12111888 121

Haining Zhuang, Shiyi Liu, Kexin Wang, Rui Zhong, Joshua Harington Aheto, Junwen Bai and Xiaoyu Tian
Characterisation of Pasting, Structural and Volatile Properties of Potato Flour
Reprinted from: *Agriculture* 2022, 12, 1974, doi:10.3390/agriculture12121974 133

Dan Li, Dong Liang, Zhonghua Li, Yang Liu, Zhonghua Guo, Zhicai Wu, et al.
Efficacy of Gas-Containing Conditioning Technology on Sterilization and Preservation of Cooked Foods
Reprinted from: *Agriculture* **2022**, *12*, 2010, doi:10.3390/agriculture12122010 . . . . **147**

About the Editor

Bengang Wu

Bengang Wu, an associate professor, is now working in the School of Food Science and Biological Engineering of Jiangsu University, and is mainly engaged in the value-added processing of food and agricultural products, research on new technologies and their mechanisms, and the development of related equipment; the technologies involved are infrared technology (dry-blanching, drying, deinsectization, sterilization, etc.), ultrasonic technology (cleaning, thawing, proteolytic enzymolysis, active ingredient extraction, etc.), and drying technologies (infrared, microwave, hot air, spray, freeze-drying, etc.). He has published more than 40 papers in domestic and international journals, and his main publications include those in *Food Chemistry*, *Food Research International*, *LWT*, *Journal of Food Engineering*, etc.

Preface to "Agricultural Products Processing and Postharvest Storage"

The research-based articles included in this Special Issue of Agriculture—Basel—entitled "Agricultural Products Processing and Postharvest Storage" focus on the main problems in the processing and preservation of agricultural products, such as high energy consumption, high cost, low efficiency, environmental pollution, low product quality, etc. These articles propose constructive new processing techniques and establish mathematical models to predict and evaluate the processing, while exploring the underlying mechanisms, with a view to reduce bottlenecks in the processing and preservation of agricultural products and promote the upgrading and renewal of the agricultural industry.

Bengang Wu
Editor

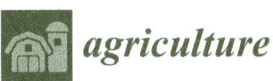

Article

Effects of Peeling, Film Packaging, and Cold Storage on the Quality of Minimally Processed Prickly Pears (*Opuntia ficus-indica* L. Mill.)

Goretti L. Díaz-Delgado [1], Elena M. Rodríguez-Rodríguez [2], Eva Dorta [1] and M. Gloria Lobo [1,*]

[1] Departamento de Producción Vegetal en Zonas Tropicales y Subtropicales, Instituto Canario de Investigaciones Agrarias, 38270 Tenerife, Spain; gdiaz@icia.es (G.L.D.-D.); edorta@icia.es (E.D.)
[2] Departamento de Ingeniería Química y Tecnología Farmacéutica, Universidad de La Laguna, 38296 Tenerife, Spain; emrguez@ull.edu.es
* Correspondence: globo@icia.es

Abstract: *Opuntia* species exhibit beneficial properties when used to treat chronic diseases, particularly obesity, diabetes, cardiovascular disease, and cancer; however, the presence of spines and glochids in the species' skin that easily stick into consumers' fingers has limited their consumption. For this study, white and orange *Opuntia ficus-indica* fruits from the Canary Islands (Spain) were minimally processed, packed in a passive atmosphere, and stored at 7 °C. The effects of peeling (by hand or with an electric peeler) and two micro-perforated films (90PPlus and 180PPlus) were evaluated. Changes in the quality parameters, gas composition, bioactive compounds, sensory features, and microbial safety of fresh-cut prickly pears were examined during 10 days of cold storage. Both varieties, hand-peeled and electrically peeled, were microbiologically safe (aerobic mesophiles < 7 log(CFU/g fresh weight)) and retained suitable nutritional quality after 8 days of storage. The yield was greater when fruits were electrically peeled than hand-peeled (70.7% vs. 44.0% and 66.5% vs. 40.8% for white and orange fruits, respectively). The concentrations of oxygen and carbon dioxide were above 15% and below 7.5%, respectively, in all the treatments over the shelf life. TSS decreased during storage independently of variety, peeling method, or film. Fructose was the most abundant sugar, followed by glucose and sucrose. The electric peeling machine improved not only the edible part of the fruit but also the contents of bioactive compounds, such as ascorbic acid and phenolic compounds.

Keywords: fresh-cut; electric peeling; gas composition; tray; micro-perforated film

1. Introduction

Opuntia fruit, also known as cactus pear fruit, prickly pear, tuna (Mexico), higo (Colombia), higo chumbo (Spain), and figue de barbarie (France), is harvested from various species of the genus *Opuntia* of the cactus family (Cactaceae). The fruit is a xerophyte, producing about 200–300 species, mainly growing in arid and semi-arid zones, and it is produced and consumed in several countries. The most important species producing edible fruit are *O. ficus-indica*, *O. robusta*, *O. streptacantha*, *O. amyclaea*, *O. megacantha*, and *O. hiptiacantha* [1]. It is native to Mexico and was introduced to Europe by the Spanish conquerors, and the Canary Islands was the first non-American territory where it was planted at different altitudes, thus enabling the extension of the commercialization period from the end of June to February [2].

Opuntia is a fruit with high contents of fiber, minerals, vitamins, and antioxidant compounds with functional properties for preventing chronic diseases [3–7]. A few studies have shown that the phytochemicals from *O. ficus-indica* help control hypoglycemic, hypolipidemic, and hypocholesterolemic diseases and are neuroprotective [8]. Moreover, a recent study confirmed that the antioxidants from red, orange, and white prickly pear varieties from the Canary Islands remain stable while traveling through the gastrointestinal

Citation: Díaz-Delgado, G.L.; Rodríguez-Rodríguez, E.M.; Dorta, E.; Lobo, M.G. Effects of Peeling, Film Packaging, and Cold Storage on the Quality of Minimally Processed Prickly Pears (*Opuntia ficus-indica* L. Mill.). *Agriculture* **2022**, *12*, 281. https://doi.org/10.3390/agriculture12020281

Academic Editor: Bengang Wu

Received: 17 December 2021
Accepted: 11 February 2022
Published: 16 February 2022

Publisher's Note: MDPI stays neutral with regard to jurisdictional claims in published maps and institutional affiliations.

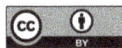

Copyright: © 2022 by the authors. Licensee MDPI, Basel, Switzerland. This article is an open access article distributed under the terms and conditions of the Creative Commons Attribution (CC BY) license (https://creativecommons.org/licenses/by/4.0/).

tract and can be easily absorbed by the human body [9]. The presence of glochids together with spines on the fruit´s surface [10] is a great disadvantage that limits its intake and commercialization in comparison to other fruits. On the other hand, modern consumers are increasingly demanding healthy and ready-to-eat products. Taking advantage of this opportunity, the prickly pear could be minimally processed (fresh-cut) to potentially increase its consumption and open new alternatives for its commercialization. The preparation of minimally processed fruits includes washing, peeling, disinfecting, packaging, and cold storing [11]. These processes cause increases in enzyme activity and the acceleration of physiological reactions, thus promoting microbial growth [12], which is usually the parameter that limits commercialization [13]. The use of bio-materials [14], surface coatings, calcium salt applications, modified atmosphere packaging, gamma radiation, and cold storage are the most used approaches used for quality retention to minimize nutritional losses, sensorial losses, and microbial growth [15]. In fact, under these conditions, one can obtain products with similar characteristics to fresh products with a shelf life of 7–10 days such as pineapple [16], kiwifruit [17], mango [18], and lychee [19].

Peeling is an extremely important step because it exposes large surface areas to air, leading to water loss, oxidation, and microorganism attacks. Moreover, peeling is usually performed by hand, thus increasing the final value of the minimally processed product. However, few studies have compared manual and mechanical peeling. Many processing innovations and automations are being implemented to reduce the amount of manual peeling in order to increase production yields [20–22]. The main factors that affect the peeling process are the mechanical and physical properties of fruit and vegetable tissues, such as skin thickness, firmness, toughness, variety, rupture force, cutting force, maximum shearing force, shear strength, tensile strength, and rupture stress [21,23]. Additionally, the peel obtained in this process is a by-product source of dietary fiber and bioactive compounds [24] that can be used to improve the profitability of manufacturing companies as a novel step in its sustainable utilization. Djeghim et al. [25] and Parafati et al. [26] reported that the use of various by-products, including prickly pear peel and prickly pear seed peel, improved the dough rheology and nutritional properties of bread. Furthermore, Morshedy et al. [27] reported that low levels of prickly pear cactus peel supplementation in the diet of lactating ewes improved the ewes' productive performance and growth, as well as the physiological status of their offspring.

The present study was aimed to cultivate ready-to-eat prickly pears with a shelf life of at least one week using simple and cheap hurdle technologies (mechanical peeling, micro-perforated films, and cold storage).

Our process flow diagram will be accessible for small and medium agro-industries to revalue this fruit in the Canary Islands and other countries in which its consumption is diminishing. Thus, manufacturers can promote the product while assuring its hygienic, nutritional, and sensorial qualities.

2. Materials and Methods

2.1. Plant Material, Sample Preparation, Packaging and Storage

Prickly pears (*O. ficus-indica* L. Mill.) were collected from a farm located in Buenavista, Tenerife, Spain (28°22'13" N, 16°51'1" W, 127 m above sea level) in December 2018. Two types of prickly pears of different colors were selected: white and orange. The white prickly pears were bigger and had thicker pericarps than the orange ones. We harvested 30 kg of both white (W) and orange (O) prickly pears, locally known as "Ariquero" and "Colorado", respectively, in the same fashion as other non-climacteric fruits when fully ripe to ensure good flavor quality and without any damage caused by decay-causing pathogens. Figure 1 shows the process flow diagram for obtaining the minimally processed prickly pears.

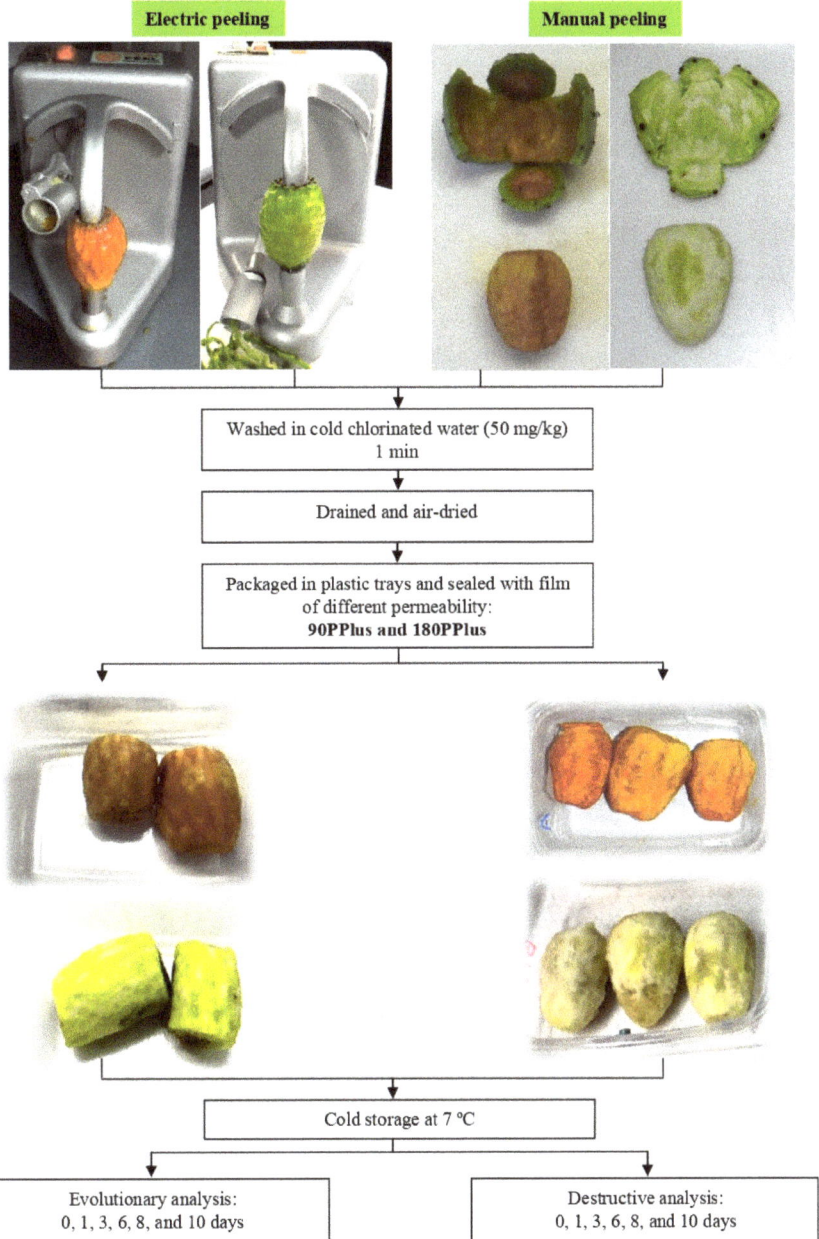

Figure 1. Process flow diagram for obtaining minimally processed prickly pears.

Fruits were washed with cold chlorinated water (200 mg/kg, pH 6.5–7.5) for 5 min and then air-dried. After washing and drying, the fruits' distal parts were removed and then peeled either by hand with a knife (H) or with an electric peeler machine (P) (Orange Peel, Pelamatic S.L, Valencia, Spain). The main difference between both peeling methods was the amount of pericarp eliminated in the process; the peel and the whole pericarp were removed in the fruits peeled with the knife (which is how it is traditionally performed by consumers; Figure 1), and the electric peeler only removed the peel (Figure 1).

Then, the peeled fruit was washed for 1 min in cold chlorinated water (50 mg/kg) before being packaged in groups of 2 or 3, depending on size, in plastic trays (polypropylene, 172 × 130 × 50 mm, supplied by Technopak Plastics S.L., Barcelona, Spain), and sealed using a heat-sealing machine (Efaman, Efabind S.L., Murcia, Spain) with a micro-perforated film (polypropylene, 52 µm, supplied by Amcor Flexibles, Burgos, Spain) of different permeability:

- Plastic 90PPlus, with low number of micro-perforations (90P) (permeability to O_2 and CO_2 of 5200 mL m^{-2} day^{-1} atm^{-1}).
- Plastic 180PPlus, with high number of micro-perforations (180P) (permeability to O_2 and CO_2 of 19,200 mL m^{-2} day^{-1} atm^{-1}).

A total of 104 trays of each variety were prepared and stored at 7 ± 1 °C; they were analyzed at the beginning of experiment and after 1, 3, 6, 8, and 10 days of storage (Figure 1).

Samples were labeled as follows: WH90P = white prickly pear, hand-peeled, packaged in 90PPlus film; OH90P = orange prickly pear, hand-peeled, packaged in 90PPlus film; WH180P = white prickly pear, hand-peeled, packaged in 180PPlus film; OH180P = orange prickly pear, hand-peeled, packaged in 180PPlus film; WE90P = white prickly pear, electrically peeled, packaged in 90PPlus film; OE90P = orange prickly pear, electrically peeled, packaged in 90PPlus film; WE180P = white prickly pear, electrically peeled, packaged in 180PPlus film; and OE180P = orange prickly pear, electrically peeled, packaged in 180PPlus film.

2.2. Technological Parameters

In order to calculate the technological parameters to determine the yield in a minimal processing industry, the following parameters were measured or calculated using 20 fruits: the whole weight, peel (residue), and edible portion. Peeling time was measured for both peeling methods and varieties, and it is expressed as the mean value of the 20 fruits in seconds. The yield of each peeling method was calculated by the following expression:

$$\text{Yield (\%)} = \left(\frac{\text{EP}}{\text{AP}}\right) \times 100$$

EP: Weight of the product after being peeled;
AP: Weight of the product as purchased.

2.3. Microbiological Analysis

Aerobic mesophiles, psychrophiles, and mold and yeast loads were evaluated to ensure microbial safety. Three trays from each treatment were analyzed in triplicate at each storage time. Six grams were homogenized in 54 mL of 0.1% peptone water (Sigma-Aldrich, Barcelona, Spain) using a homogenizer (Stomacher 80 Biomaster, Seward Limited, Worthing, United Kingdom). The serial dilutions were prepared from this original solution and finally inoculated in triplicate. Aerobic mesophiles and psychrophiles were inoculated in plate count agar (PCA) and then incubated at 30 °C for 72 h and 5 °C for 7 days, respectively, and molds and yeasts were inoculated in Glucose Chloramphenicol Agar (GCA) and incubated at 25 °C for 5 days. Microbial load is expressed as colony-forming units per gram (CFU/g) and compared with the values established by the Spanish legislation regarding minimally processed vegetables [28].

2.4. Sensorial Evaluation

Sensory evaluation was carried out by 15 panelists, who were regular consumers of prickly pears, in order to evaluate whether they were able to appreciate differences between hand-peeled (traditional method) and electrically peeled prickly pears. The number of panelists was similar to that reported by other authors [16,29–31].

Six fruits from each treatment were evaluated in terms of color, smell, taste, and overall acceptability using a linear scale from 0 (non-acceptable) to 10 (very acceptable) points. Additionally, panelists described the fruits' color (pale, normal/bright, or brown), sweetness (tasteless, normal, or very sweet), smell (unpleasant, normal, or pleasant), and texture (hard, normal, or slimy). Finally, they were asked whether they would buy the product. The trays were kept at room temperature for approximately half an hour before the tasting and opened just before it. Fruits were cut into slices between 0.5 and 1 cm thick. Three slices of each type of prickly pear were placed on plastic plates with a white background, labeled with random numbers, and served in an isolated and illuminated area at room temperature (20 °C) individually for each taster. Likewise, an unopened tray of each type was placed in the room so that the tasters could evaluate the general appearance of the packaged prickly pear. Panelists were also instructed to drink some water to rinse their palates between each sample [32].

2.5. Gas Composition

The gas composition (% CO_2 and % O_2) was determined using a compact PBI Dansensor Checkmate 9900 (Madrid, Spain), the needle of which was fed through the septum fixed on the unopened trays.

2.6. Physico-Chemical Analyses

Physico-chemical analyses were carried out for unopened trays (evolutionary analyses) and for opened trays (destructive analyses).

Color parameters (L, a*, and b*) were measured through the button of the transparent tray with a Minolta Chroma Meter CR-300 (Wheeling, WV, USA). From these data, the following parameters were calculated: hue angle (H°), chroma (C*), total color difference (ΔE), and whiteness index (WI) [33]. Thus, five trays from each treatment were analyzed in triplicate during cold storage.

$$H° = \tan^{-1}(b^*/a^*)$$

$$C^* = [(a^*)^2 + (b^*)^2]^{0.5}$$

$$WI = 100 - [(100 - L^*)^2 + (a^*)^2 + (b^*)^2]^{0.5}$$

$$\Delta E = [(L^* - L^*_i)^2 + (a^* - a^*_i)^2 + (b^* - b^*_i)^2]^{0.5}$$

In addition, three trays from each treatment were opened at each storage time, and the following parameters were analyzed in triplicate: texture (N·s/g fresh weight) using a Kramer cell (TA-HD-Plus, Aname, Madrid, Spain) to simulate chewing and hardness (expressed as °Durofel) using a durometer (Durofel, Agro-Technologie, Tarascon, France).

Finally, samples of each treatment were minced and homogenized for analysis in triplicate. Moisture was determined with the oven-drying method (P Selecta 207, Barcelona, Spain), dry matter was calculated by difference [34] (AOAC 934.06), total soluble solids (TSS) were determined using a hand refractometer (ATC-1, ATAGO, Tokyo, Japan) [20] (AOAC 932.12), pH was measured with an automatic titrator (Titralab AT1000, Germany) [34] (AOAC 981.12), and total acidity (percentage citric acid) was determined via titration with NaOH to an endpoint of pH 8.1 [20] (AOAC 942.15).

2.7. Bioactive Compounds and Antioxidant Capacity Analysis

All analyses were performed in triplicate. Ascorbic acid content was volumetrically determined with a 2,6-dichlorophenol indophenol reagent [34] (967.21). Total phenolic content (TP) is expressed as milligrams of gallic acid equivalents (GAE) per 100 g of fresh weight (f.w.) and was analyzed with a Folin–Ciocalteu assay after the extraction of 1 g of pulp with 10 mL of 80% methanol. In the same extract, the antioxidant capacity was determined using the free radical DPPH (2,2-diphenyl-1-picryl hydrazyl) [35], and the results are expressed as milligrams of Trolox (6-hydroxy-2,5,7,8-tetramethylchroman-2-carboxylic acid) equivalents (TE) per 100 g of f.w. Sugar contents were determined via high-performance liquid chromatography (HPLC) [36], with a Waters 2690 HPLC module equipped with a differential refractive index detector (Waters Corporation, Millford, MA, USA), using a Waters Carbohydrate Analysis column (3.9 × 300 mm) and acetonitrile/water (80:20) as the mobile phase. The content of each sugar is expressed as grams per 100 g of f.w.

2.8. Statistical Analysis

Data were analyzed using SPSS version 25.0 (SPSS Inc., Chicago, IL, USA) with a one-way ANOVA (Duncan's multiple range) in homogeneous groups established by the dependent variable (peeling, film type, and color of prickly pear), assuming significant differences when $p < 0.05$.

2.9. Ethical Statements

All subjects gave informed consent for inclusion before they participated in the study. The study was conducted in accordance with the Declaration of Helsinki, and the protocol was approved by the Brazilian Ethics Committee under number 845,894/2014.

3. Results and Discussion

The white prickly pears were bigger and heavier than the orange ones (140 vs. 87 g, respectively) (Figure 1). The yield was greater when fruits were electrically peeled: 70.7% (WE) versus 44.0% (WH) and 66.5% (OE) versus 40.8% (OH). The times needed by one of the regular consumer panelists to peel the white and orange prickly pear were 11.9 and 8.7 s, respectively, and the times needed by the peeler were 15.1 and 12.4 s, respectively. However, it was found to be faster to use the electric peeler to produce 1 kg of edible pulp for both varieties (214 s (WE) and 186 (OE) vs. 270 s (WH) and 213 (OH)). Thus, e.g., the production in a food processing company of 1000 trays of 250 g per day will need an operator working for 15 and 13 h using an electric peeler or 19 and 15 h using a knife for peeling white and orange prickly pears, respectively.

Moreover, electric peeling has more advantages because factory workers can operate more than one machine at the same time. In fact, using the same example, time can be reduced by 3 times when the operator places three fruits in three peelers (3 h for (WE) and 4 h for (OE)) or by 4 times (4 h for (WE) and 3 h for (OE)) when using four, which would increase company profits.

3.1. Microbiological Analysis

WE and OE presented significantly higher aerobic mesophile loads than WH and OH once prepared and after 8 days of cold storage, regardless of the type of film used, except for the white prickly pear with the 90PPlus film (Table 1). Psychrophilic values were generally higher when prickly pears were electrically peeled than those of hand-peeled pears until the 6th storage day. On the 8th day, only OE90P showed significantly higher values than the hand-peeled pears. The presence of mold and yeast was greater in orange prickly pears from day 3 than in white prickly pears. After 8 days of storage, WH showed higher levels of these microorganisms than WE under both films, and in orange prickly pear, OH90P had higher ($p < 0.05$) mold and yeast counts than OE90P.

Differences were detected in the growth of microorganisms depending on the film used (Table 1). Thus, the mesophile load was higher ($p < 0.05$) in the samples packed with 90PPlus film for WE, and it was higher in WH (except for the 8th day) and OE (from the 1st day) samples packed with the 180PPlus film. The WE and OH samples packed with 180PPlus film showed higher psychrophile loads, and the OH samples with the 90PPlus film showed significantly higher mold and yeast counts than those with the 180PPlus film. Likewise, significant increases were observed in all microorganisms' loads over time, regardless of color, peeling type, and film used. Nevertheless, the number of aerobic mesophiles in both white and orange prickly pear varieties were within the limits (7 log(CFU/g fresh weight)) regulated in Spain for ready-to-eat fruits and vegetables by the Real Decreto 3484/2000 [28] from the day of preparation until day 8 of cold storage.

Likewise, the counts of psychrophilic bacteria, molds, and yeasts were below 6 log(CFU)/g in all the treatments from the preparation until day 8 of storage (Table 1). Cefola et al. [37] detected an increase in mesophile and psychrophile growth after 13 days of storage when prickly pears were packed in a passive modified atmosphere, and the growth was higher when they were stored at 8 °C compared to 4 °C. Their final values were similar to our data. Furthermore, Palma et al. [38] and Piga et al. [12] reported a remarkable proliferation of microorganisms during storage time.

Table 1. Evolution of aerobic mesophiles, psychrophiles, and mold and yeast in white and orange minimally processed prickly pears manually or electrically peeled and packed in two films of different permeability during cold storage at 7 °C.

	Storage Period (Days)				
	0	1	3	6	8
	Aerobic mesophiles log(CFU/g f.w.)				
WH90P	2.1 ± 0.1 [a,1]	2.5 ± 0.1 [b,1]	2.9 ± 0.0 [c,1]	3.8 ± 0.1 [d,1]	4.6 ± 0.0 [e,2]
WH180P	2.1 ± 0.1 [a,1]	3.9 ± 0.1 [b,3]	4.0 ± 0.0 [c,3]	4.0 ± 0.0 [c,2]	4.4 ± 4.4 [d,1]
WE90P	2.8 ± 0.2 [a,2]	3.8 ± 0.1 [b,3]	4.0 ± 0.0 [c,3]	4.3 ± 0.0 [d,3]	4.7 ± 0.1 [e,3]
WE180P	2.8 ± 0.2 [a,2]	3.5 ± 0.1 [b,2]	3.6 ± 0.1 [b-c,2]	3.7 ± 0.1 [c,1]	4.5 ± 0.0 [d,2]
OH90P	2.3 ± 0.1 [a,1]	3.0 ± 0.0 [b,2]	3.4 ± 0.1 [c,2]	4.8 ± 0.0 [d,3]	4.1 ± 0.0 [e,1]
OH180P	2.3 ± 0.1 [a,1]	2.8 ± 0.1 [b,1]	3.5 ± 0.2 [c,2]	4.0 ± 0.2 [d,2]	4.6 ± 0.0 [e,2]
OE90P	2.8 ± 0.1 [a,2]	3.4 ± 0.0 [b,4]	3.2 ± 0.1 [c,1]	3.8 ± 0.1 [d,1]	4.7 ± 0.0 [e,3]
OE180P	2.8 ± 0.1 [a,2]	3.1 ± 0.1 [b,3]	4.1 ± 0.0 [c,3]	5.1 ± 0.1 [d,4]	5.4 ± 0.0 [e,4]
	Psychrophiles log(CFU/g f.w.)				
WH90P	1.4 ± 0.1 [a,1]	1.8 ± 0.1 [b,2]	2.3 ± 0.1 [c,1]	5.5 ± 0.1 [d,1]	5.7 ± 0.0 [e,1]
WH180P	1.4 ± 0.1 [a,1]	1.6 ± 0.1 [b,1]	2.2 ± 0.2 [c,1]	5.5 ± 0.0 [d,1]	5.7 ± 0.0 [e,1]
WE90P	2.1 ± 0.0 [a,2]	2.7 ± 0.0 [b,3]	3.8 ± 0.0 [c,2]	5.5 ± 0.1 [d,1]	5.7 ± 0.0 [e,1-2]
WE180P	2.1 ± 0.0 [a,2]	3.9 ± 0.1 [b,4]	4.5 ± 0.1 [c,3]	5.6 ± 0.0 [d,2]	5.8 ± 0.0 [e,2]
OH90P	2.1 ± 0.1 [a,2]	2.1 ± 0.1 [a,1]	2.8 ± 0.1 [b,1]	5.2 ± 0.1 [c,1]	5.4 ± 0.0 [c,1]
OH180P	2.1 ± 0.1 [a,2]	2.5 ± 0.1 [b,3]	3.4 ± 0.0 [c,2]	5.4 ± 0.0 [d,2]	5.6 ± 0.0 [e,2-3]
OE90P	1.7 ± 0.0 [a,1]	3.2 ± 0.1 [b,4]	3.3 ± 0.0 [c,2]	5.6 ± 0.0 [d,3]	5.7 ± 0.0 [e,3]
OE180P	1.7 ± 0.0 [a,1]	2.2 ± 0.0 [b,2]	3.7 ± 0.1 [c,3]	5.7 ± 0.0 [d,4]	5.6 ± 0.0 [e,2]
	Mold and yeast log(CFU/g f.w.)				
WH90P	1.9 ± 0.1 [a,1]	2.2 ± 0.1 [b,2]	2.3 ± 0.0 [c,1]	3.9 ± 0.0 [d,2]	4.7 ± 0.0 [e,1]
WH180P	1.9 ± 0.1 [a,1]	2.1 ± 0.0 [b,2]	2.3 ± 0.0 [c,1]	3.6 ± 0.1 [d,1]	4.7 ± 0.0 [e,2]
WE90P	2.0 ± 0.0 [a,1]	2.0 ± 0.0 [a,1]	2.8 ± 0.1 [b,3]	3.9 ± 0.1 [c,2]	4.7 ± 0.0 [d,2]
WE180P	2.0 ± 0.0 [a,1]	2.0 ± 0.0 [a,1]	2.5 ± 0.0 [b,2]	3.9 ± 0.0 [c,2]	4.8 ± 0.0 [d,3]
OH90P	2.0 ± 0.1 [a,2]	2.8 ± 0.0 [b,3]	2.9 ± 0.0 [c,2]	4.2 ± 0.0 [d,2]	5.2 ± 0.0 [e,4]
OH180P	2.0 ± 0.1 [a,2]	2.0 ± 0.1 [a,2]	2.8 ± 0.0 [b,1]	3.9 ± 0.0 [c,1]	5.1 ± 0.0 [d,2]
OE90P	1.8 ± 0.1 [a,1]	1.8 ± 0.1 [a,1]	3.0 ± 0.0 [b,3]	4.1 ± 0.1 [c,2]	5.2 ± 0.0 [d,3]
OE180P	1.8 ± 0.1 [a,1]	1.8 ± 0.1 [a,1]	3.2 ± 0.0 [b,4]	4.2 ± 0.0 [c,2]	5.0 ± 0.0 [d,1]

Hand-peeled (H) and electrically peeled (E) white (W) and orange (O) prickly pears packaged in 90PPlus (90P) and 180PPlus (180P) film. Different letters in a row indicate that there were significant differences between storage days ($p < 0.05$), and different numbers in a column indicate that there were significant differences between samples ($p < 0.05$).

3.2. Sensorial Evaluation

The panelists detected differences in the appearance, color, flavor, and odor at the beginning (0 days) in both prickly pear varieties, reporting higher mean values for the hand-peeled fruits ($p < 0.05$) (Table 2). No significant differences were detected in the sensory attributes at other storage times or between film packaging types.

Table 2. Mean values of the sensory attributes at the beginning.

	Initial Storage Time			
	Appearance	Color	Flavor	Odor
WH	7.5 ± 1.1 [2]	6.7 ± 0.5 [1]	7.7 ± 1.0 [2]	7.0 ± 1.4 [2]
WE	6.3 ± 0.5 [1]	7.3 ± 0.5 [2]	6.5 ± 0.8 [1]	5.8 ± 0.8 [1]
OH	8.3 ± 0.8 [2]	8.3 ± 0.5 [2]	8.5 ± 0.8 [2]	7.5 ± 1.1 [2]
OE	5.7 ± 0.8 [1]	6.5 ± 0.8 [1]	5.3 ± 0.8 [1]	5.7 ± 0.8 [1]

Hand-peeled (H) and electrically peeled (E) white (W) and orange (O) prickly pears. Different numbers in a column indicate that there were significant differences between samples ($p < 0.05$).

In general, as shown in Figure 2, tasters slightly preferred the manually peeled prickly pears to the electrically peeled ones (7.1 and 6.5 on a 10-point scale, respectively), regardless of the studied variety. WH under both packaging films at any storage time were those with the highest purchase percentages (between 75% and 100%), and the electrically peeled pears (especially those packed in 180PPlus film) were the most rejected by the tasters (only 33.3% would buy them) after 8 days of storage.

The acceptance of the minimally processed fruit did not decrease with storage time. The variable that negatively influenced the product rejection was texture, specifically when the panelists found the fruit too slimy or hard.

3.3. Gas Composition

Figure 3 shows a clear drop in the O_2 concentration and an increase in the CO_2 concentration of all the trays during cold storage, trends that were more pronounced for those sealed with 90PPlus film.

Thus, according to the film permeability, regardless of the variety and peeling method, the trays with either white or orange prickly pears packed in 180PPlus film (more micro-perforated) presented higher O_2 values and lower CO_2 values than those packed in 90PPlus film (less micro-perforated). Likewise, the accumulation of CO_2 inside the trays was greater in the OE for both packing films (90P and 180P), although these differences were not significant. Allegra et al. [39], Cefola et al. [37], and Piga et al. [12] detected significant increases and decreases ($p < 0.05$) in CO_2 and O_2 concentrations, respectively, during cold storage depending on the used film.

3.4. Physico-Chemical Analyses

3.4.1. Color

Color parameters (L, a*, and b*) were measured through the bottom of the same transparent trays during the study (Table 3).

L values were higher in white prickly pear trays than orange ones. The WE treatment led to a higher brightness (L) than the WH treatment; in the orange pears, these differences were only appreciated from day 6 in the OE180P sample. The orange prickly pears had higher a* values than the white ones, and they behaved differently during shelf life. However, the a* value increased with storage time in white prickly pears but decreased in orange pears, with only OE90P showing significantly different values. The type of peeling influenced the a* values shown by white prickly pears more than those shown by orange ones. Ultimately, WH presented a* values higher than WE during shelf life (Table A1, Appendix A). The b* parameter showed different trends depending on the studied prickly pear variety; WE showed higher values ($p < 0.05$) than those peeled manually (WH). In the orange variety from the first storage day, the highest and lowest b* values were detected in OE180P and OH90P, respectively. In addition, this parameter seemed to considerably fluctuate in the white variety during storage time, especially in WE180P, while remaining more or less constant in the orange ones, especially in OE180P (Table A1, Appendix A). The tonality (H°) decreased with storage time in the white prickly pears and remained more or less constant in the orange ones. In general, WE showed higher H° values than WH, and its trend in orange pears was similar to that described for the b* parameter. The orange variety showed lower H° values than the white variety. The type of film had little influence on the L, a*, b*, and H parameters. Electrically peeled white prickly pears showed higher chromaticity (C*) values than those peeled by hand at each storage time independently of the film used; this fact was not observed in the orange variety. Allegra et al. [39] found reported unremarkable changes in flesh color occurring during the summer storage or late, freshly cut prickly pears that were harvested either at commercial harvest time or when fully ripe.

Table 3. Color parameters of white and orange minimally processed prickly pears that were manually or electrically peeled and packed in two films of different permeability during cold storage at 7 °C.

	Storage Period (Days)				
	0	1	3	6	8
	L				
WH90P	53.9 ± 3.9 [a,1]	51.5 ± 1.9 [a,1]	49.6 ± 0.9 [a,1]	54.7 ± 3.5 [a,1]	53.3 ± 2.1 [a,1]
WH180P	56.7 ± 3.0 [b,1-2]	52.2 ± 0.6 [a,1]	52.5 ± 1.9 [a,2]	53.4 ± 2.7 [a,1]	51.9 ± 0.9 [a,1]
WE90P	60.0 ± 3.2 [b,2]	55.1 ± 2.1 [a,2]	56.5 ± 1.9 [a,3]	62.3 ± 1.6 [b,2]	61.3 ± 3.4 [b,2]
WE180P	56.2 ± 1.3 [a,1-2]	59.7 ± 1.7 [b,3]	59.9 ± 2.8 [b,4]	60.6 ± 3.2 [b,2]	61.7 ± 3.1 [b,2]
OH90P	38.5 ± 2.1 [a,1]	39.7 ± 2.3 [a,1]	41.3 ± 2.1 [a,1]	41.1 ± 4.3 [a,1]	41.5 ± 5.0 [a,1]
OH180P	40.9 ± 4.0 [a,1]	41.3 ± 3.3 [a,1]	41.0 ± 1.8 [a,1]	43.4 ± 2.7 [a,1]	43.7 ± 2.5 [a,1]
OE90P	41.2 ± 2.4 [a,1]	38.4 ± 1.5 [a,1]	41.0 ± 2.4 [a,1]	45.0 ± 5.4 [a,1]	44.5 ± 4.8 [a,1]
OE180P	41.2 ± 3.2 [a,1]	42.0 ± 3.4 [a,1]	44.2 ± 3.1 [a-b,1]	47.7 ± 2.6 [b-c,1]	49.7 ± 1.9 [c,2]
	H° (HUE)				
WH90P	110 ± 5.7 [a,1]	111 ± 4.7 [a,1]	109 ± 4.2 [a,1]	109 ± 3.2 [a,1]	105 ± 4.4 [a,1]
WH180P	111 ± 2.2 [b,1]	111 ± 1.1 [b,1]	110 ± 2.6 [b,1]	108 ± 2.1 [b,1]	106 ± 1.2 [a,1]
WE90P	115 ± 3.0 [c,1]	114 ± 1.9 [b-c,1-2]	114 ± 2.2 [b-c,2]	111 ± 2.5 [a-b,1]	109 ± 1.7 [a,1]
WE180P	115 ± 1.7 [c,1]	116 ± 1.1 [c,2]	114 ± 1.9 [b-c,2]	112 ± 1.4 [b,1]	108 ± 2.2 [a,1]
OH90P	47.1 ± 10 [a,1]	41.7 ± 7.1 [a,1]	40.1 ± 9.5 [a,1]	40.4 ± 6.9 [a,1]	40.8 ± 5.9 [a,1]
OH180P	46.3 ± 6.5 [a,1]	43.4 ± 3.4 [a,1]	43.0 ± 6.9 [a,1]	46.1 ± 8.2 [a,1]	46.8 ± 9.7 [a,1-2]
OE90P	46.6 ± 4.7 [a,1]	41.7 ± 6.6 [a,1]	45.5 ± 8.4 [a,1]	46.7 ± 9.4 [a,1]	46.8 ± 11 [a,1-2]
OE180P	61.2 ± 12 [a,2]	52.0 ± 5.9 [a,2]	52.7 ± 13 [a,1]	57.9 ± 14 [a,1]	59.8 ± 11 [a,2]
	C*				
WH90P	17.7 ± 3.6 [a,1]	15.0 ± 3.4 [a,1]	13.6 ± 3.7 [a,1]	18.3 ± 4.1 [a,1]	18.0 ± 3.9 [a,1]
WH180P	15.7 ± 3.1 [b,1]	11.8 ± 2.2 [a,1]	13.5 ± 2.3 [a-b,1]	16.0 ± 2.3 [b,1]	16.1 ± 1.2 [b,1]
WE90P	26.7 ± 3.0 [b,2]	22.2 ± 3.1 [a,2]	23.2 ± 1.9 [a-b,2]	25.7 ± 3.7 [a-b,2]	27.1 ± 2.2 [b,2]
WE180P	22.8 ± 2.2 [a,2]	23.6 ± 3.1 [a,2]	24.3 ± 2.9 [a,2]	25.8 ± 2.8 [a,2]	28.6 ± 4.0 [a,2]
OH90P	28.0 ± 3.4 [b,1]	21.0 ± 4.9 [a,1]	20.6 ± 3.7 [a,1]	19.9 ± 5.2 [a,1]	20.7 ± 4.9 [a,1]
OH180P	26.0 ± 5.7 [a,1]	26.5 ± 1.8 [a,1]	24.7 ± 2.2 [a,1]	23.8 ± 4.2 [a,1]	22.3 ± 1.7 [a,1]
OE90P	36.2 ± 3.1 [b,2]	20.1 ± 3.8 [a,1]	21.2 ± 4.9 [a,1]	24.7 ± 2.3 [a,1]	22.4 ± 2.1 [a,1]
OE180P	23.1 ± 4.9 [a,1]	26.0 ± 5.2 [a,1]	24.2 ± 4.6 [a,1]	25.0 ± 1.6 [a,1]	24.9 ± 2.2 [a,1]
	ΔE				
WH90P		5.81 ± 2.1 [b,1]	6.16 ± 0.9 [b,1]	4.70 ± 1.2 [a-b,1]	3.20 ± 0.3 [a,1]
WH180P		5.44 ± 1.3 [a,1]	5.32 ± 3.8 [a,1]	5.69 ± 1.1 [a,1]	6.49 ± 1.6 [a,2-3]
WE90P		7.08 ± 1.8 [a,1]	6.67 ± 2.3 [a,1]	5.85 ± 1.6 [a,1]	5.60 ± 2.7 [a,1-2]
WE180P		4.40 ± 1.2 [a,1]	4.90 ± 1.4 [a,1]	6.47 ± 1.4 [a-b,1]	8.43 ± 2.3 [b,3]
OH90P		8.38 ± 1.3 [a,1]	7.82 ± 1.6 [a,2]	9.46 ± 2.3 [a,1]	9.26 ± 3.0 [a,1]
OH180P		6.46 ± 4.0 [a,1]	6.65 ± 2.1 [a,1-2]	8.45 ± 5.0 [a,1]	8.98 ± 3.7 [a,1]
OE90P		14.7 ± 1.9 [a,2]	15.0 ± 2.9 [a,3]	16.6 ± 0.7 [a,2]	17.7 ± 0.6 [a,2]
OE180P		6.17 ± 0.9 [a-b,1]	4.90 ± 0.9 [a,1]	7.48 ± 1.3 [b-c,1]	8.14 ± 1.2 [c,1]
	WI				
WH90P	50.4 ± 2.6 [a,1]	49.1 ± 1.1 [a,1]	47.7 ± 1.0 [a,1]	51.0 ± 2.2 [a,1]	49.7 ± 1.4 [a,1]
WH180P	53.9 ± 3.2 [b,1]	50.6 ± 0.4 [a,1]	50.5 ± 1.4 [a,1-2]	50.7 ± 2.1 [a,1]	49.3 ± 0.9 [a,1]
WE90P	51.8 ± 3.0 [a,1]	49.8 ± 1.4 [a,1]	50.7 ± 1.8 [a,1-2]	54.3 ± 2.1 [a,1]	52.8 ± 3.5 [a,1]
WE180P	50.6 ± 1.5 [a,1]	53.3 ± 1.9 [a,2]	53.1 ± 3.5 [a,2]	52.8 ± 3.4 [a,1]	52.0 ± 2.6 [a,1]
OH90P	32.3 ± 1.3 [a,1]	36.0 ± 1.1 [b,1]	37.7 ± 1.2 [b,1]	37.6 ± 2.8 [b,1]	37.8 ± 3.6 [b,1]
OH180P	34.9 ± 2.0 [a,2]	35.9 ± 3.3 [a-b,1]	36.0 ± 2.1 [a-b,1]	38.4 ± 1.7 [bc,1-2]	39.4 ± 1.7 [c,1-2]
OE90P	30.9 ± 1.4 [a,1]	34.9 ± 0.5 [b,1]	37.2 ± 2.5 [b,1]	41.2 ± 2.9 [c,2-3]	41.5 ± 2.7 [c,2-3]
OE180P	36.5 ± 12 [a-b,2]	36.2 ± 2.4 [a,1]	39.1 ± 1.8 [b,1]	42.0 ± 2.3 [c,3]	43.8 ± 1.2 [c,3]

Hand-peeled (H) and electrically peeled (E) white (W) and orange (O) prickly pears packaged in 90PPlus (90P) and 180PPlus (180P) film. Different letters in a row indicate that there were significant differences between storage days ($p < 0.05$), and different numbers in a column indicate that there were significant differences between samples ($p < 0.05$).

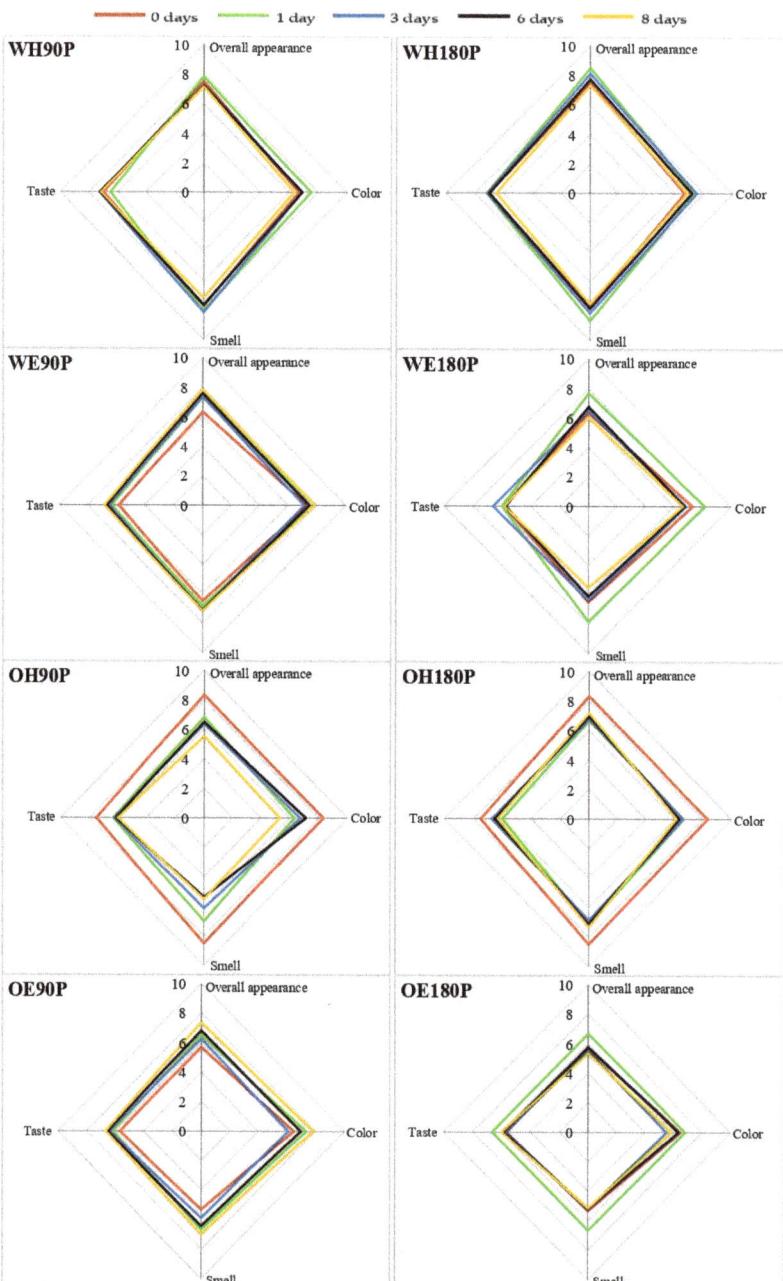

Figure 2. Taster evaluation of the color, smell, taste, and overall appearance of hand-peeled (H) and electrically peeled (E) white (W) and orange (O) prickly pears packaged in 90PPlus (90P) and 180PPlus (180P) film.

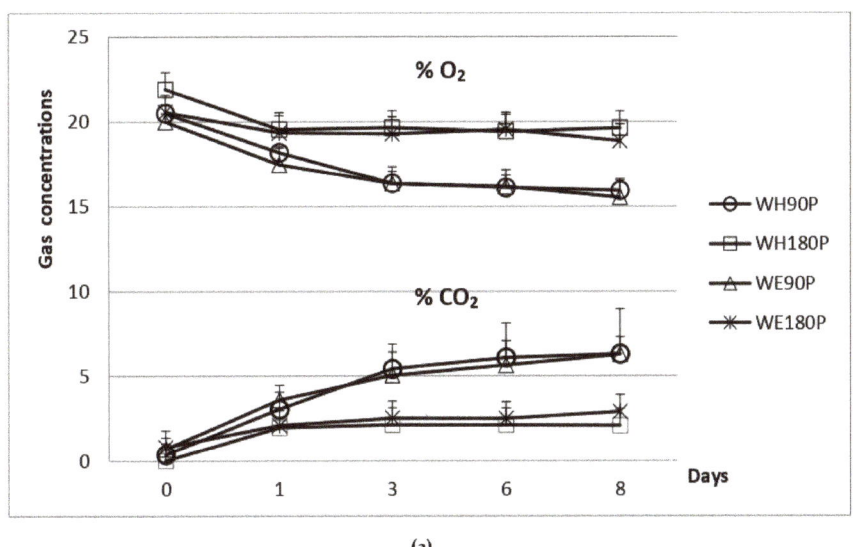

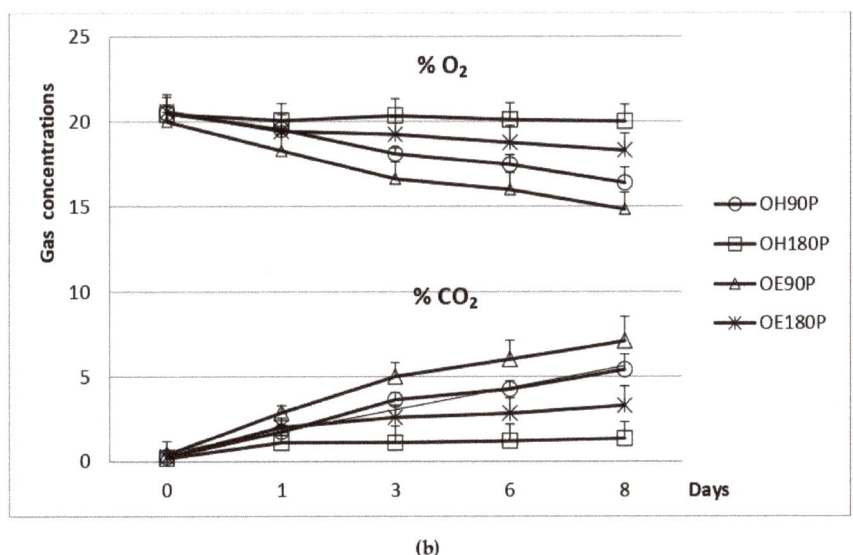

Figure 3. (a) CO_2 and O_2 concentration (%) evolutions inside white prickly pear trays; (b) CO_2 and O_2 concentration (%) evolutions inside orange prickly pear trays. Hand-peeled (H) and electrically peeled (E) white (W) and orange (O) prickly pears were packaged in 90PPlus (90P) and 180PPlus (180P) film.

In general, loss of color (ΔE) (Table 3) was only observed in electrically peeled prickly pears packed with 180PPlus film, though this parameter was not affected by storage time in the other types of prickly pears, even showing improvement in the case of WH90P. Allegra et al. [39] also reported losses of color, especially after 7 days of storage, as did Ochoa-Velasco and Guerrero-Beltrán [40]. Film type did not influence color loss, with the exception of the OE packed with 90P film that presented higher losses than those packed in 180PPlus film. The whiteness index (WI) significantly increased with the storage time in all types of studied orange prickly pears, though it did not change over time in the white ones, except in WH180P in which it decreased. Likewise, the WI was much higher in white prickly pears than in the orange ones. The types of peeling and film did not significantly affect this parameter.

3.4.2. Hardness and Texture

The hardness (Table A1, Appendix A) did not significantly change over the 8 days of cold storage in the studied varieties, except when the white ones were electrically peeled and packed in either of the two films. The hardness of the electrically peeled white and orange prickly pears was higher (50.8 and 42.9 °Durofel for white and orange varieties, respectively) than that of the manually peeled pears (32.1 and 31.3 °Durofel for white and orange varieties, respectively) for all storage times and both types of film. Hardness presented significantly different values during the entire shelf life of the white prickly pears, but the hardness values stopped showing differences by day 3 for the orange prickly pears. The influence of the type of film used was negligible, especially in the orange prickly pears; it was only detected that WH180P showed higher ($p < 0.05$) hardness values than WH90P from day 1 to day 6 of packaging. Another interesting parameter was texture, which was evaluated with a Kramer cell that simulated mastication (Table A1, Appendix A). We found that texture significantly increased during the 8 days of storage, except in WH90P, OE180P, and OE90P, for which it decreased ($p < 0.05$). White prickly pears showed higher texture values than the orange ones during shelf life (10.6 and 6.1 N s/g f.w., respectively). In addition, the texture values were significantly higher when the white prickly pears were peeled by hand than with the electric peeler (11.7 and 9.5 N s/g f.w., respectively). In the orange variety, the electrically peeled fruits presented significantly higher values than the manually peeled ones at the beginning of cold storage. The type of film used in packaging did not influence this parameter.

3.4.3. Dry Matter, pH, and Acidity

At the beginning of storage, the dry matter content (data not shown) was higher in the white prickly pears than in the orange ones (19.8% and 17.5%, respectively), and it was higher in those white fruits peeled by hand than with the electric peeler (21.1% and 18.5%, respectively). Thus, WH were the prickly pears with the highest dry matter values ($\geq$20.5%), and the OE showed the lowest values (<16.5%). Likewise, the dry matter contents of both varieties, regardless of the type of film and peeling, remained almost constant throughout cold storage, which was similar to the results reported by Piga et al. [12] for the "Gialla" variety. The hand-peeled prickly pears showed higher pH values and lower acidity values than the electrically peeled pears (data not shown). It was observed that the pH significantly decreased after 8 days of storage in WH180P, OH180P, and OE180P, and the acidity significantly increased in WH180P, OH90P, and OE180P. In the other treatments, both pH and acidity remained constant over time. Accordingly, the lowest pH value was detected in OE180P at 8 days of storage (pH = 5.39), and pH values lower than 6 were also observed in OE90P. The film used in packaging had little impact on the values of these two parameters in the studied varieties. Piga et al. [12] analyzed prickly pears of the "Gialla" variety and reported similar results (decreases in pH during storage) when fruits were manually peeled and stored at 4° C for 9 days. Ochoa-Velasco and Guerrero-Beltrán [40] detected decreases in pH with storage time (16 days at 4° C) in white prickly pears of the *O. albicarpa* species. However, Palma et al. [38] reported that pH and acidity significantly decreased with storage time (at 4 °C/10 days) in the orange "Gialla" variety, though they remained constant in the white "Bianca" variety.

3.4.4. Sugars

In general, the TSS content was higher in the white prickly pears than in the orange ones (Table 4). However, Palma et al. [38] did not observe that the prickly pears of the "Bianca" variety were sweeter than those of the "Gialla" variety. The prickly pears with the highest and lowest TSS were WH and OE, respectively, which coincided with the results already indicated for dry matter content. In all cases, a decrease in TSS was observed with storage time, as was also observed by Palma et al. [38] in the "Gialla" variety but not in the "Bianca" variety. Piga et al. [12] detected that TSS content did not significantly change over storage time in the "Gialla" variety (13.5 TSS). Nevertheless, Ochoa-Velasco and Guerrero-Beltrán [40] reported an increase in TSS (from 13.6 to 17.4 in the white variety and from 13.9 to 18.0 in the red variety). It was observed that this decrease was not significant in OE (from 12.3 to ≈11.0). In WH, the TSS decreased ($p < 0.05$) from an initial value of 17.7 to 13.1 (WH90P) and 13.9 (WH180P). No significant differences were detected in TSS depending on the type of packaging film used with the exception of WE, for which those packed in 180PPlus film showed higher values than those packed in 90PPlus film between 1 and 6 storage days. Fructose (Table 4) was the sugar with the highest concentration in all treatments, with the exception of OE at the beginning and the first day of storage, followed by glucose and lastly sucrose, which presented values lower than 1% except in WE. Fructose content in WE and OE increased with storage time, and glucose content in OE decreased with time.

Table 4. Total soluble solids, fructose, glucose, and sucrose contents in white and orange minimally processed prickly pears peeled by hand or with an electric peeler and packed in two films of different permeability during cold storage at 7 °C.

	Storage Period (Days)				
	0	1	3	6	8
	TSS (°Brix)				
WH90P	17.7 ± 1.9 [b,1]	17.1 ± 0.4 [b,3]	17.0 ± 0.9 [b,3]	15.7 ± 1.2 [b,2]	13.1 ± 0.3 [a,1]
WH180P	17.7 ± 1.9 [b,1]	17.3 ± 0.8 [b,3]	15.5 ± 1.7 [a-b,2-3]	16.9 ± 0.6 [b,2]	13.9 ± 0.4 [a,1]
WE90P	16.0 ± 0.9 [c,1]	13.3 ± 0.3 [a-b,1]	12.3 ± 1.2 [a,1]	13.0 ± 0.2 [a-b,1]	13.9 ± 0.4 [a,1]
WE180P	16.0 ± 0.9 [b,1]	15.5 ± 1.1 [b,2]	14.0 ± 0.0 [a,1-2]	16.2 ± 0.2 [b,2]	14.1 ± 0.6 [a,1]
OH90P	15.1 ± 1.1 [b,2]	14.3 ± 1.0 [b,1]	14.7 ± 1.3 [b,1]	12.2 ± 0.2 [a,1]	11.9 ± 0.3 [a,1]
OH180P	15.1 ± 1.1 [b,2]	12.3 ± 1.4 [a,1]	12.7 ± 1.1 [a,1]	11.9 ± 1.1 [a,1]	13.0 ± 0.2 [a,1]
OE90P	12.3 ± 1.3 [a,1]	11.4 ± 1.1 [a,1]	12.7 ± 0.5 [a,1]	11.5 ± 0.6 [a,1]	11.1 ± 0.7 [a,1]
OE180P	12.3 ± 1.3 [a,1]	13.2 ± 1.1 [a,1]	11.1 ± 0.8 [a,1]	11.4 ± 0.9 [a,1]	11.3 ± 0.4 [a,1]
	Fructose (g/100 g f.w.)				
WH90P	6.56 ± 0.0 [b,2]	6.04 ± 0.2 [a,3]	6.12 ± 0.2 [a,3]	6.43 ± 0.2 [b,2]	6.02 ± 0.0 [a,1-2]
WH180P	6.56 ± 0.0 [b,2]	6.44 ± 0.1 [b,4]	5.67 ± 0.1 [a,1-2]	6.57 ± 0.1 [b,2]	6.41 ± 0.4 [b,2]
WE90P	5.11 ± 0.1 [a,1]	5.47 ± 0.2 [b,2]	5.53 ± 0.2 [b,1]	6.47 ± 0.0 [c,2]	5.71 ± 0.0 [b,1]
WE180P	5.11 ± 0.1 [a,1]	5.18 ± 0.1 [a,1]	5.94 ± 0.2 [b,2-3]	6.00 ± 0.1 [b,1]	5.75 ± 0.3 [b,1]
OH90P	6.56 ± 0.1 [c,2]	5.16 ± 0.25 [a,2]	5.81 ± 0.4 [b,1-2]	6.54 ± 0.1 [c,3]	6.21 ± 0.2 [b-c,3]
OH180P	6.56 ± 0.1 [a,2]	5.94 ± 0.3 [a,3]	6.08 ± 0.2 [a,2]	6.22 ± 0.3 [a,2]	6.27 ± 0.1 [a,3]
OE90P	4.75 ± 0.2 [b,1]	4.29 ± 0.1 [a,1]	5.30 ± 0.5 [c,1]	5.97 ± 0.1 [d,2]	5.15 ± 0.1 [b-c,1]
OE180P	4.75 ± 0.2 [a,1]	4.75 ± 0.2 [a,2]	5.36 ± 0.2 [b,1]	5.16 ± 0.1 [b,1]	5.90 ± 0.2 [c,2]
	Glucose (g/100 g f.w.)				
WH90P	4.84 ± 0.1 [b,2]	4.23 ± 0.2 [a,2]	4.04 ± 0.1 [a,2]	4.24 ± 0.1 [a,2]	4.15 ± 0.0 [a,2-3]
WH180P	4.84 ± 0.1 [c,2]	4.70 ± 0.0 [c,3]	4.11 ± 0.1 [a,2]	4.37 ± 0.0 [b,3]	4.36 ± 0.2 [b,2]
WE90P	3.94 ± 0.2 [b-c,1]	3.96 ± 0.2 [bc,1]	3.60 ± 0.1 [a,1]	4.15 ± 0.0 [c,2]	3.82 ± 0.0 [a-b,1]
WE180P	3.94 ± 0.2 [a,1]	3.75 ± 0.1 [a,1]	3.99 ± 0.1 [a,2]	3.79 ± 0.1 [a,1]	4.08 ± 0.2 [a,1-2]
OH90P	4.85 ± 0.0 [c,2]	3.95 ± 0.1 [a,2]	3.72 ± 0.2 [a,1]	4.87 ± 0.2 [c,3]	4.38 ± 0.2 [b,2]
OH180P	4.85 ± 0.0 [c,2]	4.22 ± 0.2 [b,2]	3.87 ± 0.2 [a,1]	4.20 ± 0.2 [b,2]	4.59 ± 0.1 [c,2]
OE90P	4.02 ± 0.2 [b,1]	3.46 ± 0.0 [a,1]	3.65 ± 0.3 [a,1]	4.23 ± 0.0 [b,2]	3.65 ± 0.1 [a,1]
OE180P	4.02 ± 0.2 [b,1]	3.62 ± 0.1 [a,1]	3.63 ± 0.1 [a,1]	3.56 ± 0.0 [a,1]	3.68 ± 0.1 [a,1]
	Sucrose (g/100 g f.w.)				
WH90P	0.72 ± 0.0 [d,1]	0.67 ± 0.0 [c,1]	0.58 ± 0.0 [b,1]	0.67 ± 0.0 [c,1]	0.46 ± 0.0 [a,1]
WH180P	0.72 ± 0.0 [c,1]	0.84 ± 0.0 [d,2]	0.60 ± 0.0 [b,1]	0.63 ± 0.0 [b,1]	0.53 ± 0.0 [a,2]
WE90P	1.20 ± 0.1 [b,2]	1.58 ± 0.1 [c,4]	1.25 ± 0.1 [b,3]	0.69 ± 0.0 [a,1]	0.65 ± 0.0 [a,3]
WE180P	1.20 ± 0.1 [c,2]	0.93 ± 0.0 [b,3]	0.67 ± 0.0 [a,2]	0.73 ± 0.1 [a,1]	0.96 ± 0.0 [b,4]
OH90P	0.52 ± 0.0 [d,2]	0.33 ± 0.0 [c,2-3]	0.33 ± 0.0 [c,4]	0.23 ± 0.0 [a,1]	0.28 ± 0.0 [b,2]
OH180P	0.52 ± 0.0 [a,2]	0.35 ± 0.0 [b,3]	0.29 ± 0.0 [a,2]	0.29 ± 0.0 [a,2]	0.26 ± 0.0 [a,2]
OE90P	0.36 ± 0.0 [c,1]	0.31 ± 0.0 [b,1-2]	0.22 ± 0.0 [a,1]	0.23 ± 0.0 [a,1]	0.21 ± 0.0 [a,1]
OE180P	0.36 ± 0.0 [c,1]	0.30 ± 0.0 [b,1]	0.30 ± 0.0 [b,3]	0.25 ± 0.0 [a,1]	0.35 ± 0.0 [c,3]

Hand-peeled (H) and electrically peeled (E) white (W) and orange (O) prickly pears packaged in 90PPlus (90P) and 180PPlus (180P) film. Different letters in a row indicate that there were significant differences between storage days ($p < 0.05$), and different numbers in a column indicate that there were significant differences between samples ($p < 0.05$).

3.4.5. Bioactive Compound and Antioxidant Capacity Analyses

The ascorbic acid content considerably varied depending on the variety, storage time, and type of peeling (Table 5), but the type of film showed little influence. A decrease in ascorbic acid during storage was observed, and it was more pronounced in the electrically peeled pears. Palma et al. [38] reported a decrease in ascorbic acid content during the storage of the "Bianca" and "Gialla" varieties. In contrast, Piga et al. [12] did not describe any significant differences in the content of this vitamin during the storage of the minimally processed "Gialla" variety. However, it should be noted that after 8 days of storage at 7 °C in this study, the ascorbic acid content ranged between 15 and 21 mg/100 g of fresh weight, with losses relative to the initial time ranging between 8% and 38%. Significant differences were also detected between the white prickly pear treatments for each day of storage, and we obtained different results for the orange variety. WE showed higher values ($p < 0.05$) of ascorbic acid for all storage days than WH, but those differences in the orange ones were not significant ($p > 0.05$) (except on day 3, in which OH showed higher values than OE).

Table 5. Ascorbic acid, total phenolics, and antioxidant capacity (DPPH) in white and orange minimally processed prickly pears peeled by hand or with an electric peeler and packed in two films of different permeability during cold storage at 7 °C.

	Storage Period (Days)				
	0	1	3	6	8
	Ascorbic acid (mg/100 g f.w.)				
WH90P	16.4 ± 0.5 [a-b,1]	17.8 ± 1.3 [b,1]	15.1 ± 0.5 [a,1]	17.6 ± 0.1 [b,1]	15.1 ± 1.6 [a,1]
WH180P	16.4 ± 0.5 [b,1]	18.5 ± 0.7 [c,1]	15.5 ± 0.1 [a-b,1]	16.8 ± 1.0 [b,1]	14.9 ± 1.0 [a,1]
WE90P	24.9 ± 0.3 [b,2]	27.3 ± 1.3 [b,2]	21.4 ± 3.3 [a,2]	21.5 ± 0.4 [a,2]	18.4 ± 0.7 [a,2]
WE180P	24.9 ± 0.3 [b,2]	25.2 ± 2.4 [b,2]	21.9 ± 2.7 [a-b,2]	24.4 ± 0.9 [b,2]	21.1 ± 0.7 [a,3]
OH90P	25.2 ± 0.4 [e,1]	24.2 ± 0.8 [d,1]	20.9 ± 0.2 [c,3]	18.2 ± 0.4 [a,1]	19.1 ± 0.4 [b,1]
OH180P	25.2 ± 0.4 [b,1]	24.6 ± 0.4 [b,1]	19.1 ± 1.2 [a,2]	18.6 ± 0.7 [a,1]	18.4 ± 0.8 [a,1]
OE90P	28.0 ± 2.1 [c,1]	24.8 ± 1.0 [b,1]	17.9 ± 0.9 [a,1-2]	17.1 ± 2.0 [a,1]	17.4 ± 1.1 [a,1]
OE180P	28.0 ± 2.1 [c,1]	24.3 ± 2.2 [b,1]	17.0 ± 0.8 [a,1]	18.3 ± 0.4 [a,1]	19.7 ± 1.7 [a,1]
	Total phenolics (mg GAE/100 g f.w.)				
WH90P	66.9 ± 5.7 [a-b,1]	65.4 ± 2.4 [a,1]	77.5 ± 4.4 [b-c,1]	85.0 ± 0.6 [c,2]	80.9 ± 11 [c,1]
WH180P	66.9 ± 5.7 [a-b,1]	61.0 ± 0.6 [a,1]	79.5 ± 7.5 [c,1]	71.6 ± 5.5 [b-c,1]	78.6 ± 6.0 [c,1]
WE90P	60.7 ± 6.3 [a,1]	79.9 ± 19 [b,1-2]	120 ± 1.0 [d,3]	98.6 ± 4.9 [c,3]	122 ± 1.1 [d,2]
WE180P	60.7 ± 6.3 [a,1]	86.5 ± 7.5 [b,2]	98.7 ± 5.4 [c,2]	94.9 ± 6.4 [b-c,3]	121 ± 6.1 [d,2]
OH90P	59.6 ± 2.4 [a,1]	105 ± 13 [c,2]	96.6 ± 5.4 [b-c,1]	84.0 ± 9.2 [b,1]	91.9 ± 4.6 [b-c,1]
OH180P	59.6 ± 2.4 [a,1]	73.0 ± 9.3 [b,1]	97.6 ± 3.5 [d,1]	91.8 ± 2.2 [c-d,1]	86.3 ± 2.2 [c,1]
OE90P	85.7 ± 5.6 [a,2]	111 ± 6.9 [b-c,2]	117 ± 20 [b-c,1]	102 ± 2.6 [a-b,2]	127 ± 9.2 [c,2]
OE180P	85.7 ± 5.6 [a,2]	137 ± 3.4 [c,3]	106 ± 14 [b,1]	147 ± 0.9 [c-d,3]	152 ± 5.7 [d,3]
	Antioxidant capacity (DPPH) (mg TE/100 g f. w.)				
WH90P	2.2 ± 0.1 [a,2]	2.1 ± 0.4 [a,1]	2.1 ± 0.4 [a,1]	1.7 ± 0.3 [a,1]	1.6 ± 0.6 [a,1]
WH180P	2.2 ± 0.1 [b,2]	2.1 ± 0.1 [b,1]	1.7 ± 0.2 [a,1]	1.5 ± 0.2 [a,1]	1.5 ± 0.3 [a,1]
WE90P	1.8 ± 0.2 [a,1]	2.2 ± 0.4 [a,1]	1.8 ± 0.3 [a,1]	1.8 ± 0.3 [a,1]	1.4 ± 0.3 [a,1]
WE180P	1.8 ± 0.2 [a,1]	2.0 ± 0.1 [a,1]	2.0 ± 0.1 [a,1]	1.5 ± 0.4 [a,1]	1.7 ± 0.7 [a,1]
OH90P	1.9 ± 0.4 [a,1]	2.0 ± 0.6 [a,1]	1.8 ± 0.5 [a,1]	1.8 ± 0.4 [a,1]	1.8 ± 0.7 [a,1]
OH180P	1.9 ± 0.4 [a,1]	2.1 ± 0.7 [a,1]	1.8 ± 0.5 [a,1]	1.8 ± 0.4 [a,1]	1.7 ± 0.3 [a,1]
OE90P	1.9 ± 0.2 [a-b,1]	2.4 ± 0.2 [c,1]	2.2 ± 0.1 [b-c,1]	1.9 ± 0.3 [a-b,1]	1.6 ± 0.4 [a,1]
OE180P	1.9 ± 0.2 [a-b,1]	2.2 ± 0.5 [b,1]	2.2 ± 0.2 [b,1]	1.8 ± 0.2 [a-b,1]	1.4 ± 0.2 [a,1]

Hand-peeled (H) and electrically peeled (E) white (W) and orange (O) prickly pears packaged in 90PPlus (90P) and 180PPlus (180P) film. Different letters in a row indicate that there were significant differences between storage days ($p < 0.05$), and different numbers in a column indicate that there were significant differences between samples ($p < 0.05$).

Total phenolic content increased with storage time (Table 5). Ochoa-Velasco and Guerrero-Beltrán [40] found that the phenolic content in white prickly pears slightly decreased during storage but significantly increased in red prickly pears after 4 days of storage. In contrast, Palma et al. [38] reported decreases in the contents of these compounds over storage time in the "Bianca" and "Gialla" varieties and Piga et al. [12] described a decrease after 3 days of storage at 4 °C in the "Gialla" variety. In our study, the white and orange varieties suffered more noticeable increases from days 3 and 1 of storage, respectively. It was also observed that the peeling method influenced the antioxidant compound contents; the electrically peeled pears showed higher values than the hand-peeled pears. Significant differences were observed in OE depending on the type of film, with the exception of days 0 and 3. In contrast to total phenolic content, as storage time progresses, a decrease in antioxidant capacity (DPPH) was observed for both varieties. These results were similar to those obtained by Palma et al. [38] in the "Bianca" variety but not in the "Gialla" variety, as well as those of Piga et al. [12]. No significant differences were detected in antioxidant capacity (DPPH) depending on the type of film used or the type of peeling performed, except for WH fruits that presented higher values than WE at the moment of processing.

4. Conclusions

In this study, minimally processed white and orange prickly pears maintained suitable microbial and nutritional quality after 8 days of storage at 7 °C. Throughout storage, the counts of microorganisms increased regardless of the variety, peeling method, or micro-perforated film used. However, the counts of aerobic mesophiles bacteria remained below the limits established by the Spanish legislation (<7 log(CFU/g f.w.) until day 8. Similarly, the counts of psychrophiles, molds, and yeasts did not exceed values of 6 log(CFU/g f.w.).

Electrically peeled prickly pears presented interesting characteristics from a technological and nutritional point of view. Moreover, the contents of bioactive compounds such as ascorbic acid and total phenolic compounds were higher in the electrically peeled fruits.

Fresh-cut orange prickly pears were well evaluated independently of the peeling method and the micro-perforated film used from the beginning to the end of the experiment. White prickly pears were initially evaluated less well when peeled with the electric peeler than with the knife because the electrically peeled pears presented part of the thick pericarp characteristic of this variety.

We recommend using the 180PPlus film and adjusting the electric peeling method depending on the thickness of the prickly pear pericarp to prevent consumers from perceiving any unpleasant sensation, as occurred with the white prickly pears used in this study.

Electrically peeled minimally processed prickly pears could be a value-added healthy alternative because of their high nutritional quality, thus facilitating their consumption. The by-products generated in the agro-industries can be used for animal feeding or as sources of antioxidants, fiber, natural colorants, mucilage, etc.

Author Contributions: Conceptualization, M.G.L. and G.L.D.-D.; methodology, M.G.L., G.L.D.-D., E.M.R.-R. and E.D.; software, E.M.R.-R. and G.L.D.-D.; validation, E.M.R.-R., G.L.D.-D. and M.G.L.; formal analysis, G.L.D.-D. and E.M.R.-R.; investigation, G.L.D.-D., M.G.L., E.M.R.-R. and E.D.; resources, M.G.L.; data curation, G.L.D.-D. and E.M.R.-R.; writing—original draft preparation, G.L.D.-D.; writing—review and editing, M.G.L., E.M.R.-R. and E.D.; visualization, G.L.D.-D., M.G.L., E.M.R.-R. and E.D.; supervision, M.G.L. and E.M.R.-R.; project administration, M.G.L.; funding acquisition, M.G.L. All authors have read and agreed to the published version of the manuscript.

Funding: This research was funded by "Instituto Nacional de Investigación y Tecnología Agraria y Alimentaria (INIA)", grant number RTA 2015-00044-C02 "Estudio integral de aprovechamiento de Opuntia (Tuna o Higo Chumbo) para la obtención de derivados e ingredientes funcionales mediante la aplicación de tecnologías innovadoras".

Institutional Review Board Statement: Not applicable.

Informed Consent Statement: Informed consent was obtained from all subjects involved in the sensorial evaluation.

Data Availability Statement: Data will be made available on reasonable request.

Acknowledgments: The authors would like to acknowledge the support and collaboration given by the orchard farmers.

Conflicts of Interest: The authors declare no conflict of interest.

Appendix A

Table A1. Color, hardness, and texture of manually or electrically peeled white and orange minimally processed prickly pears packed in two films of different permeability during cold storage at 7 °C.

	Storage Period (Days)				
	0	1	3	6	8
a*					
WH90P	−4.50 ± 1.98 [a,2]	−4.10 ± 1.21 [a,2]	−3.63 ± 0.74 [a,2]	−3.78 ± 1.00 [a,2]	−3.62 ± 1.36 [a,2]
WH180P	−3.89 ± 0.92 [a,2]	−3.05 ± 0.29 [a,3]	−3.16 ± 0.76 [a,2]	−3.17 ± 0.39 [a,2]	−2.95 ± 0.35 [a,2]
WE90P	−8.08 ± 1.01 [a,1]	−6.71 ± 0.74 [a,1]	−6.68 ± 0.52 [a,1]	−6.71 ± 1.23 [a,1]	−6.42 ± 1.00 [a,1]
WE180P	−7.16 ± 0.37 [a,1]	−7.09 ± 0.42 [a,1]	−7.10 ± 0.72 [a,1]	−6.89 ± 0.56 [a,1]	−6.36 ± 1.39 [a,1]
OH90P	15.1 ± 3.58 [a,2]	13.8 ± 1.41 [a,1]	12.8 ± 3.08 [a,1]	12.1 ± 2.54 [a,1]	12.0 ± 2.63 [a,1]
OH180P	15.9 ± 3.46 [a,2]	15.4 ± 1.65 [a,1]	14.6 ± 2.64 [a,1]	13.2 ± 3.39 [a,1]	12.0 ± 2.75 [a,1]
OE90P	20.8 ± 2.00 [b,3]	12.4 ± 0.76 [a,1]	11.6 ± 2.51 [a,1]	12.6 ± 1.80 [a,1]	11.9 ± 2.73 [a,1]
OE180P	8.92 ± 0.47 [a,1]	12.9 ± 2.39 [a,1]	11.0 ± 3.87 [a,1]	9.92 ± 4.48 [a,1]	9.21 ± 3.29 [a,1]
b*					
WH90P	17.1 ± 3.22 [a,1]	14.5 ± 3.17 [a,1]	13.2 ± 3.51 [a,1]	17.8 ± 3.93 [a,1]	17.7 ± 3.74 [a,1]
WH180P	15.2 ± 3.05 [b,1]	12.1 ± 1.58 [a,1]	13.1 ± 2.25 [a-b,1]	15.6 ± 2.20 [b,1]	15.8 ± 1.15 [b,1]
WE90P	25.4 ± 2.95 [b-c,2]	21.1 ± 3.13 [a,2]	22.2 ± 1.88 [a-b,2]	24.8 ± 3.56 [a-c,2]	26.3 ± 2.02 [c,2]
WE180P	21.7 ± 2.17 [a,2]	22.4 ± 2.88 [a,2]	23.2 ± 2.79 [a,2]	24.8 ± 2.76 [a-b,2]	27.9 ± 3.80 [b,2]
OH90P	23.2 ± 4.38 [a,1]	15.5 ± 6.00 [a,1]	15.8 ± 3.91 [a,1]	15.6 ± 5.04 [a,1]	16.3 ± 4.40 [a,1]
OH180P	21.1 ± 5.02 [a,1]	20.7 ± 1.80 [a,1]	19.7 ± 2.29 [a,1]	19.6 ± 3.88 [a,1]	18.5 ± 2.50 [a,1-2]
OE90P	29.6 ± 3.43 [b,2]	16.8 ± 3.95 [a,1]	17.6 ± 4.99 [a,1]	20.6 ± 3.49 [a,1]	18.6 ± 3.16 [a,1-2]
OE180P	21.6 ± 5.39 [a,1]	22.4 ± 5.33 [a,1]	21.1 ± 5.23 [a,1]	22.5 ± 2.68 [a,1]	22.8 ± 2.80 [a,2]
Hardness (°Durofel)					
WH90P	31.0 ± 2.0 [a,1]	28.0 ± 1.7 [a,1]	28.0 ± 3.0 [a,1]	24.7 ± 3.2 [a,1]	27.5 ± 1.5 [a,1]
WH180P	31.0 ± 2.0 [a,1]	38.5 ± 0.5 [a,2]	40.0 ± 1.0 [a,2]	41.0 ± 4.6 [a,2]	31.5 ± 9.5 [a,1]
WE90P	57.0 ± 1.0 [b,2]	51.3 ± 5.5 [a,3]	45.5 ± 5.5 [a,2-3]	53.5 ± 0.5 [b,3]	55.0 ± 4.6 [b,2]
WE180P	57.0 ± 1.0 [c,2]	41.0 ± 1.0 [a,2]	49.5 ± 2.5 [b,3]	50.3 ± 3.1 [b,3]	48.3 ± 6.0 [b,2]
OH90P	38.0 ± 2.0 [a,1]	32.0 ± 5.2 [a,1]	29.8 ± 3.0 [a,1]	30.3 ± 7.1 [a,1]	27.0 ± 5.3 [a,1]
OH180P	38.0 ± 2.0 [a,1]	28.3 ± 4.0 [a,1]	29.5 ± 3.0 [a,1]	29.5 ± 3.0 [a,1]	30.7 ± 6.4 [a,1]
OE90P	48.7 ± 4.2 [a,2]	41.7 ± 3.8 [a,2]	43.3 ± 8.0 [a,2]	39.3 ± 9.6 [a,1]	34.6 ± 10.1 [a,1]
OE180P	48.7 ± 4.2 [a,2]	42.1 ± 1.0 [a,2]	42.5 ± 0.5 [a,2]	44.4 ± 9.0 [a,1]	43.8 ± 2.7 [a,1]
Texture (N s/g fresh weight)					
WH90P	10.4 ± 1.5 [a,2]	12.1 ± 2.3 [a,1]	11.4 ± 2.5 [a,2-3]	10.3 ± 2.2 [a,1]	10.0 ± 0.4 [a,1]
WH180P	10.4 ± 1.5 [a,2]	11.1 ± 1.8 [a-b,1]	13.5 ± 0.6 [b,3]	13.7 ± 2.0 [b,1]	13.6 ± 0.4 [b,3]
WE90P	7.5 ± 0.8 [a,1]	8.3 ± 0.4 [a-b,1]	8.5 ± 0.3 [b,1]	9.6 ± 0.7 [c,1]	11.6 ± 0.3 [d,2]
WE180P	7.5 ± 0.8 [a,1]	10.1 ± 2.0 [b,1]	10.8 ± 0.7 [b,1-2]	11.8 ± 0.8 [b,1]	9.8 ± 0.5 [b,1]
OH90P	3.6 ± 0.6 [a,1]	3.6 ± 0.9 [a,1]	5.7 ± 0.6 [b,1]	5.1 ± 1.0 [a-b,1]	5.6 ± 1.3 [b,1]
OH180P	3.6 ± 0.6 [a,1]	5.2 ± 2.0 [a-b,1-2]	6.5 ± 0.3 [b,1]	5.7 ± 0.2 [b,1]	6.6 ± 0.2 [b,1]
OE90P	7.7 ± 0.5 [b,2]	7.3 ± 0.3 [b,2]	6.2 ± 0.8 [a,1]	6.1 ± 0.4 [a,1]	5.6 ± 0.2 [a,1]
OE180P	7.7 ± 0.5 [a,2]	5.7 ± 0.3 [a,12]	8.9 ± 2.3 [a,1]	8.3 ± 0.7 [a,2]	7.6 ± 1.2 [a,1]

Hand-peeled (H) and electrically peeled (E) white (W) and orange (O) prickly pears packaged in 90PPlus (90P) and 180PPlus (180P) film. Different letters in a row indicate that there were significant differences between storage days ($p < 0.05$), and different numbers in a column indicate that there were significant differences between samples ($p < 0.05$).

References

1. Yahia, E.M. *Fruit and Vegetable Phytochemicals: Chemistry and Human Health*; John Wiley & Sons: Hoboken, NJ, USA, 2017; Volume 2, ISBN 978-1-119-15794-6.
2. Paz, P.L.P.; de Padrón, C.E.H. *Plantas Medicinales o Útiles en la Flora Canaria: Aplicaciones Populares*; Detalles Del Producto: La Laguna, Spain, 1999; ISBN 978-84-87973-12-3.
3. Cano, M.P.; Gómez-Maqueo, A.; García-Cayuela, T.; Welti-Chanes, J. Characterization of Carotenoid Profile of Spanish Sanguinos and Verdal Prickly Pear (*Opuntia ficus-indica*, spp.) Tissues. *Food Chem.* **2017**, *237*, 612–622. [CrossRef] [PubMed]
4. Kossori, R.L.; Villaume, C.; Boustani, E.; Sauvaire, Y.; Méjean, L. Composition of Pulp, Skin and Seeds of Prickly Pears Fruit (*Opuntia ficus-indica*, sp.). *Plant Foods Hum. Nutr.* **1998**, *52*, 263–270. [CrossRef] [PubMed]
5. Hernández-Pérez, T.; Carrillo-López, A.; Guevara-Lara, F.; Cruz-Hernández, A.; Paredes-López, O. Biochemical and Nutritional Characterization of Three Prickly Pear Species with Different Ripening Behavior. *Plant Foods Hum. Nutr.* **2005**, *60*, 195–200. [CrossRef] [PubMed]
6. Silva, M.A.; Albuquerque, T.G.; Pereira, P.; Ramalho, R.; Vicente, F.; Oliveira, M.B.P.P.; Costa, H.S. *Opuntia ficus-indica* (L.) Mill.: A Multi-Benefit Potential to Be Exploited. *Molecules* **2021**, *26*, 951. [CrossRef]
7. Gómez-Maqueo, A.; Steurer, D.; Welti-Chanes, J.; Cano, M.P. Bioaccesibility of Antioxidants in Prickly Pear Fruits Treated with High Hydrostatic Pressure: An Application for Healthier Foods. *Molecules* **2021**, *26*, 5252. [CrossRef]

8. Osuna-Martínez, L.; Reyes Esparza, J.; Rodríguez-Fragoso, L. Cactus (*Opuntia ficus-indica*): A Review on Its Antioxidants Properties and Potential Pharmacological Use in Chronic Diseases. *Nat. Prod. Chem. Res.* **2014**, *2*, 153–160. [CrossRef]
9. Gómez-Maqueo, A.; Antunes-Ricardo, M.; Welti-Chanes, J.; Cano, M.P. Digestive Stability and Bioaccessibility of Antioxidants in Prickly Pear Fruits from the Canary Islands: Healthy Foods and Ingredients. *Antioxidants* **2020**, *9*, 164. [CrossRef]
10. Flores, C.A.; de Luna, J.M.; Ramirez, P.P. *Mercado Mundial Del Nopalito*; Servicios a la Comercialización Agropecuaria (ASERCA)/Universidad Autónoma Chapingo (UACh)/Centro de Investigaciones Económicas, Sociales y Tecnológicas de la Agroindustria y la Agricultura Mundial (CIESTAAM): Chapingo, México, 1995; 177p.
11. Artés, F.; Allende, A. Minimal Fresh Processing of Vegetables, Fruits and Juices. In *Emerging Technologies for Food Processing*; Elsevier: Amsterdam, The Netherlands, 2005; Volume 26, pp. 677–716, ISBN 978-0-12-676757-5.
12. Piga, A.; Caro, A.D.; Pinna, I.; Agabbio, M. Changes in Ascorbic Acid, Polyphenol Content and Antioxidant Activity in Minimally Processed Cactus Pear Fruits. *LWT Food Sci. Technol.* **2003**, *2*, 257–262. [CrossRef]
13. Abadias, M.; Usall, J.; Anguera, M.; Solsona, C.; Viñas, I. Microbiological Quality of Fresh, Minimally-Processed Fruit and Vegetables, and Sprouts from Retail Establishments. *Int. J. Food Microbiol.* **2008**, *123*, 121–129. [CrossRef]
14. Kahramanoglu, I.; Usanmaz, S.; Okatan, V.; Wan, C. Preserving Postharvest Storage Quality of Fresh-Cut Cactus Pears by Using Different Bio-Materials. *CABI Agric. Biosci.* **2020**, *1*, 7. [CrossRef]
15. Troyo, R.; Acedo, A.J. Effects of Calcium Ascorbate and Calcium Lactate on Quality of Fresh-Cut Pineapple (Ananas Comosus). *Int. J. Agric. For. Life Sci.* **2019**, *3*, 143–150.
16. Padrón Mederos, M.A.; Rodríguez-Galdón, B.; Díaz-Romero, C.; Lobo, G.; Rodríguez-Rodríguez, E. Quality Evaluation of Minimally Fresh-Cut Processed Pineapples. *LWT* **2020**, *129*, 109607. [CrossRef]
17. Agar, I.; Massantini, R.; Hess-Pierce, B.; Kader, A. Postharvest CO_2 and Ethylene Production and Quality Maintenance of Fresh-Cut Kiwi fruit Slices. *J. Food Sci.* **2006**, *64*, 433–440. [CrossRef]
18. Silva, F.A.; Finkler, L.; Finkler, C.L.L. Effect of Edible Coatings Based on Alginate/Pectin on Quality Preservation of Minimally Processed "Espada" Mangoes. *J. Food Sci. Technol.* **2018**, *55*, 5055–5063. [CrossRef] [PubMed]
19. Mphahlele, R.R.; Caleb, O.J.; Ngcobo, M.E.K. Effects of Packaging and Duration on Quality of Minimally Processed and Unpitted Litchi Cv. "Mauritius" under Low Storage Temperature. *Heliyon* **2020**, *6*, e03229. [CrossRef] [PubMed]
20. Kohli, D.; Champawat, P.S.; Mudgal, V.D.; Jain, S.K.; Tiwari, B.K. Advances in Peeling Techniques for Fresh Produce. *J. Food Process Eng.* **2021**, *44*, e13826. [CrossRef]
21. Tapia, M.; Gutiérrez-Pacheco, M.M.; Vázquez Armenta, F.J.; González Aguilar, G.A.; Ayala-Zavala, J.F.; Rahman, M.S.; Siddiqui, M.W. Washing, Peeling and Cutting of Fresh-Cut Fruits and Vegetables. In *Minimally Processed Foods*; Springer: Berlin/Heidelberg, Germany, 2015; pp. 57–78, ISBN 978-3-319-10677-9.
22. Emadi, B.; Yarlagadda, P. Peeling Pumpkin Using Rotary Cutter. In *Proceedings, Global Congress on Manufacturing and Management, GCMM 2006*; Ciampi, M., da Rocha Brito, C., Eds.; COPEC—Council of Researches in Education and Sciences: Santos, Brazil, 2006; pp. 114–118, ISBN 978-85-89120-38-8.
23. Shirmohammadi, M.; Yarlagadda, P.; Kosse, V.; Gu, Y.T. Study of Mechanical Deformations on Tough Skinned Vegetables during Mechanical Peeling Process (A Review). *GSTF J. Eng. Technol.* **2012**, *1*, 31–37. [CrossRef]
24. Alexandre, E.M.C.; Coelho, M.C.; Ozcan, K.; Pinto, C.A.; Teixeira, J.A.; Saraiva, J.A.; Pintado, M. Emergent Technologies for the Extraction of Antioxidants from Prickly Pear Peel and Their Antimicrobial Activity. *Foods* **2021**, *10*, 570. [CrossRef]
25. Djeghim, F.; Bourekoua, H.; Różyło, R.; Bieńczak, A.; Tanaś, W.; Zidoune, M.N. Effect of By-Products from Selected Fruits and Vegetables on Gluten-Free Dough Rheology and Bread Properties. *Appl. Sci.* **2021**, *11*, 4605. [CrossRef]
26. Parafati, L.; Restuccia, C.; Palmeri, R.; Fallico, B.; Arena, E. Characterization of Prickly Pear Peel Flour as a Bioactive and Functional Ingredient in Bread Preparation. *Foods* **2020**, *9*, 1189. [CrossRef]
27. Morshedy, S.A.; Abdal Mohsen, A.E.; Basyony, M.M.; Almeer, R.; Abdel-Daim, M.M.; El-Gindy, Y.M. Effect of Prickly Pear Cactus Peel Supplementation on Milk Production, Nutrient Digestibility and Rumen Fermentation of Sheep and the Maternal Effects on Growth and Physiological Performance of Suckling Offspring. *Animals* **2020**, *10*, 1476. [CrossRef] [PubMed]
28. Ministerio de la Presidencia. *Real Decreto 3484/2000, de 29 de Diciembre, por el que se Establecen las Normas de Higiene para la Elaboración, Distribución y Comercio de Comidas Preparadas*; Ministerio de la Presidencia: Madrid, Spain, 2001; Volume BOE-A-2001-809, pp. 1435–1441.
29. Escalona, V.H.; Aguayo, E.; Artés, F. Quality and Physiological Changes of Fresh-Cut Kohlrabi. *HortScience* **2003**, *38*, 1148–1152. [CrossRef]
30. Karacay, E.; Ayhan, Z. Microbial, Physical, Chemical and Sensory Qualities of Minimally Processed and Modified Atmosphere Packaged "Ready To Eat" Orange Segments. *Int. J. Food Prop.* **2010**, *13*, 960–971. [CrossRef]
31. Panadés, G.; Chiralt, A.; Fito, P.; Rodríguez, I.; Nuñez, M.; Albors, A.; Jiménez, R. Influence of Operating Conditions on Sensory Quality of Minimally Processed Osmotically Dehydrated Guava. *J. Food Qual.* **2003**, *26*, 91–103. [CrossRef]
32. Obenland, D.; Collin, S.; Sievert, J.; Negm, F.; Arpaia, M. Influence of Maturity and Ripening on Aroma Volatiles and Flavor in 'Hass' Avocado. *Postharvest Biol. Technol.* **2012**, *71*, 41–50. [CrossRef]
33. Aguayo, E.; Allende, A.; Artés, F. Keeping Quality and Safety of Minimal Fresh Processed Melon. *Eur. Food Res. Technol.* **2003**, *216*, 494–499. [CrossRef]
34. Horwitz, W.; Latimer, G.W. *Association of Official Analytical Chemists International Official Methods of Analysis of AOAC International*; AOAC International: Gaithersburg, MD, USA, 2006; ISBN 978-0-935584-77-6.

35. Bondet, V.; Brand-Williams, W.; Berset, C. Kinetics and Mechanisms of Antioxidant Activity Using the DPPH.Free Radical Method. *LWT -Food Sci. Technol.* **1997**, *30*, 609–615. [CrossRef]
36. Rodríguez-Galdón, B.; Tascón-Rodríguez, C.; Rodríguez-Rodríguez, E.M.; Díaz-Romero, C. Fructans and Major Compounds in Onion Cultivars (*Allium cepa*). *J. Food Compos. Anal.* **2009**, *22*, 25–32. [CrossRef]
37. Cefola, M.; Renna, M.; Pace, B. Marketability of Ready-to-Eat Cactus Pear as Affected by Temperature and Modified Atmosphere. *J. Food Sci. Technol.* **2014**, *51*, 25–33. [CrossRef]
38. Palma, A.; Continella, A.; Malfa, S.; D'Aquino, S. Changes in Physiological and Some Nutritional, Nutraceuticals, Chemical-Physical, Microbiological and Sensory Quality Minimally Processed Cactus Pears Cvs "Bianca", "Gialla" and "Rossa" Stored under Passive Modified Atmosphere. *J. Sci. Food Agric.* **2017**, *98*, 1839–1849. [CrossRef]
39. Allegra, A.; Sortino, G.; Miciletta, G.; Riotto, M.; Fasciana, T.; Inglese, P. The Influence of Harvest Period and Fruit Ripeness at Harvest on Minimally Processed Cactus Pears (*Opuntia ficus-indica* L. Mill.) Stored under Passive Atmosphere. *Postharvest Biol. Technol.* **2015**, *104*, 57–62. [CrossRef]
40. Ochoa Velasco, C.E.; Guerrero-Beltran, J. Postharvest Quality of Peeled Prickly Pear Fruit Treated with Acetic Acid and Chitosan. *Postharvest Biol. Technol.* **2014**, *92*, 139–145. [CrossRef]

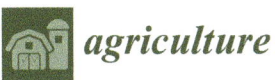

Article

The Variation of Rice Quality and Relevant Starch Structure during Long-Term Storage

Hao Hu [1], Shipeng Li [1], Danjie Pan [2], Kaijun Wang [2], Mingming Qiu [1], Zhuzhu Qiu [1], Xingquan Liu [1] and Jiaojiao Zhang [1,*]

[1] College of Food and Health, Zhejiang Agriculture and Forest University, Hangzhou 311300, China
[2] Hangzhou Food Security Service Center, Hangzhou 310016, China
* Correspondence: jjzhang@zafu.edu.cn; Tel.: +86-13564440954

Abstract: The main substances of rice are starches, which vary their metabolism during storage. We conducted a series of tests including rice physicochemical properties, edible quality, starch content and chain length distribution along with starch structure variation to disclose the shift of rice quality by observing the changes of rice during storage. The results showed that: (1) the rice deterioration occurred as time passed, and the germination rate decreased from 70.8% to 29.4% during the storage; (2) fatty acid values increased significantly during long-term storage; (3) electrical conductivity increased as time passed; and (4) the two-year-storage rice showed significantly decreased viscosity and edible quality after sensory evaluation, decreased hardness and damaged surface area of starch granules as storage time passed. Additionally, the damaged surface area of starch granules increased with storage time. Fourier transform infrared spectroscopy (FTIR) showed that the short-range order and spiral degree of rice starch first decreased in the first year and then increased over the storage time. Furthermore, X-ray diffraction showed that the main starch of rice was A-type crystalline. Meanwhile, apparent amylose content increased from 31.00% to 33.85%, then decreased to 31.75%. The peak viscosity reduced from 2735.00 mPa·s to 2163.67 mPa·s and the disintegration value was brought down from 1377.67 mPa·s to 850.33 mPa·s. Based on the results, rice should not be stored for more than 2 years under suitable granary conditions to maintain it at a good quality.

Keywords: rice; starch structure; physicochemical quality; storage

Citation: Hu, H.; Li, S.; Pan, D.; Wang, K.; Qiu, M.; Qiu, Z.; Liu, X.; Zhang, J. The Variation of Rice Quality and Relevant Starch Structure during Long-Term Storage. *Agriculture* **2022**, *12*, 1211. https://doi.org/10.3390/agriculture12081211

Academic Editor: Bengang Wu

Received: 8 July 2022
Accepted: 9 August 2022
Published: 12 August 2022

Publisher's Note: MDPI stays neutral with regard to jurisdictional claims in published maps and institutional affiliations.

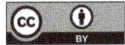

Copyright: © 2022 by the authors. Licensee MDPI, Basel, Switzerland. This article is an open access article distributed under the terms and conditions of the Creative Commons Attribution (CC BY) license (https://creativecommons.org/licenses/by/4.0/).

1. Introduction

Rice is a staple food for half of the world's population and plays an important role in daily diet [1]. The COVID-19 pandemic and the outbreak of conflict between Russia and Ukraine had disrupted world food production and supplication, making food storage more important than before [2]. The storage quality of rice is usually affected by temperature, humidity, atmosphere and storage time, so its physical, chemical and physiological characteristics will undergo a variation during long-term storage. When rice ages in storage, its color and flavor will change obviously [3]. Compared with fresh rice, aged rice usually turns dark and yellow and develops unpleasant odors due to the rancidity of fatty acids. Additionally, the processing characteristics of aged rice vary greatly, such as decreased viscosity and gelatinization temperature, along with increased hardness [4,5] Based on the effect of storage conditions and aging phenomenon on rice quality, it is quite important to control the aging rate of rice and develop methods to maintain the storage and edible quality of rice.

Starch, as the most important component of rice, accounts for about 80% of rice dry weight, which is closely related with rice aging and its quality variation [6]. Starch is a kind of polysaccharide polymer which is mainly composed of α-D-glucopyranosyl units linked by glycosidic bonds [7]. It contains linear amyloses linked by α-1, 4-glycosidic bond and highly branched amylopectins linked by α-1, 6-glycosidic [8]. The short side chains of branched starch are stacked in the double helix structure to form the crystalline region in starch. The alternative distribution of the crystalline region and the amorphous region constitutes the growth ring of starch granules [9]. The starch function usually changes accordingly with the structural transforms, like the straight-chain starch content is correlated with the pasting property of rice [10]. The higher straight chain amylose content, the harder the edible quality of the rice will be [11]. For the amylopectin, the longer branched chain can form a longer double helix structure in the semi-crystalline layer, leading to a higher gelatinization temperature of rice. The vice versa is also true. Meanwhile, the interaction between amylose and the outer chain of amylopectin in the crystal lamella also has a crucial impact on rice gelatinization [12]. Many studies have shown that the multi-scale structure and physicochemical property of starch have a significant influence on the texture, processing and nutritional properties of rice [13]. Starch retrogradation is the main reason for the hardening of rice after cooking and cooling [14]. When straight-chain starch content is increased, it will facilitate the starch retrogradation. What's more, the rice with higher straight-chain starch content and long-chain branched starch content tends to contain more slow-digesting starch (SDS) and resistant starch (RS) and possess more functional properties [15,16].

To improve the storage quality of rice, it is important to figure out the effect of the transformation of the starch structure and physicochemical properties on the taste quality of rice during storage. Although many research studies have explored this relationship in the laboratory conditions, there is still a lack of studies on the long-term storage at the granary level [17]. Compared with the previous related studies, in this paper, we mainly focus on the rice from granary and investigate the variation in the rice quality and starch structure and their interaction, so as to provide practical suggestions for maintaining rice with a desirable quality in granary.

2. Materials and Methods

2.1. Materials

The samples belong to indica rice (Zhongzheyou 8), which are stored for 0, 1 and 2 years in Quzhou grain depot in Zhejiang Province under the temperature of 20–25 °C in summer and 10–15 °C in other seasons. The conditions were maintained by air conditioner to keep the rice at a quasi-low temperature. The rice stored for different years were set as different treatments. Each treatment was composed of five samples from five different silos, for a total of 15 samples in this study.

2.2. Physicochemical Properties' Variation of Rice

Rice germination rate was tested according to Hu's method with appropriate modifications [18]. One hundred pellets of rice seeds were soaked in 0.5% sodium hypochlorite for 30 s, and then rinsed 3 times using distilled water. The cleaned rice seeds were placed into a sterile germination box (20 × 20 cm), followed by being incubated under the condition of 60% relative humidity at 30 °C for 10 d. The germinated seeds were taken to calculate the germination rate. The rice conductivity was determined using Qu's method [19]. The determination of fatty acid values was carried out with Zhai's test method [20]. The protein content was determined by the method in Daiana deSouza's research [21].

2.3. Rice Edible Quality Evaluation

Rice edible quality was tested using a previous method with a slight modification [20]. Ten grams of cleaned rice seeds with different storage times were soaked for 30 min and cooked in a steamer for 40 min for a tasting test. The tasting test was conducted by artificial oral tasting combined with tasting apparatus (STA1B style, Sasake Co., Toshima, Japan).

2.4. Rice Starch Isolation

Rice was soaked overnight with five-time volumes of distilled water, after which it was pulped by a 200-mesh sieve and washed with distilled water. After centrifugation at

4000 rpm for 10 min, the suspension was collected by removing the upper layer of protein. Then, it was dried at 42 °C and filtrated through a 100-mesh sieve for the further analysis.

2.5. Starch Content Determination

2.5.1. Amylose and Total Starch Content Analysis

The straight-chain amylose content of rice starch was determined by iodine colorimetric method. It was calculated from the standard curves drawn with different proportions of straight-chain starch and branched-chain starch blends [22].

2.5.2. Distribution of Starch Chain Length

Based on Ren's method, the distribution of starch chain length in rice was tested [23]. The starch (10 mg) was dissolved in 5 mL water and then placed in a boiling water bath for 60 min. Afterwards, sodium azide solution (10 µL 2% w/v), acetate buffer (50 µL, 0.6 M, pH 4.4) and isoamylase (10 µL, 1400 U) were added to the starch dispersion, and the mixture was incubated at 37 °C for 24 h. The hydroxyl groups of the debranched glucans were reduced with 0.5% (w/v) of sodium borohydride under alkaline conditions for 20 h. Then, the solution was diluted with 570 µL of distilled water. The sample extracts were analyzed using high-performance anion-exchange chromatography (HPAEC) equipped with a CarboPac PA-200 anion-exchange column (4.0 × 250 mm; Dionex) and a pulsed amperometric detector (PAD; Dionex ICS 5000 system). Data were acquired on the ICS5000 (Thermo Scientific, Waltham, MA, USA) and processed using chromeleon 7.2 CDS (Thermo Scientific).

2.6. Starch X-ray Diffraction Analysis (XRD)

The crystal structure of rice starch was analyzed by a X'Pert3 Powder (PANalytical, Almelo, The Netherlands). The machine was equipped with a Cu-Kα target ray and the wavelength was 0.15406 nm. The starch was detected at the voltage of 40 kV and the tube flow was 200 mA. The diffraction ranged from 4° to 40° (2θ) with the 4°/min step length. The degree of relative crystallinity was calculated based on the two-phase hypohypothes according to the method reported by Lopez-Rubio et al. [24].

2.7. Starch Fourier Transform Infrared Spectroscopy Anlysis (FTIR)

The rice starch samples were ground with KBr at the ratio of 1:100. Then, the mixed power was tableted by a tablet machine to form flakes. The short-range structure was observed by FTIR (Brucker GMBH, Berlin, Germany) at the range of 4000–400 cm^{-1}. The operation was executed at the frequency of 4 cm^{-1} for 16 times.

2.8. Starch Rapid Viscosity Analysis (RVA)

The pasting property of starch flour was determined using a rapid viscosity analyzer and performed on the parboiled starch flour. The previously isolated starch was weighted around 2.58 g and mixed with distilled water to the total weight of 28 g. The suspension was maintained at 50 °C for 1 min, then it was heated to 95 °C at a rate of 12 °C/min and was held for 5 min. The rice paste was cooled to 50 °C at a rate of 12 °C/min and was maintained for 2 min. The pasting curve of rice stored for different times was obtained by RVA equipment (Newport Scientific Instruments inc. Fyshwick, Austrilia).

2.9. Differential Scanning Calorimetry (DSC) Analysis of Starch

The thermal stability of starch was evaluated by DSC calorimeter (METTLER TOLEDO, Inc. New York, NY, USA). The rice starch (3 mg) and distilled water (1:3, w/w) were sealed in an aluminum crucible and then equilibrated overnight. The measurement temperature was raised from 30 °C to 130 °C at the ratio of 10 °C/min.

2.10. Scanning Electron Microscope Analysis of Starch (SEM)

The rice starch was fixed with 2.5% glutaraldehyde overnight and then eluted with gradient ethanol (30, 50, 70, 90, and 95%) for 20 min to preserve the rice morphology. After this treatment, a piece of fixed samples was coated with a thin layer gold and placed in the SEM to observe with the resolution of 2000× and 6000×.

2.11. Data Statistics and Analysis

The single treatment of each test had three replicates, and each test was conducted twice. Statistical analysis, one-way analysis of variance (ANOVA), Duncan's test and a post-hoc test were conducted using SPSS statistical software (Version 22.0, IBM, Armonk, New York, NY, USA). All the figures were plotted using Origin Pro software(Originlab 2020 student edition, Northampton, MA, USA).

3. Results and Discussion

3.1. Rice Physicochemical Properties Variation of Different Storage Time

Physical and chemical indexes are important characteristics of rice quality. Germination rate is a specific manifestation of seed vigor, which is usually affected by storage time. The longer the storage time, the lower the germination rate would be. In this study, as shown in Figure 1a, rice germination rate decreased significantly after being stored for two years, with a decrease of 41.4%, which means its vitality and nutritional quality decreased obviously. Additionally, fatty acid value is a key indicator of rice freshness and aging. The accumulation of excessive fatty acid can lead to rice rancidity, thus decreasing its edible quality [25]. Compared with fresh ones, the fatty acid value of rice became significantly higher after one year storage, whereas there was no difference after two years storage (Figure 1b), which may be due to the reduced lipase activity with longer storage time. Furthermore, cell membrane permeability is related to the nutrient supply of the rice embryo, so the rice cell membrane spoilage can be used to evaluate rice quality, which can be assessed by measuring conductivity [26]. The rice conductivity increased from 50 μs/(cm·g) to 73.6 μs/(cm·g) with storage time, indicating the rice quality decreased obviously (Figure 1c), which is consistent with the previous report [1]. However, the protein content is less affected by storage time, so it slightly decreased without evident difference in this study (Figure 1d).

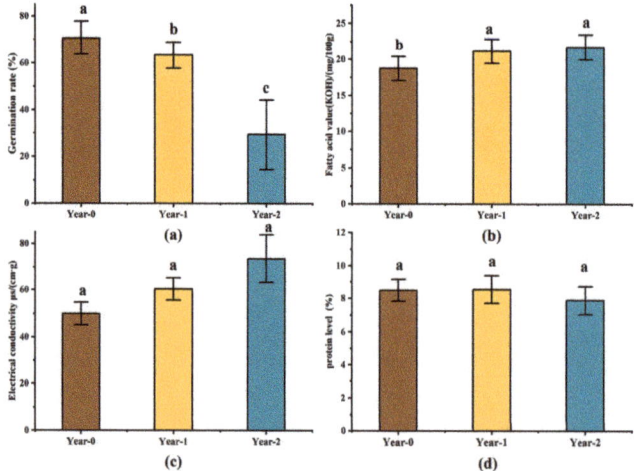

Figure 1. The changes in physical and chemical indexes of rice. (**a**) Germination rate, (**b**) fatty acid value, (**c**) electrical conductivity, (**d**) protein content. Different letters in this figure indicate there are significant differences among them. ($p < 0.05$).

3.2. Rice Taste Quality Eveluation

Sensory evaluation is the most classical and direct method to measure the taste quality of rice, which is also an important factor to influence consumers' purchase desire [27]. Rice characteristics, including hardness, stickiness, elasticity, color, odor and cold rice texture, are the expressions of rice taste quality. As shown in Table 1, the variation of rice sensory scores indicated that rice edible quality had significant decrease after being stored two years, especially rice luster, viscosity, elasticity and hardness. In a specific range, higher fat content of rice could make it more lustrous, so when the fat oxidation and decomposition happened in rice storage, its fatty acid value would increase, resulting in rice luster spoilage and the decreased flavor score [28]. The same phenomenon occurred in this study (Table 1). Additionally, firmness and stickiness are two key factors to assess the rice texture [29,30].

Table 1. Rice edible quality variation during different storage time.

Organoleptic Indicator	Year-0	Year-1	Year-2
Color	6.00 ± 0.00 [a]	6.00 ± 0.00 [a]	6.00 ± 0.00 [a]
Luster	5.20 ± 1.30 [a]	4.80 ± 0.84 [a]	4.60 ± 0.55 [b]
Grain integrity	3.00 ± 0.00 [a]	3.00 ± 0.00 [a]	3.00 ± 0.00 [a]
Viscosity	6.80 ± 0.45 [a]	6.20 ± 0.45 [a]	5.60 ± 0.55 [b]
Elasticity	6.20 ± 0.84 [a]	5.80 ± 0.84 [a]	5.60 ± 1.34 [b]
Hardness	7.20 ± 0.45 [a]	6.80 ± 0.84 [a]	6.60 ± 0.55 [b]
Taste	18.0 ± 1.73 [a]	17.00 ± 0.00 [a]	16.80 ± 0.45 [a]
Cold rice texture	3.00 ± 0.00 [a]	3.00 ± 0.00 [a]	3.00 ± 0.00 [a]

Notes: Different letter values in the same line were significantly different ($p < 0.05$).

The straight-chain starch content normally affects the hardness and viscosity of rice, which is on account of its leaching out and the formation of a web-like structure around the swollen granules during the cooking process. The long B-chain of branched starch can also form a double helix structure with straight-chain starch, which makes rice water absorption capacity decline and then results in rice hardness increasing [31]. Although the protein content did not have significant difference in this study, the increase in rice hardness indicated that the protein structure, especially the interaction between disulfide bonds, was strengthened [32]. Interestingly, the highest straight-chain amylose content was found in the rice stored for 1 year (Table 2), but the hardness score decreased significantly after 2-year storage. It manifested that rice hardness was not only affected by the straight-chain amylose content, but also by other factors, such as the soluble branched-chain starch content, molecular size and the interaction force between them [33]. As shown in Tables 2 and 3, rice stored for one year had the highest straight-chain starch content, but it didn't have an evident effect on rice viscosity. With the storage time extending, the straight-chain starch content decreased in the rice stored for two years, along with a declined viscosity, which might be due to the integrity breakdown of rice starch granules (Figure 2).

Table 2. Order degree of rice starch from different storage time.

Samples	Relative Crystalline (%)	995/1022	1047/1022
Year-0	34.23 ± 0.93 [a]	1.3871 ± 0.0139 [a]	1.3656 ± 0.0046 [a]
Year-1	34.95 ± 1.29 [a]	1.3192 ± 0.0117 [c]	1.3001 ± 0.0028 [c]
Year-2	35.25 ± 0.52 [a]	1.3616 ± 0.0136 [b]	1.3488 ± 0.0039 [b]

Notes: Values in the same column with different letters are significantly different ($p < 0.05$).

Table 3. Chain length distribution variation of rice amylopectin in storage.

Samples	AAC(%)	A(%)	B1(%)	B2(%)	B3(%)	ACL(DP)
Year-0	31.00 ± 0.73 [b]	24.67 ± 0.09 [a]	53.24 ± 0.06 [b]	11.16 ± 0.04 [b]	10.92 ± 0.10 [b]	20.15 ± 0.04 [b]
Year-1	33.85 ± 0.28 [a]	24.64 ± 0.02 [a]	51.08 ± 0.03 [c]	13.31 ± 0.03 [a]	11.00 ± 0.01 [b]	20.18 ± 0.01 [b]
Year-2	31.73 ± 0.48 [b]	23.63 ± 0.10 [b]	54.01 ± 0.05 [a]	11.19 ± 0.04 [b]	11.16 ± 0.04 [a]	20.32 ± 0.03 [a]

Notes: Apparent amylose content (AAC); A, B1, B2, B3 and average chain length (ACL) refer to DP ranges of 6–12, 13–24, 25–36, DP ≥ 37 and average chain length, respectively. Values in the same column with different letters are significantly different ($p < 0.05$).

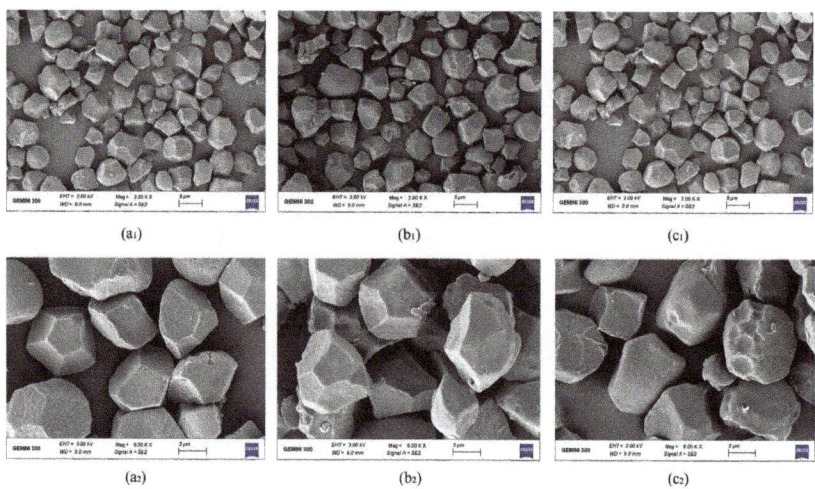

Figure 2. Scanning electron microscope photos of rice starch granules with different storage times; (**a1,a2**) are starch granules under storage year-0 2K, 6K lens; (**b1,b2**) are starch granules under storage year-1 2K, 6K lens; (**c1,c2**) are starch granules under storage year-2 2K, 6K lens.

3.3. Rice Starch Structure Variation of Different Storage Time

Natural starch granules mainly have three types of structure, including A, B and C. A-type crystalline structure has characteristic diffraction peaks at 2θ around 15.33°, 17.33°, 18.15° and 23.22°; B-type crystalline structure has characteristic diffraction peaks at 2θ around 5.59°, 17.2°, 23.2° and 24°; C-type crystalline structure has characteristic diffraction peaks at 2θ around 5.73°, 15.3°, 17.3°, 18.3° and 23.3°. Meanwhile, the main characteristic diffraction peaks of V-type crystalline structure are at 2θ of 7.36°, 13.1° and 20.1°. The rice starch structure generally belongs to A-type crystal texture [34].

As shown in Figure 3a, the starch isolated from rice had specific monomorphic diffraction peaks at 15.33° and 23.5°. The starches from rice with different times all belonged to A-type crystal structure, indicating that the storage time had no effect on rice crystal configuration, whereas the peak intensities were different at 2θ of 18.15°, 20.17° and 23.22°. The peak intensity decreased after 1 year of storage but increased after 2 years, which was consistent with the variation of A-type starch crystals. According to the results in Figure 3a and Table 3, the straight-chain starch content in rice samples stored for 2 years decreased significantly, which suggested that the free short straight-chain starch was bound to form a double-helix structure and this led to an increase in A-type crystals. The peak intensity at 20.1° represents the decreased content of V-type crystals, which are usually composed of single-helix straight-chain starch and lipids [35]. The tendency was related to the fat oxidative decomposition, which promoted the increase in straight-chain starch content. However, the B-type crystals gradually increased based on the diffraction intensity up to 23.22°. The composition of B-type crystals is often related to the content of branched starch B-chains. As shown in Table 3, the content of longer B-chains (B2, B3) increased with storage time extending, which was the principal reason for the B-type crystals' accession.

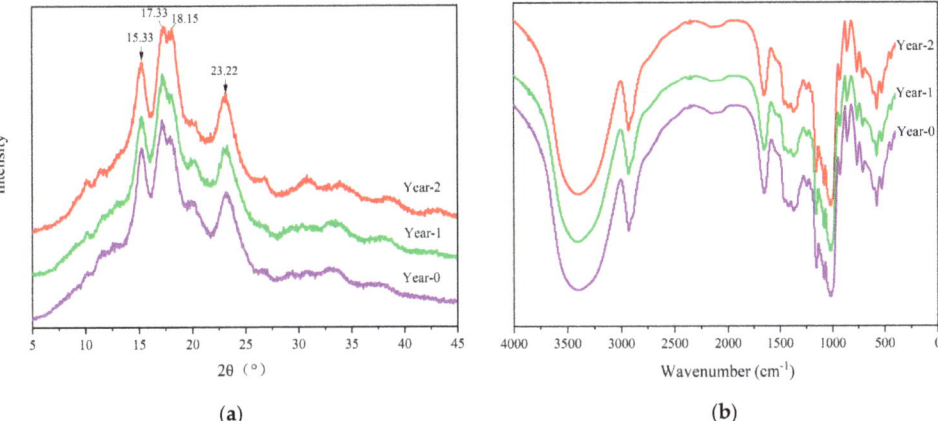

Figure 3. Rice starch variation during storage. (**a**) X-ray diffraction patterns of rice starch at different storage periods; (**b**) Fourier spectra of rice starch at different storage periods.

In addition to the variation of crystal types, we also calculated the relative crystallinity of starch isolated from rice and evaluated its helical structure and short-range ordering. As shown in Figure 3b, there was no new peaks appearing in rice with different storage times, indicating that the storage can only affect the physical structure of starch. As shown in Table 3, there was no significant difference in the relative crystallinity. The light transmission of freshly harvested rice starch was at 3410 cm^{-1}, which indicated the hydrogen bonds between starch molecules were the most solid helical structure. When the storage time was extended, the light transmittance decreased, manifesting that the quantity of hydrogen bonds decreased and the interaction force between starch molecules became weak. Besides, the density ratios of peaks at 1047 cm^{-1}/1022 cm^{-1} and 995 cm^{-1}/1022 cm^{-1} were used to determine the degree of short-range orderliness and double helix structure in starch, respectively [36,37]. As shown in Table 3, the starch of fresh rice had the highest 1047/1022 ratio and 995/1022 ratio, with 1.39 and 1.37, respectively. This means that the starch of fresh rice had the most stable helical structure and the highest short-range orderliness. With the storage process prolonging, the helical structure and short-range orderliness started to decrease and then increase. The decrease in helical structure and orderliness was mainly related with the disruption of branched chains in branched starch, and the increase in helical structure might be due to the fact that apparent amylose was involved in the amorphous region and then formed a new double helical structure, which was supported by the previous results in Table 2.

3.4. Pasting and Thermal Properties Variation of Rice in Storage

Generally, the variation of starch granules can cause different rice pasting and thermal properties. Here, we evaluated these two properties to uncover the quality transformation of rice, in which pasting refers to the process of turning the starch structure from ordered to disordered. The rapid viscosity analysis (RVA) is usually used to test rice pasting property, including the expansion, destruction and reorganization of starch [38]. As shown in Table 4 and Figure 4a, compared with the starch in fresh rice, the peak viscosity of stored rice starch continued to decrease prominently during the storage, especially in the second year, which is consistent with the results of the sensory evaluation (Table 1). Unlike other studies that showed a positive correlation between the peak viscosity and the straight-chain starch content [39], the results in this study indicated that there was not simply a positive relationship between them. The straight-chain starch content increased, whereas the peak viscosity decreased after two years of storage. Combined with the SEM images of starch granules (Figure 2), the starch granules were severely damaged at the same time. The incompleteness of starch granules limited the starch expansion, leading to the decline of peak viscosity. Starch pasting is the water blending in the starch cluster crystallization area under heating, which disassembles the intermolecular state of starch and causes starch molecules to lose their original arrangement; for example, the hydrogen bonds between the ordered (crystalline) and disordered (amorphous) molecules of starch granules are broken and dispersed in water to become a colloidal solution [40].

Table 4. Rice pasting properties variation in storage.

Samples	PV (mPa·s)	TV (mPa·s)	BD (mPa·s)	FV (mPa·s)	PT (°C)	SB (mPa·s)
Year-0	2735.00 ± 84.18 [a]	1357.33 ± 27.93 [b]	1377.67 ± 59.65 [a]	2918.00 ± 37.36 [a]	83.83 ± 0.78 [ab]	1560.67 ± 32.65 [c]
Year-1	2622.00 ± 24.27 [a]	1586.33 ± 13.65 [a]	1035.67 ± 26.54 [b]	3519.00 ± 83.47 [b]	82.62 ± 0.28 [b]	1932.67 ± 91.48 [a]
Year-2	2163.67 ± 88.79 [b]	1313.33 ± 37.07 [b]	850.33 ± 51.73 [c]	3003.00 ± 45.90 [a]	84.63 ± 0.81 [a]	1689.67 ± 23.71 [b]

The letters PV represent the peak viscosity; TV represents the trough viscosity; BD represents the breakdown viscosity; FV represents the final viscosity; SB represents the setback viscosity; PT represents the pasting temperature. Values in the same column with different letters are significantly different ($p < 0.05$).

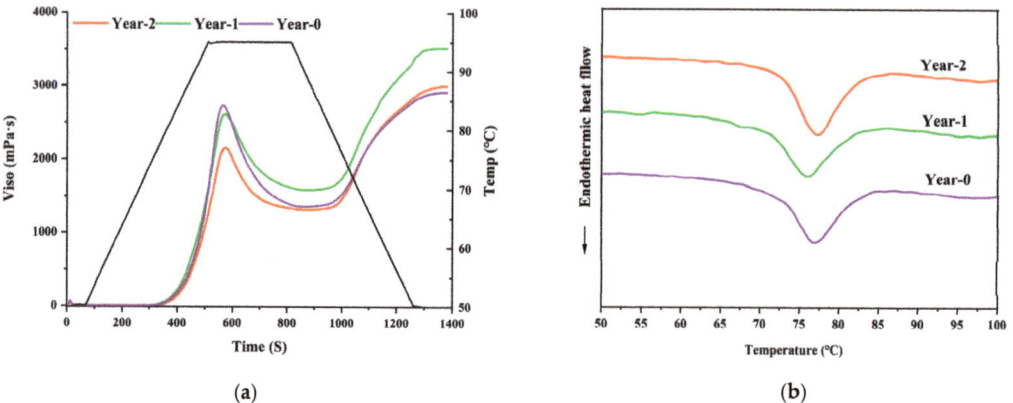

Figure 4. Rice pasting and thermal property variation during storage. (a) Rice starch RVA diagram; (b) Rice DSC diagram.

As shown in Figure 4b, the pasting temperature showed a tendency of first decreasing and then increasing during storage. There was no significant difference between the pasting temperature of fresh rice and one-year stored rice, but it increased significantly in the second year. The thermal stability was related to the double helix structure, which was consistent with the trend of pasting temperature variation. The disintegration value reflects the stability of the starch, like shearing resistance and heating resistance. The larger branched starch molecules will be more likely to intertwine with each other, allowing to maintain the integrity of the starch granules [41]. The results mentioned above showed that the proportion of longer branched starch increased with storage time extending, which led to the improved disintegration values of starch. It was reported that the decrease in the solubility of denatured protein resulted in the limitation of starch swelling and the enhancement of starch granule integrity, which might be another reason for the decrease in starch disintegration value [42]. When the dextrinized starch solution is cooled slowly, the starch molecules will automatically get together and form insoluble crystal bundles through the intermolecular hydrogen bond interaction, which is recognized as retrogradation [43]. The results showed that rice starch retrogradation value increased from 1560.67 mPa·s to

1932.67 mPa·s after being stored for one year, whereas it decreased to 1689.67 mPa·s after 2-year storage. It is consistent with our findings in the straight-chain content variation.

The pasting parameters of starch includes the onset temperature (To), peak temperature (Tp), resultant temperature (Tc) and enthalpy (ΔH). According to Figure 4b and Table 5, the To of starch from freshly harvested rice was about 71.78 °C, which became lower after one-year storage, indicating that the thermal stability of rice starch declined after being stored for the same time. This tendency was caused by the decrease in the content of the branched chain starch, the disruption of the double helix structure and the decline of the short-range ordering (Tables 2 and 3). The To increased with the storage time increasing to 2 years, indicating that long storage time could make rice possess high thermal stability. The results are consistent with the increase in short-range ordering and the decrease in straight-chain starch content. The ΔH value reflects the heat energy associated with crystal melt and the quantity of double helices in starch. The enthalpy of starch decreased after 1 year storage and then kept level off in the rest of storage time, whereas its thermal stability first increased and then decreased during storage.

Table 5. Gelatinization parameters of rice starch during storage.

Samples	To (°C)	Tp (°C)	Tc (°C)	ΔH (J/g)
Year-0	71.78 ± 0.15 [b]	76.28 ± 0.12 [b]	81.82 ± 0.28 [a]	3.29 ± 0.16 [a]
Year-1	70.55 ± 0.25 [c]	75.40 ± 0.10 [c]	80.67 ± 0.23 [b]	3.23 ± 0.07 [a]
Year-2	72.44 ± 0.17 [a]	76.72 ± 0.09 [a]	81.53 ± 0.16 [a]	3.39 ± 0.08 [a]

Notes: The letter ΔH represents the endothermic enthalpy; To represents the onset temperature; Tp represents the peak temperature; Tc represents the conclusion temperature. Values in the same column with different letters are significantly different ($p < 0.05$).

3.5. Morphological Structure Variation of Rice Starch

The effect of long-term storage on the starch granules morphology was investigated by scanning electron microscopy (SEM). The morphological characteristics of starch granules from fresh and stored rice are shown in Figure 2. The fresh rice starch granules were uniform in size, polygonal in shape, regular in shape and smooth on the surface, which is agreeable with other studies [44]. The stored rice starch granules were polygonal, irregular in shape and rough on the surface. There was no significant difference between fresh rice starch and rice stored for 1 year, but the proportion of broken starch granules increased after 2-year storage. Besides, the areas of wrinkles and roughness increased significantly, and the surface of starch granules showed obvious pits. It indicated that starch granules were damaged, thus leading to the declined integrity with the extension of storage time. Furthermore, the moisture is more likely to make water blend in the starch granules from the broken area, which provides more chances to contact with the double helix structure of branched starch. As a result, it is easier to destroy the orderly structure of starch under the heating condition and then lead to decreasing the pasting temperature.

4. Conclusions

In this paper, we investigated the effect of the long-term storage on the multiscale structure and physicochemical properties of rice under granary conditions. The results showed that the fatty acid value and the electrical conductivity of rice increased, whereas its germination rate decreased significantly. The straight-chain starch content first increased and then decreased with the storage time extending. The same tendency occurred in the long-branched chain of branched starch, the short-range orderliness and the degree of double helix structure. However, the pasting temperature had an opposite trend. Simultaneously, the starch granule suffered from breakage, along with the peak viscosity and disintegration value of rice starch decreasing. Some other indicators, such as relative crystallinity, enthalpy, hardness, viscosity and luster, also exerted the corresponding variation. All the results indicates that the structure of rice starch changed significantly after 2-year storage, accompanied by the transformed physicochemical properties. Therefore, to maintain rice with a fair quality, it should be stored under suitable granary conditions for no more than two years. However, most of the results are the description of rice quality and starch variation; they are not the deep mechanism. Thus, if we want to know the reason of the transformation, the changes of their biochemicals, genes and chemical bonds should also be studied in the next studies.

Author Contributions: Methodology, S.L.; software, S.L.; validation, D.P.; formal analysis, K.W.; investigation, M.Q.; resources, Z.Q.; data curation, X.L.; writing—original draft preparation, H.H.; writing—review and editing, J.Z.; visualization, S.L.; supervision, X.L.; project administration, H.H.; funding acquisition, J.Z. All authors have read and agreed to the published version of the manuscript.

Funding: Please add: This research was funded by National Natural Science Foundation of China, youth program, grant number is No. 32102103; Science and Technology Department of Zhejiang Province, Zhejiang Lingyan Research Plan Program, grant number is No. 2022C020202.

Institutional Review Board Statement: Not applicable.

Informed Consent Statement: Not applicable.

Data Availability Statement: Not applicable.

Conflicts of Interest: The authors declare no conflict of interest.

References

1. Kim, D.-S.; Kim, Q.W.; Kim, H.; Kim, H.-J. Changes in the Chemical, Physical, and Sensory Properties of Rice According to Its Germination Rate. *Food Chem.* **2022**, *388*, 133060. [CrossRef] [PubMed]
2. Kemmerling, B.; Schetter, C.; Wirkus, L. The Logics of War and Food (in) Security. *Glob. Food Secur.* **2022**, *33*, 100634. [CrossRef]
3. Park, C.-E.; Kim, Y.-S.; Park, K.-J.; Kim, B.-K. Changes in Physicochemical Characteristics of Rice during Storage at Different Temperatures. *J. Stored Prod. Res.* **2012**, *48*, 25–29. [CrossRef]
4. Sung, J.; Kim, B.-K.; Kim, B.-S.; Kim, Y. Mass Spectrometry-Based Electric Nose System for Assessing Rice Quality during Storage at Different Temperatures. *J. Stored Prod. Res.* **2014**, *59*, 204–208. [CrossRef]
5. Tulyathan, V.; Srisupattarawanich, N.; Suwanagul, A. Effect of Rice Flour Coating on 2-Acetyl-1-Pyrroline and n-Hexanal in Brown Rice Cv. Jao Hom Supanburi during Storage. *Postharvest Biol. Technol.* **2008**, *47*, 367–372. [CrossRef]
6. Wani, A.A.; Singh, P.; Shah, M.A.; Schweiggert-Weisz, U.; Gul, K.; Wani, I.A. Rice Starch Diversity: Effects on Structural, Morphological, Thermal, and Physicochemical Properties-A Review. *Compr. Rev. Food Sci. Food Saf.* **2012**, *11*, 417–436. [CrossRef]
7. Gu, F.; Gong, B.; Gilbert, R.G.; Yu, W.; Li, E.; Li, C. Relations between Changes in Starch Molecular Fine Structure and in Thermal Properties during Rice Grain Storage. *Food Chem.* **2019**, *295*, 484–492. [CrossRef]
8. Nakamura, Y.; Kainuma, K. On the Cluster Structure of Amylopectin. *Plant Mol. Biol.* **2022**, *108*, 291–306. [CrossRef]
9. Chi, C.; Li, X.; Huang, S.; Chen, L.; Zhang, Y.; Li, L.; Miao, S. Basic Principles in Starch Multi-Scale Structuration to Mitigate Digestibility: A Review. *Trends Food Sci. Technol.* **2021**, *109*, 154–168. [CrossRef]
10. Li, H.; Dhital, S.; Slade, A.J.; Yu, W.; Gilbert, R.G.; Gidley, M.J. Altering Starch Branching Enzymes in Wheat Generates High-Amylose Starch with Novel Molecular Structure and Functional Properties. *Food Hydrocoll.* **2019**, *92*, 51–59. [CrossRef]
11. Takeda, Y.; Shitaozono, T.; Hizukuri, S. Structures of Sub-Fractions of Corn Amylose. *Carbohydr. Res.* **1990**, *199*, 207–214. [CrossRef]
12. Li, C.; Gong, B. Insights into Chain-Length Distributions of Amylopectin and Amylose Molecules on the Gelatinization Property of Rice Starches. *Int. J. Biol. Macromol.* **2020**, *155*, 721–729. [CrossRef] [PubMed]
13. Zhu, L.; Zhang, H.; Wu, G.; Qi, X.; Wang, L.; Qian, H. Effect of Structure Evolution of Starch in Rice on the Textural Formation of Cooked Rice. *Food Chem.* **2021**, *342*, 128205. [CrossRef] [PubMed]
14. Huang, S.; Chao, C.; Yu, J.; Copeland, L.; Wang, S. New Insight into Starch Retrogradation: The Effect of Short-Range Molecular Order in Gelatinized Starch. *Food Hydrocoll.* **2021**, *120*, 106921. [CrossRef]
15. Gani, A.; Ashwar, B.A.; Akhter, G.; Shah, A.; Wani, I.A.; Masoodi, F.A. Physico-Chemical, Structural, Pasting and Thermal Properties of Starches of Fourteen Himalayan Rice Cultivars. *Int. J. Biol. Macromol.* **2017**, *95*, 1101–1107. [CrossRef] [PubMed]
16. Shen, S.; Chi, C.; Zhang, Y.; Li, L.; Chen, L.; Li, X. New Insights into How Starch Structure Synergistically Affects the Starch Digestibility, Texture, and Flavor Quality of Rice Noodles. *Int. J. Biol. Macromol.* **2021**, *184*, 731–738. [CrossRef] [PubMed]
17. Wang, H.; Wang, Y.; Wang, R.; Liu, X.; Zhang, Y.; Zhang, H.; Chi, C. Impact of Long-Term Storage on Multi-Scale Structures and Physicochemical Properties of Starch Isolated from Rice Grains. *Food Hydrocoll.* **2022**, *124*, 107255. [CrossRef]
18. Hu, Y.; Bai, J.; Xia, Y.; Lin, Y.; Ma, L.; Xu, Y.; Ding, Y.; Chen, L. Increasing SnRK1 Activity with the AMPK Activator A-769662 Accelerates Seed Germination in Rice. *Plant Physiol. Biochem.* **2022**, *185*, 155–166. [CrossRef] [PubMed]
19. Qu, J.; Wang, M.; Liu, Z.; Jiang, S.; Xia, X.; Cao, J.; Lin, Q.; Wang, L. Preliminary Study on Quality and Storability of Giant Hybrid Rice Grain. *J. Cereal Sci.* **2020**, *95*, 103078. [CrossRef]

20. Zhai, Y.; Pan, L.; Luo, X.; Zhang, Y.; Wang, R.; Chen, Z. Effect of Electron Beam Irradiation on Storage, Moisture and Eating Properties of High-Moisture Rice during Storage. *J. Cereal Sci.* **2022**, *103*, 103407. [CrossRef]
21. de Souza, D.; Sbardelotto, A.F.; Ziegler, D.R.; Marczak, L.D.F.; Tessaro, I.C. Characterization of Rice Starch and Protein Obtained by a Fast Alkaline Extraction Method. *Food Chem.* **2016**, *191*, 36–44. [CrossRef] [PubMed]
22. Kong, X.; Zhu, P.; Sui, Z.; Bao, J. Physicochemical Properties of Starches from Diverse Rice Cultivars Varying in Apparent Amylose Content and Gelatinisation Temperature Combinations. *Food Chem.* **2015**, *172*, 433–440. [CrossRef] [PubMed]
23. Ren, Z.; He, S.; Zhao, N.; Zhai, H.; Liu, Q. A Sucrose Non-Fermenting-1-Related Protein Kinase-1 Gene, *IbSnRK1*, Improves Starch Content, Composition, Granule Size, Degree of Crystallinity and Gelatinization in Transgenic Sweet Potato. *Plant Biotechnol. J.* **2019**, *17*, 21–32. [CrossRef] [PubMed]
24. Lopez-Rubio, A.; Flanagan, B.M.; Gilbert, E.P.; Gidley, M.J. A Novel Approach for Calculating Starch Crystallinity and Its Correlation with Double Helix Content: A Combined XRD and NMR Study. *Biopolymers* **2008**, *89*, 761–768. [CrossRef]
25. Wang, T.; She, N.; Wang, M.; Zhang, B.; Qin, J.; Dong, J.; Fang, G.; Wang, S. Changes in Physicochemical Properties and Qualities of Red Brown Rice at Different Storage Temperatures. *Foods* **2021**, *10*, 2658. [CrossRef]
26. Mitra, A.; Li, Y.-F.; Klämpfl, T.G.; Shimizu, T.; Jeon, J.; Morfill, G.E.; Zimmermann, J.L. Inactivation of Surface-Borne Microorganisms and Increased Germination of Seed Specimen by Cold Atmospheric Plasma. *Food Bioprocess Technol.* **2014**, *7*, 645–653. [CrossRef]
27. Charoenthaikij, P.; Chaovanalikit, A.; Uan-On, T.; Waimaleongora-ek, P. Quality of Different Rice Cultivars and Factors Influencing Consumer Willingness-to-purchase Rice. *Int. J. Food Sci. Technol.* **2021**, *56*, 2452–2461. [CrossRef]
28. Xia, D.; Zhou, H.; Wang, Y.; Ao, Y.; Li, Y.; Huang, J.; Wu, B.; Li, X.; Wang, G.; Xiao, J.; et al. QFC6, a Major Gene for Crude Fat Content and Quality in Rice. *Theor. Appl. Genet.* **2022**, *135*, 2675–2685. [CrossRef] [PubMed]
29. Peng, Y.; Mao, B.; Zhang, C.; Shao, Y.; Wu, T.; Hu, L.; Hu, Y.; Tang, L.; Li, Y.; Tang, W.; et al. Influence of Physicochemical Properties and Starch Fine Structure on the Eating Quality of Hybrid Rice with Similar Apparent Amylose Content. *Food Chem.* **2021**, *353*, 129461. [CrossRef] [PubMed]
30. Li, C.; Li, E.; Gong, B. Main Starch Molecular Structures Controlling the Textural Attributes of Cooked Instant Rice. *Food Hydrocoll.* **2022**, *132*, 107866. [CrossRef]
31. Li, C.; Luo, J.-X.; Zhang, C.-Q.; Yu, W.-W. Causal Relations among Starch Chain-Length Distributions, Short-Term Retrogradation and Cooked Rice Texture. *Food Hydrocoll.* **2020**, *108*, 106064. [CrossRef]
32. Mariotti, M.; Sinelli, N.; Catenacci, F.; Pagani, M.A.; Lucisano, M. Retrogradation Behaviour of Milled and Brown Rice Pastes during Ageing. *J. Cereal Sci.* **2009**, *49*, 171–177. [CrossRef]
33. Li, H.; Fitzgerald, M.A.; Prakash, S.; Nicholson, T.M.; Gilbert, R.G. The Molecular Structural Features Controlling Stickiness in Cooked Rice, a Major Palatability Determinant. *Sci. Rep.* **2017**, *7*, 43713. [CrossRef] [PubMed]
34. Junejo, S.A.; Flanagan, B.M.; Zhang, B.; Dhital, S. Starch Structure and Nutritional Functionality—Past Revelations and Future Prospects. *Carbohydr. Polym.* **2022**, *277*, 118837. [CrossRef] [PubMed]
35. Dhital, S.; Brennan, C.; Gidley, M.J. Location and Interactions of Starches in Planta: Effects on Food and Nutritional Functionality. *Trends Food Sci. Technol.* **2019**, *93*, 158–166. [CrossRef]
36. Warren, F.J.; Gidley, M.J.; Flanagan, B.M. Infrared Spectroscopy as a Tool to Characterise Starch Ordered Structure—A Joint FTIR–ATR, NMR, XRD and DSC Study. *Carbohydr. Polym.* **2016**, *139*, 35–42. [CrossRef]
37. Deng, F.; Yang, F.; Li, Q.; Zeng, Y.; Li, B.; Zhong, X.; Lu, H.; Wang, L.; Chen, H.; Chen, Y.; et al. Differences in Starch Structural and Physicochemical Properties and Texture Characteristics of Cooked Rice between the Main Crop and Ratoon Rice. *Food Hydrocoll.* **2021**, *116*, 106643. [CrossRef]
38. Zhou, Z.; Robards, K.; Helliwell, S.; Blanchard, C. Effect of Storage Temperature on Rice Thermal Properties. *Food Res. Int.* **2010**, *43*, 709–715. [CrossRef]
39. Tao, K.; Li, C.; Yu, W.; Gilbert, R.G.; Li, E. How Amylose Molecular Fine Structure of Rice Starch Affects Functional Properties. *Carbohydr. Polym.* **2019**, *204*, 24–31. [CrossRef]
40. Singh, N.; Kaur, L.; Sandhu, K.S.; Kaur, J.; Nishinari, K. Relationships between Physicochemical, Morphological, Thermal, Rheological Properties of Rice Starches. *Food Hydrocoll.* **2006**, *20*, 532–542. [CrossRef]
41. Vamadevan, V.; Bertoft, E. Observations on the Impact of Amylopectin and Amylose Structure on the Swelling of Starch Granules. *Food Hydrocoll.* **2020**, *103*, 105663. [CrossRef]
42. Oppong Siaw, M.; Wang, Y.-J.; McClung, A.M.; Mauromoustakos, A. Effect of Protein Denaturation and Lipid Removal on Rice Physicochemical Properties. *LWT* **2021**, *150*, 112015. [CrossRef]
43. Al-Attar, H.; Ahmed, J.; Thomas, L. Rheological, Pasting and Textural Properties of Corn Flour as Influenced by the Addition of Rice and Lentil Flour. *LWT* **2022**, *160*, 113231. [CrossRef]
44. Wang, H.; Liu, Y.; Chen, L.; Li, X.; Wang, J.; Xie, F. Insights into the Multi-Scale Structure and Digestibility of Heat-Moisture Treated Rice Starch. *Food Chem.* **2018**, *242*, 323–329. [CrossRef] [PubMed]

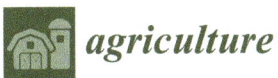

Article

Application of Mathematical Models and Thermodynamic Properties in the Drying of Jambu Leaves

Francileni Pompeu Gomes [1,*], Osvaldo Resende [1], Elisabete Piancó de Sousa [2], Juliana Aparecida Célia [1] and Kênia Borges de Oliveira [1]

1 Federal Institute of Education, Science and Technology of Goiano-Campus of Rio Verde, Rio Verde 75900-000, Goiás, Brazil
2 Federal Institute of Education, Science and Technology of Rio Grande do Norte–Campus Pau dos Ferros, Pau dos Ferros 59900-000, Rio Grande do Norte, Brazil
* Correspondence: francileni.gomes@ifap.edu.br

Abstract: Jambu is a vegetable originally from the northern region of Brazil, has bioactive properties, being little explored by other regions, due to its high peresivity. And one of the methods to increase the shelf life of plant products is the removal of water. The objective of this work was to evaluate the drying kinetics of jambu leaf mass. Two treatments were carried out: The mass of fresh jambu leaves and the mass of fresh jambu leaves with the addition of drying foam, both submitted in an oven with forced air circulation at temperatures (50, 60 and 70 °C and thickness of 1.0 cm). The proximate composition of the materials was performed before and after drying. Twelve mathematical models were tested on drying kinetics data and thermodynamic properties were calculated. The parameters of the proximate composition for the mass of leaves and foam after drying were: Moisture content of (2 to 7%), ash content of (13 to 17%), protein content of (22 to 30%), lipids of (0.6 to 4%) and total titratable acidity (0.20 to 0.28%) of tartaric acid. The models that best fit the experimental data to describe the drying kinetics of jambu masses were: Wang & Singh. The use of foam mat presented higher values of effective diffusion coefficient and activation energy and lower values of enthalpy and entropy, reducing the drying time.

Keywords: *Acmella oleracea*; foam mat; drying kinetics

1. Introduction

Several vegetables are limited to some regions; consequently, they are not well known and are little consumed in other regions of Brazil, and many of them contain higher levels of micro and macro nutrients when compared to conventional vegetable [1,2]. Studies show that there is a large amount of vegetables that are little explored and known in the country, and their scientific dissemination can contribute to food security. [1]. Jambu (*Acmella oleracea*) is an abundant vegetable in the Northern region of Brazil, where its different plant organs (flowers, leaves and stems) are consumed in preparations of typical foods of the Amazon region and as traditional medicinal herb in the treatment of diseases of mouth and throat [2–4].

The species *Acmella oleracea* is investigated for several applications, including evaluation of larvicidal activity of different crude extracts of leaves, as well as antioxidant and immunomodulatory properties, and many studies have focused on its use for centuries in the treatment of oral pain due to its analgesic properties [4–6].

Jambu is a perishable vegetable and requires post-harvest treatment in order to prevent and minimize losses that occur during its marketing, seeking to reduce to a minimum the losses of the active ingredients of interest and compounds aimed at adding flavor or aroma to food [7,8]. Conservation processes include artificial drying by hot air convection, one of the oldest used methods [9].

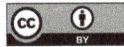

The temperature and drying time must be appropriate for each vegetable, in order to preserve its physical characteristics, nutritional and sensory properties. It is necessary to use drying techniques that better preserve the qualities of the food [10].

The foam mat drying process in can be carried out on liquid or semi-liquid foods, the foam is incorporated by means of aeration with a foaming agent and then dried [11]. Due to the foam structure, which generates a larger area exposed to the drying air, there is a higher mass transfer rate and shorter dehydration time [12].

Drying of agricultural products can be organized in several ways in which drying kinetics data can be represented by theoretical, semi-theoretical and empirical mathematical models [13]. The drying kinetics process presents important information about the characteristics of the typical drying behavior, heating, the period of fast drying due to the constant rate and the falling rate periods [14]. Drying curves are extremely important for the development of processes and equipment sizing; from the curves it is possible to estimate the necessary drying time of a certain amount of products and the time for production, obtaining an estimate of energy expenditure that reflects in the processing cost and influences the final price of the product.

Therefore, *Acmella oleracea* is a plant of commercial interest, due to its pharmacological properties, but there are few studies assessing its processing and application of conservation methods [15,16]. Thus, the objective of the present work was to perform the drying kinetics of jambu leaf mass and jambu leaf mass with foam, at different temperatures (50, 60 and 70 °C) in a thickness of 1.0 cm. determine thermodynamic properties and evaluate its physicochemical characterization.

2. Material and Methods

2.1. Obtaining of Raw Material and Drying

Jambu vegetable were collected on october the 2020 on a family farm in the municipality of Macapá, AP (0°01′26.0″ South and 51°06′53.5″ West of Greenwich), and the experiment it was made at the Food Laboratory of the Federal Institute of Amapá-IFAP (0°05′12.3″ North and 51°05′31.0″ West of Greenwich).

Jambu leaves were washed in chlorinated water, sanitized (solution composed of 2.5% sodium hypochlorite, for 15 min) and crushed (without adding water, for 2 min) in processor to obtain a homogeneous mass.

The foam was prepared by the mixture and aeration for 15 min in a domestic mixer (Mundial Chantilly, São Paulo, Brazil) of the mass of jambu leaves, 1% of a stabilizing agent (Super Liga Neutra®) combined with 2% of an emulsifier (Emustab®). The mass of leaves and the foam were subjected to thin-layer convective drying.

Drying was carried out in a forced air circulation oven (Lucadema), at temperatures of 50, 60 and 70 °C and air velocity of 1.0 ms^{-1} (measured in a digital anemometer Homis Mod 489). The materials (mass of leaves and foam) were spread evenly in rectangular stainless steel trays (25.5 × 13.5 cm), forming a thin layer of 1.0 cm thickness measured with a digital caliper (King Tools).

During drying, the trays were weighed at regular intervals until they reached constant mass. The experiment was carried out in triplicate. The dehydrated material was removed from the tray with a spatula and crushed in a household food processor (Black Decker, Brazil) for 1 min to obtain the powder, which were subsequently stored in laminated packaging composed of two layers (Pet-Low-density polyethylene terephthalate and metallized PET-metallized polyethylene terephthalate).

Physicochemical Characterization

The mass of leaves, foam and powder were evaluated for the following physicochemical parameters: moisture content 103 °C/24 h; ash content determined by muffle incineration at 550 °C; Lipid content the soxlet was used; Protein was determined by kjedahl and total acidity by titration [17].

2.2. Mathematical Modeling

From the experimental data of drying kinetics, the values of the moisture content ratio were calculated according to Equation (1).

$$RX = \frac{X - X_e}{X_i - X_e} \qquad (1)$$

where: RX: moisture content ratio of the product, dimensionless; X; moisture content of the product (d.b.); X_i: initial moisture content of the product (d.b.); X_e: equilibrium moisture content of the product (d.b.).

Table 1 presents the mathematical models widely used to describe drying kinetics of vegetables. The models were fitted by nonlinear regression analysis using the Gauss-Newton method.

Table 1. Empirical and semi-empirical equations used to represent drying kinetics.

	Model Designation	Model	Equation
1	Page	$RX = \exp\exp(-k*t^n)$	(2)
2	Midilli	$RX = a*\exp\exp(-k*t^n) + b*t$	(3)
3	Henderson & Pabis	$RX = a*\exp\exp(-k*t)$	(4)
4	Approximation of Diffusion	$RX = a*\exp\exp(-k*t) + (1-a)*\exp\exp(-k*b*t)$	(5)
5	Two Terms	$RX = a*\exp\exp(-k_0*t) + b*\exp\exp(-k_1*t)$	(6)
6	Two-Term Exponential	$RX = a*\exp\exp(-k*t) + (1-a)*\exp\exp(-k*a*t)$	(7)
7	Logarithmic	$RX = a*\exp\exp(-k*t^n) + c$	(8)
8	Thompson	$RX = \frac{(-a - (a^2 + 4*b*t)^{0.5})}{2} * b$	(9)
9	Newton	$RX = \exp\exp(-k*t)$	(10)
10	Verma	$RX = a*\exp\exp(-k*t) + (1-a)*\exp\exp(-k_1*t)$	(11)
11	Wang & Singh	$RX = 1 + a*t + b*t^2$	(12)
12	Valcam	$RX = a + b*t + c*t^{1.5} + d*t^2$	(13)

RX-Moisture content ratio of the product, dimensionless; k, k_0, k_1-Drying constants; h^{-1}; a, b, c, n-Coefficients of the models; t-Drying time, h.

The preliminary criteria to select the model with best fit were: coefficient of determination (R^2), relative mean error (P), estimated mean error (SE) and the mean chi-square (χ^2).

$$\chi^2 = \sum \frac{(Y - \hat{Y})^2}{DF} \qquad (14)$$

$$P = \frac{100}{n} \sum \frac{|Y - \hat{Y}|}{Y} \qquad (15)$$

$$SE = \sqrt{\frac{\sum (Y - \hat{Y})^2}{DF}} \qquad (16)$$

where: Y: experimental RX value; $\hat{Y}$: RX value estimated by the model; n: number of observations; DF: degrees of freedom of the model (observations minus the number of model parameters).

In order to select a single model to describe the drying process under each condition, those models that preliminarily select (according to the criteria R^2, P and SE) were subjected to the selection criteria of Akaike Information (AIC) and Schwarz's Bayesian Information (BIC).

The information criteria were determined by the following Equations:

$$AIC = -2\log L + 2p \qquad (17)$$

$$BIC = -2\log L + p\log(N - r) \qquad (18)$$

where: p: number of model parameters; logL: logarithm of the likelihood function considering the estimates of the parameters; N: total observations; r: matrix X rank (incidence matrix for fixed effects).

Fick's diffusive model was fitted to the drying data considering the geometric shape of flat plate [18], with eight-terms approximation [19], according to Equation (19), for the determination of effective diffusivity.

$$RX = \left(\frac{8}{\pi^2}\right) \sum_{n=0}^{\infty} \frac{1}{(2n+1)^2} \exp\left(-(2n+1)^2 \pi^2 D \frac{t}{4L_0^2} \frac{S}{V}\right) \quad (19)$$

where: RX: moisture content ratio, dimensionless; D: effective diffusion coefficient, m^2 s^{-1}; S: equivalent plate area, m^2; V: equivalent plate volume, m^3; L$_0$: mass thickness, m; n: number of terms of the Equation; t: time, s.

The expression described by Arrhenius Equation (20) was applied, relating the dependence of effective diffusivity as a function of temperature.

$$D = D_0 \exp\left(\frac{-E_a}{RT_a}\right) \quad (20)$$

where: Do: pre-exponential factor; Ea: activation energy, kJ mol^{-1}; R: universal constant of gases, 8.314 kJ kmol^{-1}. K^{-1}; Ta: absolute temperature, K.

The linearization of the coefficients of the equationthe Arrhenius was used to calculate the activation energy from, applying the logarithm as follows:

$$\text{Ln } D = \text{LnD}_0 - \frac{E_a}{R} \cdot \frac{1}{T_a} \quad (21)$$

2.3. Thermodynamic Properties

The thermodynamic properties of the drying process of the mass of leaves and foam determined were: enthalpy, entropy and Gibbs free energy, according to Equations (22)–(24), respectively.

$$\Delta H = E_a - R \cdot T_a \quad (22)$$

$$\Delta S = R \cdot [\text{Ln}(D_0) - \text{Ln}\left(\frac{K_B}{h_p}\right) - \text{Ln}(T_a)] \quad (23)$$

$$\Delta G = \Delta H - T_a \cdot \Delta S \quad (24)$$

where: ΔH-specific enthalpy, J mol^{-1}; ΔS-specific entropy, J mol^{-1} K^{-1}; ΔG-Gibbs free energy, J mol^{-1}; KB-Boltzmann constant, 1.38×10^{-23} J K^{-1}; hp-Planck constant, 6.626×10^{-34} J s^{-1}; T-temperature, °C.

3. Results and Discussion

3.1. Physicochemical Characterization

Table 2 shows the means of the evaluations of physicochemical composition of the mass of jambu leaves, foam and powder obtained at different temperatures.

The results found for the fresh mass of jambu leaves and foam showed that they have a significant contents of moisture and protein and reduced contents of lipids, ash and total titratable acidity. These contents are close to those described by Neves et al. [1], who found moisture content of 89% w.b., ash of 1.11%, lipids of 0.16%, proteins of 2.44%. The moisture contents obtained in the drying of the mass of jambu leaves ranged from 5.70 to 2.21% w.b. and showed a non-significant decrease with the increase in temperature. For the drying of the foam, there was a higher moisture retention, significant at temperatures of 60 and 70 °C when compared with the dried mass of leaves, with no significant influence of the increase in temperature.

Table 2. Mean values of the physicochemical composition of the mass of jambu leaves, foam and powder obtained under different drying conditions.

Material	Temperature °C	Analyses				
		Moisture Content (% w.b.)	Protein %	Lipids %	Ash %	Total Titratable Acidity * %
Fresh mass of jambu leaves	—	92.71 ± 0.29	3.39 ± 0.23	0.24 ± 0.08	1.34 ± 0.04	0.03 ± 0.0
Foam	—	90.31 ± 0.05	3.30 ± 0.22	0.26 ± 0.07	1.31 ± 0.01	0.04 ± 0.0
Dried mass of jambu leaves	50	5.70 aA	28.33 aA	0.78 aB	17.18 aA	0.26 aA
	60	3.79 aB	30.44 aA	0.68 aB	16.28 aA	0.29 aA
	70	2.21 aB	28.48 aA	0.69 aB	16.32 aA	0.27 aA
Dried foam	50	6.29 aA	24.75 aA	4.72 aA	14.20 aB	0.24 aA
	60	7.67 aA	22.98 aB	4.71 aA	13.74 aA	0.24 aA
	70	6.58 aA	23.37 aA	4.09 aA	13.00 aB	0.20 aB

Lowercase letters in the column refer to the comparison between the different temperatures for the same material, and uppercase letters in the column refer to the comparison of the same temperature between the two materials, and the same letters do not differ from each other by Tukey test ($p < 0.05$). * Tartaric Acid.

However, the fresh mass of leaves and foam of jambu showed relevant contents of protein (3.39% and 3.3%, respectively) and lipids (0.24 and 0.26%, respectively), so drying led to a reduction in moisture content that contributed to a significant increase in the contents of proteins and lipids, and the lipid content found in the foam after drying was higher than that found in the mass of leaves. Values similar to those obtained here were reported by Gomes et al. [16], who found that jambu powder had moisture contents between 4 and 6% w.b. and lipid and protein parameters of 7% and 27%, respectively, with no significant degradation under the studied conditions.

For the ash content of the fresh mass of jambu leaves and foam, there was no variation with the increase in temperature. It was found that the mass of leaves had higher percentages of ash, with values between 16 and 17%. The total acidity levels of the mass of leaves (0.26–0.29% tartaric acid) and foam (0.20–0.24 tartaric acid) after drying showed an acidic character compared with the fresh material (0.03 and 0.04% tartaric acid). The acidity content increased when temperature drying was applied, possibly due to the conversion of sugars into organic acids [11]. In the comparison of the materials before and after drying, there was a reduction in moisture content, while the protein and lipid contents increased, and the dried foam stood out with higher, values, differ dried mass of leaves. This increase may be linked to the addition of stabilizer and emulsifier used to obtain the foam.

Convective drying with forced air circulation is a method recommended for drying leaves because it helps reduce heat losses and improves drying quality [20]. The physicochemical parameters evaluated showed that the addition of stabilizers and emulsifiers did not cause significant changes in the mass of jambu composition. And foaming was a positive factor in the process as it reduced drying time, since this is a limiting factor for the drying conditions (temperature, speed and relative humidity of the air, as well as thickness), which must be controlled to maintain the quality of the final product and reduce moisture content [12].

3.2. Mathematical Modeling

To better understand the drying kinetics of the crushed mass of jambu leaves and foam, different mathematical models were evaluated. Table 3 shows the values of the estimated mean error (SE), relative mean error (P), coefficient of determination (R^2) and chi-square test (χ^2) for the mathematical models fitted to the experimental data of the drying kinetics of the mass of jambu leaves and foam at temperatures of 50, 60 and 70 °C and thickness of 1.0 cm Table 3.

Table 3. Estimated mean error (SE), relative mean error (P), coefficient of determination (R^2) and chi-square test (χ^2) for the twelve models analyzed in the drying of crushed mass of jambu leaves.

Mass of Leaves

Model	50 °C				60 °C				70 °C			
	SE (Decimal)	P (%)	χ^2 (Decimal) $\times 10^{-3}$	R^2 (%)	SE (Decimal)	P (%)	χ^2 (Decimal) $\times 10^{-3}$	R^2 (%)	SE (Decimal)	P (%)	χ^2 (Decimal) $\times 10^{-3}$	R^2 (%)
Wang & Singh	0.0074	6.90	0.055	99.94	0.009	7.075	0.09	99.91	0.011	4.2	0.13	99.87
Verma	0.0881	75.95	7.7532	91.79	0.180	167.9	32.51	68.31	0.012	4.9	0.15	99.85
Valcam	0.0363	35.56	1.3184	98.60	0.047	54.3	2.19	97.86	0.042	10.7	1.77	97.19
Thompson	0.0528	46.59	2.7902	96.96	0.051	56.8	2.65	97.33	0.060	27.5	3.54	96.36
Page	0.0234	20.44	0.5494	99.40	0.024	26.2	0.56	99.44	0.021	10.1	0.46	99.53
Newton	0.0521	46.58	2.7099	96.96	0.051	56.8	2.57	97.33	0.058	27.5	3.42	96.36
Midilli	0.0069	6.13	0.0480	99.95	0.009	8.2	0.07	99.93	0.006	2.4	0.03	99.97
Logarithmic	0.0083	8.22	0.0686	99.93	0.009	9.3	0.08	99.92	0.008	3.6	0.07	99.93
Henderson & Pabis	0.0460	41.13	2.1155	97.69	0.043	49.5	1.88	98.11	0.049	22.9	2.39	97.54
Two-term exponential	0.0528	46.58	2.7896	96.96	0.051	56.8	2.65	97.33	0.060	27.5	3.54	96.36
Two terms	0.0236	21.84	0.5576	99.43	0.045	49.5	2.01	98.11	0.024	11.5	0.57	99.46
Approximation of diffusion	0.0094	8.98	0.0882	99.91	0.011	10.6	0.13	99.87	0.012	4.9	0.15	99.85

Foam

Model	50 °C				60 °C				70 °C			
	SE (decimal)	P (%)	χ^2 (decimal) $\times 10^{-3}$	R^2 (%)	SE (decimal)	P (%)	χ^2 (decimal) $\times 10^{-3}$	R^2 (%)	SE (decimal)	P (%)	χ^2 (decimal) $\times 10^{-3}$	R^2 (%)
Wang & Singh	0.006	4.1	0.03	99.97	0.010	6.2	0.10	99.90	0.016	7.3	0.27	99.77
Verma	0.242	154.6	58.38	44.48	0.346	217.0	119.56	0.00	0.439	313.1	192.32	0.00
Valcam	0.050	37.2	2.50	97.62	0.043	29.4	1.83	98.40	0.052	38.2	2.72	97.80
Thompson	0.049	35.8	2.43	97.61	0.060	39.8	3.59	96.73	0.064	46.4	4.08	96.52
Page	0.022	15.6	0.50	99.50	0.023	15.0	0.52	99.52	0.020	15.2	0.39	99.67
Newton	0.048	35.8	2.35	97.61	0.059	39.8	3.44	96.73	0.062	46.4	3.87	96.52
Midilli	0.008	5.0	0.06	99.95	0.007	4.8	0.05	99.95	0.008	4.3	0.06	99.95
Logarithmic	0.010	7.2	0.09	99.91	0.010	7.0	0.10	99.91	0.013	7.5	0.16	99.87
Henderson & Pabis	0.043	31.5	1.86	98.17	0.050	33.6	2.48	97.74	0.050	37.5	2.47	97.89
Two-term exponential	0.049	35.8	2.43	97.61	0.060	39.8	3.59	96.73	0.064	46.4	4.07	96.52
Two terms	0.021	15.8	0.46	99.58	0.025	17.0	0.62	99.48	0.053	37.5	2.76	97.89
Approximation of diffusion	0.010	7.4	0.10	99.91	0.013	8.3	0.17	99.86	0.019	10.4	0.37	99.70

Wang & Singh, Midilli and Logarithmic models showed the best fits under all drying conditions according to the preliminary criteria of evaluation: R^2 higher than 99%, lower estimated mean error (SE) and chi-square test (χ^2), as well as relative mean error (P) lower than 10%, which is considered as an adequate representation of the model [21].

Together with the previous statistical parameters (Table 3), the Akaike information criterion (AIC) and Schwarz's Bayesian Information criterion (BIC) were adopted as additional criteria to select the best model. The results of AIC and BIC for Wang & Singh, Midilli and Logarithmic models are described in Table 4.

Table 4. Akaike Information criterion (AIC) and Schwarz's Bayesian Information criterion (BIC) for the models that best fitted to the drying data of the crushed mass of jambu leaves.

Model		Wang & Singh		Midilli		Logarithmic	
Drying	Temperature °C	BIC	AIC	BIC	AIC	BIC	AIC
Mass of Leaves	50	−242.58	−247.33	−242.15	−250.07	−231.76	−238.10
	60	−205.62	−210.11	−207.35	−214.83	−207.87	−213.86
	70	−150.17	−154.48	−173.45	−180.62	−147.70	−153.43
Foam	50	−224.32	−228.62	−189.15	−194.88	−189.15	−194.88
	60	−156.83	−160.61	−169.75	−176.04	−154.81	−159.84
	70	−106.23	−109.36	−133.10	−138.32	−114.71	−118.88

Considering the lower values of the AIC and BIC information criteria as indication of better fit, Wang & Singh model showed the best fit to the experimental data for temperature of 50 °C of thin-layer and foam-mat drying. For the other treatment conditions, Midilli model obtained better fit to the experimental data. These results indicate that, regardless of the drying method used, the mathematical models fitted well to the data. Logarithmic and Midilli models were indicated as those with better fit to the experimental data of drying kinetics of the mass of jambu leaves [22].

Data of drying kinetics at different temperatures were analyzed in terms of moisture content ratio (RX), as shown in Figure 1. The moisture content ratio decreases continuously until the equilibrium is reached. The increase in air temperature resulted in a reduction in the time required to reach the equilibrium moisture content for the different conditions studied.

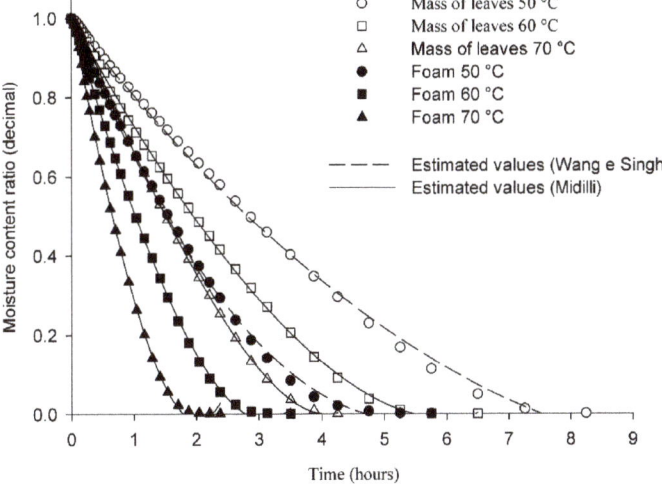

Figure 1. Moisture content ratio in the drying of crushed mass of jambu leaves, obtained experimentally and estimated by the Wang & Singh and Midilli models for the different drying conditions.

The moisture content ratio curve has been considered the best way to explain the behavior during the drying process [23]. Combined with the adequate model for drying kinetics, it is used to explain the total drying behavior [14]. As the model describes the mechanisms of heat and mass transport, it can be used to simulate other process conditions such as variation in thickness, foam composition and temperature, velocity and relative humidity of the air, among others [12].

The results indicated that just as air temperature played an important role in reducing drying time, the use of foam mat enhanced this reduction. The drying time was between 4 and 7 h in the drying of the mass of leaves and showed a considerable reduction in the drying of the foam, being 2 and 5 h.

Increase in drying temperature reduces the drying time due to molecular movement, thus increasing the rate of moisture content removal from the sample, which results in the reduction of drying time [11]. Franco et al. [12] report that the porous structure of the foam and the large surface area in contact with the drying air cause higher mass transfer rates, thus leading to a reduction in drying time and, therefore, a final product with better quality. The coefficients of fits of the mathematical equations obtained under the different experimental conditions of drying kinetics are presented in Table 5.

Table 5. Coefficients of the models that best fitted to the drying data of crushed mass of jambu leaves and foam.

Model	Temperature (°C)	Mass of Leaves				Foam			
		a	b	k	n	a	b	k	n
Midilli	50	0.997247	−0.014930	0.073879	1.142397	0.990898	−0.017696	0.157579	1.160437
	60	1.006883	−0.019378	0.127761	1.088324	0.998051	−0.032604	0.242910	1.185451
	70	1.003061	−0.031494	0.143453	1.178146	1.008538	−0.038754	0.444715	1.204884
Wang & Singh	50	−0.099148	0.002023	—	—	−0.186675	0.008153	—	—
	60	−0.146170	0.004782	—	—	−0.275789	0.016182	—	—
	70	−0.181939	0.005765	—	—	−0.435303	0.041703	—	—

The constant "k" increases with increasing temperature, since higher temperatures lead to higher drying rates [24], a behavior also observed. Considering that the parameter n is related to the internal resistance of the material to drying [25], with the addition of temperature the constant n of the Midilli and Wang and Sing model showed a tendency to increase with increasing temperature.

Figure 2 shows the values of the effective diffusion coefficient during the drying of the crushed mass of jambu leaves and foam. The effective diffusion coefficient showed higher values at the higher drying temperatures and with application of the foam mat.

The effective diffusion coefficient showed a trend of linear increase as the drying air temperature increased. The use of foam promoted higher values of the effective diffusion coefficient compared to the material without foam mat for the three temperatures analyzed. The same was observed for the hot air drying of mint leaves, whose effective diffusivity was slightly higher when the air temperature was increased from 60 °C to 70 °C [26]. Gomes et al. [22] described a trend of increase in diffusion coefficient with the increase in drying air temperature and material layer thickness when studying the mass of jambu leaves.

The increasing values of effective diffusivity with the increase in temperature can be attributed to the fact that water molecules are more weakly bound to the food matrix at higher temperatures, requiring less energy for diffusion [27].

The activation energy increased with the application of the foam mat, from 31 kJ mol^{-1} (samples without foam mat) to 43–48 kJ mol^{-1} (samples with foam mat). These differences in activation energy may result from the variation in effective diffusivity, depending on the variability and physical structure of the sample, chemical composition, geometry and air drying temperature [28].

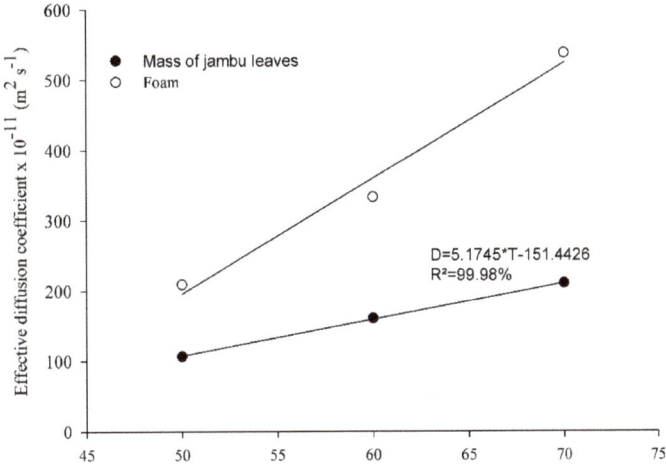

Figure 2. Mean value of the effective diffusion coefficient (D) obtained in the drying of the crushed mass of jambu leaves and foam at temperatures of 50, 60 and 70 °C.

3.3. Thermodynamic Properties

The enthalpy values decreased with the increase in drying air temperature, and compared to the mass of jambu leaves, the smallest magnitudes are obtained with foam mat (Table 6). The lowest enthalpy value was observed with increased temperature, which indicates that the amount of energy needed to remove water bound to the product during drying was lower [27], showing that the foam-mat drying process required lower energy expenditure for water removal.

Table 6. Mean values of enthalpy (ΔH), entropy (ΔS) and Gibbs free energy (ΔG) obtained in the drying of the crushed mass of jambu leaves with and without foam mat at temperatures of 50, 60 and 70 °C.

	Mass of Jambu Leaves		
Temperature (°C)	ΔH (KJ mol^{-1})	ΔS (KJ mol^{-1} K^{-1})	ΔG (KJ mol^{-1})
50	40.79223	−0.27725	130.3847
60	40.70909	−0.2775	133.1584
70	40.62595	−0.27775	135.9347
	Foam		
Temperature (°C)	ΔH (KJ mol^{-1})	ΔS (KJ mol^{-1} K^{-1})	ΔG (KJ mol^{-1})
50	28.62219	−0.32029	132.1241
60	28.53905	−0.32054	135.3282
70	28.45591	−0.32079	138.5349

Entropy was consistent with enthalpy, showing lower values for foam-mat drying. Such reduction indicates a lower excitation of water molecules and an increase in the degree of order of the water-foam system [29]. Regarding Gibbs free energy, the values were positive for both dried materials. According to Chen et al. [30], positive values of Gibbs free energy are characteristic of endergonic reaction, which indicates that the drying and absorption processes under the studied conditions were not spontaneous [27].

In a comparison of the thermodynamic properties for the different drying conditions, it is possible to observe that foam-mat drying shows a better performance. Drying is one of the most energy-consuming processes and is widely used in food industries, so increasing efficiency has the potential to reduce the energy demand of drying operations and, consequently, of the industry [31].

4. Conclusions

In the comparison of the material before and after drying, there was a reduction in moisture content, while protein and lipid contents increased. The addition of stabilizers and emulsifiers for foaming did not cause significant changes in the physicochemical composition of the material. Foaming was a positive factor in the drying process as it reduced the time required to achieve the equilibrium moisture content, also shown by the effective diffusion coefficients, which increased with the application of the foam mat, as well as the thermodynamic properties evaluated, which also pointed to this enhancing effect, with reduction of enthalpy and entropy and higher values of Gibbs free energy. The selection criteria indicated Wang & Singh and Midilli models to describe the drying kinetics of the mass of jambu leaves and foam. We suggest carrying out studies of the bioactive compounds present in the powder material.

Author Contributions: F.P.G.: data collection, data analysis and interpretation, performing the analysis, drafting the article. O.R.: conception or design of the work, critical revision, final approval of the version to be published. E.P.d.S.: data analysis and interpretation, conception or design of the work, critical revision. J.A.C. and K.B.d.O. Review and formatting of work. All authors have read and agreed to the published version of the manuscript.

Funding: This research received no external funding.

Acknowledgments: To the Food Laboratory of IFAP, Embrapa–AP, IF Goiano, CAPES, FAPEG, FINEP and CNPq for their support, which was indispensable to the execution of this study.

Conflicts of Interest: The authors report there are no competing interests to declare.

References

1. Neves, D.A.; Schmiele, M.; Pallone, J.; Orlando, E.A.; Risso, E.M.; Cunha, E.C.E.; Godoy, H.T. Chemical and nutritional characterization of raw and hydrothermal processed jambu (*Acmella oleracea* (L.) R.K. Jansen). *Food Res. Int.* **2019**, *116*, 1144–1152. [CrossRef] [PubMed]
2. Nascimento, A.M.; de Souza, L.M.; Baggio, C.H.; Werner, M.F.D.P.; Maria-Ferreira, D.; da Silva, L.M.; Sassaki, G.L.; Gorin, P.A.; Iacomini, M.; Cipriani, T.R. Gastroprotective effect and structure of a rhamnogalacturonan from *Acmella oleracea*. *Phytochemistry* **2013**, *85*, 137–142. [CrossRef] [PubMed]
3. Nascimento, L.E.S.; Arriola, N.D.A.; da Silva, L.A.L.; Faqueti, L.G.; Sandjo, L.P.; de Araújo, C.E.S.; Biavatti, M.W.; Barcelos-Oliveira, J.L.; Amboni, R.D.D.M.C. Phytochemical profile of different anatomical parts of jambu (*Acmella oleracea* (L.) R.K. Jansen): A comparison between hydroponic and conventional cultivation using PCA and cluster analysis. *Food Chem.* **2020**, *332*, 127393. [CrossRef] [PubMed]
4. Rondanelli, M.; Fossari, F.; Vecchio, V.; Braschi, V.; Riva, A.; Allegrini, P.; Petrangolini, G.; Iannello, G.; Faliva, M.A.; Peroni, G.; et al. Fitoterapia *Acmella oleracea* for pain management. *Fitoterapia* **2020**, *140*, 104419. [CrossRef]
5. Araújo, I.F.; Loureiro, H.A.; Marinho, V.H.; Neves, F.B.; Sarquis, R.S.; Faustino, S.M.; Yoshioka, S.A.; Ferreira, R.M.; Souto, R.N.; Ferreira, I.M. Biocatalysis and Agricultural Biotechnology Larvicidal activity of the methanolic, hydroethanolic and hexanic extracts from *Acmella oleracea*, solubilized with silk fibroin, against Aedes aegypti. *Biocatal. Agric. Biotechnol.* **2020**, *24*, 101550. [CrossRef]
6. Nipate, S.S.; Tiwari, A.H. Journal of Ayurveda and Integrative Medicine Antioxidant and immunomodulatory properties of Spilanthes oleracea with potential effect in chronic fatigue syndrome in fi rmity. *J. Ayurveda Integr. Med.* **2020**, *11*, 124–130. [CrossRef]
7. Martinazzo, A.P.; Melo, E.C.; Corrêa, P.C.; Santos, R.H.S. Modelagem matemática e parâmetros qualitativos da secagem de folhas de capim-limão [Cymbopogon citratus (DC.) Stapf]. *Rev. Bras. Plantas Med.* **2010**, *12*, 488–498. [CrossRef]
8. Oliveira, M.T.R.; Berbert, P.A.; Martinazzo, A.P. Avaliação de modelos matemáticos na descrição das curvas de secagem por convecção de Pectis brevipedunculata (Gardner) Sch. Bip. *Rev. Bras. Plantas Med.* **2013**, *15*, 1–12. [CrossRef]
9. Zarein, M.; Samadi, S.H.; Ghobadian, B. Investigation of microwave dryer effect on energy efficiency during drying of apple slices. *J. Saudi Soc. Agric. Sci.* **2015**, *14*, 41–47. [CrossRef]
10. Influência da Secagem Nas Propriedades Funcionais de Biopolímeros Alimentares_ Das Técnicas Tradicionais Às Novas técnicas de Desidratação Pdf. Available online: https://ainfo.cnptia.embrapa.br/digital/bitstream/item/77765/1/doc-276.pdf (accessed on 20 May 2022).

11. Abbasi, E.; Azizpour, M. Evaluation of physicochemical properties of foam mat dried sour cherry powder. *LWT—Food Sci. Technol.* **2016**, *68*, 105–110. [CrossRef]
12. Franco, T.S.; Perussello, C.A.; Ellendersen, L.D.S.N.; Masson, M.L. Foam mat drying of yacon juice: Experimental analysis and computer simulation. *J. Food Eng.* **2015**, *158*, 48–57. [CrossRef]
13. Santos, N.C.; Almeida, R.L.J.; Pereira, T.D.S.; De Queiroga, A.P.R.; Silva, V.M.D.A.; Amaral, D.S.D.; Almeida, R.D.; Ribeiro, V.H.D.A.; Barros, E.R.; Da Silva, L.R.I. Modelagem matemática aplicada a cinética de secagem das cascas de pitomba (*Talisia esculenta*). *Res. Soc. Dev.* **2020**, *9*, e46921986. [CrossRef]
14. Pinar, H.; Çetin, N.; Ciftci, B.; Karaman, K.; Kaplan, M. Biochemical composition, drying kinetics and chromatic parameters of red pepper as affected by cultivars and drying methods. *J. Food Compos. Anal.* **2021**, *102*, 103976. [CrossRef]
15. Balieiro, O.C.; Pinheiro, M.S.D.S.; Silva, S.Y.; Oliveira, M.N.; Silva, S.C.; Gomes, A.A.; Pinto, L. Analytical and preparative chromatographic approaches for extraction of spilanthol from *Acmella oleracea* flowers. *Microchem. J.* **2020**, *157*, 105035. [CrossRef]
16. Gomes, F.P.; Resende, O.; Sousa, E.P.; Damasceno, L.F. Comparison of powdered and fresh jambu (*Acmella oleracea*). *Heliyon* **2020**, *6*, e05349. [CrossRef]
17. Instituto Adolfo Lutz. *Métodos Físico-Químicos Para Análise de Alimentos*, 4th ed.; 1° edição digital: São Paulo, Brazil, 2008.
18. Brooker, C.W.; Bakker-Arkema, D.B.; Hall, F.W. *Drying and Storage of Grains and Oilseeds*; The Avi Publishing Company: Westport, CT, USA, 1992.
19. Afonso, P.C. Paulo Cesar e Corrêa, Comparação de modelos matemáticos para descrição da cinética de secagem em camada fina de sementes de feijão. *Rev. Bras. Eng. Agrícola e Ambient.* **1999**, *3*, 349–353. [CrossRef]
20. Babu, A.K.; Kumaresan, G.; Raj, V.A.A.; Velraj, R. Review of leaf drying: Mechanism and influencing parameters, drying methods, nutrient preservation, and mathematical models. *Renew. Sustain. Energy Rev.* **2018**, *90*, 536–556. [CrossRef]
21. Mohapatra, D.; Rao, P.S. A thin layer drying model of parboiled wheat. *J. Food Eng.* **2005**, *66*, 513–518. [CrossRef]
22. Gomes, F.P.; Resende, O.; Sousa, E.P.; de Oliveira, D.E.C.; Neto, F.R.d. Drying kinetics of crushed mass of 'jambu': Effective diffusivity and activation energy. *Rev. Bras. Eng. Agric. e Ambient.* **2018**, *22*, 499–505. [CrossRef]
23. Tunde-Akintunde, T.Y. Mathematical modeling of sun and solar drying of chilli pepper. *Renew. Energy* **2011**, *36*, 2139–2145. [CrossRef]
24. Corrêa, P.C.; Oliveira, G.H.H.; Botelho, F.M.; Goneli, A.L.D.; Carvalho, F.M. Modelagem matemática e determinação das propriedades termodinâmicas do café (*Coffea arabica* L.) durante o processo de secagem. *Rev. Ceres* **2010**, *57*, 595–601. [CrossRef]
25. Perez, L.G.; de Oliveira, F.M.N.; Andrade, J.S.; Filho, M.M. Cintica de secagem da polpa cupuau (*Theobroma grandiflorum*) prdesidratada por imerso-impregnao. *Rev. Cienc. Agron.* **2013**, *44*, 102–106. [CrossRef]
26. Therdthai, N.; Zhou, W. Characterization of microwave vacuum drying and hot air drying of mint leaves (*Mentha cordifolia* Opiz ex Fresen). *J. Food Eng.* **2009**, *91*, 482–489. [CrossRef]
27. Lisboa, H.M.; Araujo, H.; Paiva, G.; Oriente, S.; Pasquali, M.A.D.B.; Duarte, M.E.; Mata, M.E.C. Determination of characteristic properties of mulatto beans (*Phaseolus vulgaris* L.) during convective drying. *J. Agric. Food Res.* **2019**, *1*, 100003. [CrossRef]
28. Zhao, C.C.; Ameer, K.; Eun, J.B. Effects of various drying conditions and methods on drying kinetics and retention of bioactive compounds in sliced persimmon. *LWT* **2021**, *143*, 111149. [CrossRef]
29. Jideani, V.A.; Mpotokwana, S.M. Modeling of water absorption of Botswana bambara varieties using Peleg's equation. *J. Food Eng.* **2009**, *92*, 182–188. [CrossRef]
30. Chen, X.; Li, X.; Mao, X.; Huang, H.; Wang, T.; Qu, Z.; Miao, J.; Gao, W. Effects of drying processes on starch-related physicochemical properties, bioactive components and antioxidant properties of yam flours. *Food Chem.* **2017**, *224*, 224–232. [CrossRef]
31. Acar, C.; Dincer, I.; Mujumdar, A. A comprehensive review of recent advances in renewable-based drying technologies for a sustainable future. *Dry Technol.* **2020**, *40*, 1029–1050. [CrossRef]

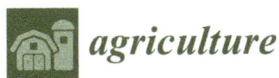

Article

Biomechanical Characterization of Bionic Mechanical Harvesting of Tea Buds

Kun Luo [1], Zhengmin Wu [2], Chengmao Cao [1,*], Kuan Qin [1], Xuechen Zhang [1] and Minhui An [1]

[1] School of Engineering, Anhui Agricultural University, Hefei 230036, China
[2] State Key Laboratory of Tea Plant Biology and Utilization, Anhui Agricultural University, Hefei 230036, China
* Correspondence: ccm@ahau.edu.cn

Abstract: To date, mechanized picking of famous tea (bud, one bud one leaf) causes a lot of damage. Manual picking results in high-quality tea but the process is inefficient. Therefore, in order to improve the quality of mechanically harvested tea buds, the study of bionic picking is beneficial to reduce the damage rate of mechanical picking. In this paper, the manual flexible picking process is studied, and a bionic bladeless mechanical picking mechanics model is developed. The relationship between the mechanical properties and structural deformation of tea stalks is obtained by microstructural observation and mechanical experimental analysis and determination of the bud bionic picking mechanics flow by combined loading tests is carried out. The results show that the key factor for low damage in tea picking is the precise flexible force applied to different parts of the shoot tip during pinching, upward, and picking. The biological force of tea stalks is closely related to the stalk diameter and maturity of stalk tissue development. The larger the xylem of the tea stalk, the stronger its resistance to bending, stretching, and deformation. The stalks at the tender end of the tea are more resilient than the lower stalks and will not break under the action of large angle bending. Additionally, the stalks at the shoot tip have significantly lower pull-off force than the stalks at other places. By simulating the manual picking process, the mechanical picking mechanical parameters were determined to be a clamping pressure of 340 kPa, bending force of 0.134 N, and pull-off force of 5.1 N. These findings help the design of low-damage pickers for famous tea and provide a reference for low-damage bionic picking of tea.

Keywords: bending force; bionic finger; damage; elasticity coefficient; force loading; low-loss picking; microstructure; pressure; tea buds; tension

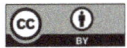

1. Introduction

Tea is one of the main cash crops in China [1]. The global tea cultivation area is 4.89 million hectares [2]. Most premium teas are not harvested by dedicated mechanical equipment but by manual picking. The low efficiency of manual harvesting has hindered the development of the tea industry [3]. When machinery is used to harvest fine tea, the non-selective picking method can cause considerable damage and breakage of tea buds. Most mechanical tea-bud pickers are discontinuous and rigid shear pickers that can damage and alter tea quality [4].

Manually harvested tea is high-quality tea. However, studies have not investigated the harvesting mechanism in depth by taking into consideration the finger flexibility forces, stalk structure, and interactions between multiple forces during manual picking. There is flexible contact between the fingers and shoots during manual picking. Additionally, no adverse chemical changes occur at the bud breakage point upon contact with fingers. Here, we studied a low-damage mechanical harvesting technique for tea buds, based on the imitation ability of artificial flexibility forces and mechanisms for low-damage tea picking. Bionic picking can reduce the damage from mechanical tea picking and thereby considerably improve the picking efficiency.

Tea buds are easily damaged by external forces, and the mechanical properties of different parts of tea stalks vary considerably. Moreover, the bending resistance and shear strength of tea stalks significantly correlate with the structures of the xylem and pith [5,6]. Further, Du et al. [7] combined grey relations with multiple linear regression to identify the correlations between the cellulose content, flexural strength, shear strength, stem diameter, and moment of inertia of tea stalks. In turn, Jia et al. [8] observed a normal distribution of the tea stalk pull-off force. Meanwhile, Hao [9] determined the pull-off and pinch-off forces of tea shoots, and, using hyperspectral techniques, Du et al. [10] observed that the neutral and acid detergent fiber contents of tea stalks directly affected the magnitude of the shear strength. Furthermore, the average modulus of elasticity, compression, and shear of the fourth node stalk of new tea tree tips were calculated as 31.81, 10.12, and 9.19 MPa, respectively [11]. As for the control of flexible forces during picking, Miao and Zheng [12] established a flexible-force control algorithm that can provide low-damage picking for different fruit types. In turn, Zou et al. [13] established a rheological constitutive equation for leafy greens, analyzed the force–displacement relationship, and obtained a low-damage flexible clamping model for leafy greens. Finally, Hou et al. [14] established a link between the soft contact mechanical index of the finger and the mechanical structure of the finger tissue to obtain a bionic flexible-finger mechanical model.

Therefore, here, we studied the mechanics of manual harvesting of premium tea buds to identify the reasons for the high quality that characterizes hand-picked buds. The principles of bionic low-damage picking mechanics were determined by analyzing the finger flexibility forces, tea stalk mechanical properties (flexible clamping force, compression force, pull-off force, bending force), and tea-bud picking paths. Multiple mechanical modes for individual loading modes were designed for the experiments using tea stalks. On this basis, the finger flexibility forces, tender tip-bending forces, clamping forces, and breakage forces were analyzed. Mechanical low-damage picking mechanisms were obtained by analyzing the manual picking path of tea buds under a coupled loading mode.

2. Materials and Methods

2.1. Bionic Picking Analysis

Bionic picking of tea buds simulates the respective hand-picking movements. As shown in Figure 1a, tea buds are manually picked using the index finger and the thumb to grip the tea stalk. The flexible subcutaneous tissue allows the picking point to be tightly wrapped. The solid red box in the diagram shows the distribution area of the picking points, which is generally within 10–15 mm. The area of contact between the index finger and the thumb is the intermeshing region. After clamping the picking point in the intermeshing region, the wrist rotates to drive the finger to rotate, and the finger rotates at a certain angle to pick the shoots off.

As Figure 1b shows, in manual tea picking, the thumb and forefinger are used to pinch the stalk from the lower part of the bud. The diameter of the tea stalk gradually increases from the top to the bottom of the tea stalk. The engaged fingers remain in a flexible state as they gradually move upwards from the lower section. As the fingers pass through the stalk nodes, they relax under increased stress, thereby ensuring the passage of older leaves. When the fingers pass over a node, they fit around the stalk again. The tea stalks are then pinched once the intermeshing region reaches the picking point. The wrist drives the thumb and forefinger, and the tea bud is bent and broken.

2.2. Preparation of Experimental Material

Tea buds are newly sprouted tissues borne of stalks that have not become lignified. The water content in the shoots and stalks is high, and tea shoots are susceptible to damage upon harvesting [15]. The mechanical properties of tea stalks reportedly improve with increasing lignification [16] depending on the forces applied to tea during the picking process. This study focused on the mechanical properties of the stalks between the buds and leaves (BIS), one and two leaf interstitial stalks (OTS), and stalks between the second and third leaves (STS). The structure and morphology of the tea tissues (BIS, OTS, and STS) analyzed in this study are shown in Figure 2. The mechanical properties of tea stalks vary according to their position on the plant. Therefore, the mechanical mechanisms during manual picking of tea stalks should be analyzed for different stem positions.

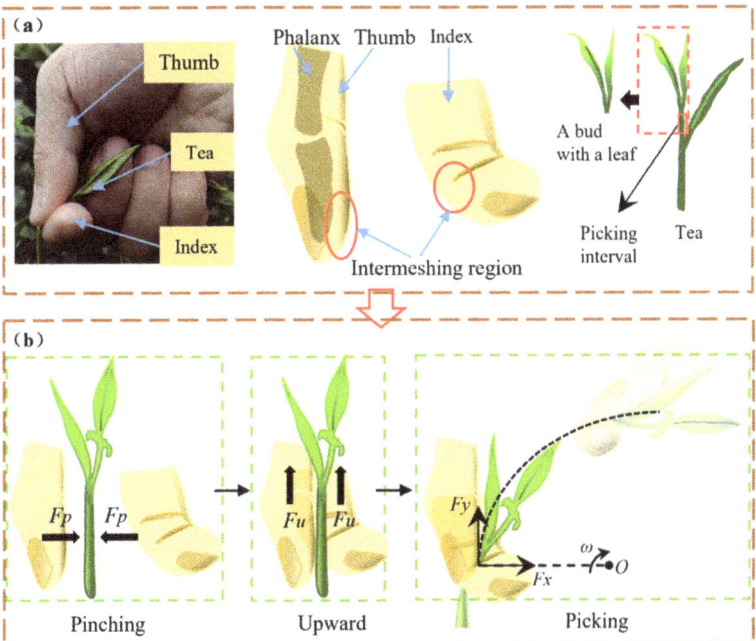

Figure 1. Analysis of tea-bud manual picking. (**a**) Hand-picked objects. (**b**) Manual picking process. Fp—Clamping force, Fu—Tensile force, Fy—y-axis component force, Fx—x-axis component force, ω—Tensile force, O—Tensile force.

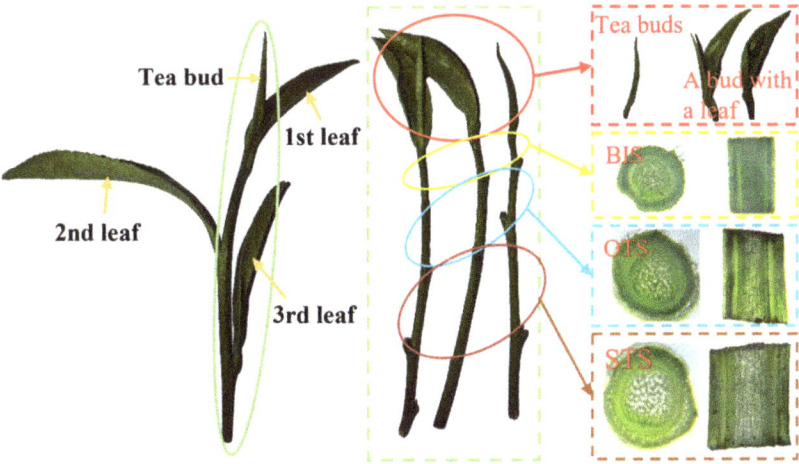

Figure 2. Structure of analyzed tea samples. BIS: stalks between buds and leaves; OTS: one and two leaves interstitial stalks; STS: stalks between the second and third leaves.

The tea samples selected for this study were obtained from the Agricultural Park of Anhui Agricultural University in Hefei, Anhui Province, China. The tea variety used was 'Shu Cha Zao', and the samples were predominantly grown during April. The average bud length of the samples was 25 ± 2 mm, and the average total length of the tea stalks was 70 ± 2 mm. Because the water content of tea leaves considerably affects the mechanical properties of stalks, the experiment was completed within 5 min from the picking of the samples. In this paper, 500 test samples were prepared for analysis of the stems. It is crucial to understand the deformation and mechanical parameters of the plant tissues at the point where the thumb and the forefinger engage to properly determine the characteristics required by bionic picking. To identify the mechanical properties of the fingers at the point of engagement with the tea, the thumb and the forefinger were placed on separate fixation blocks. The respective force changes were measured according to the displacement of the different fingers. The ballast structure was designed according to the shape of the tea stalk.

2.3. Measurements of Tea Mechanics

Tea is picked off at BIS because of the mechanical properties of the tea stalks [7] and the amount and type of force applied by the flexible fingers at different positions. A mechanical measurement platform with different loading modes was used to measure the mechanical properties of the tea stalks. As shown in Figure 3, the computer software (LabVIEW) recorded the force and time data in real time, and the loaded parts moved at a speed of 0.4 mm s^{-1}. One sensor (ZNLBS-G-10KG) measured force within a range of 100 N with a sensitivity of 2.0 mv v^{-1} while the other sensor (JLBS-M2-500G) measured force within a range of 0–5 N with a sensitivity of 2.0 mv v^{-1} (Bengbu Zhongnuo Sensor Co., Ltd., Bengbu, China).

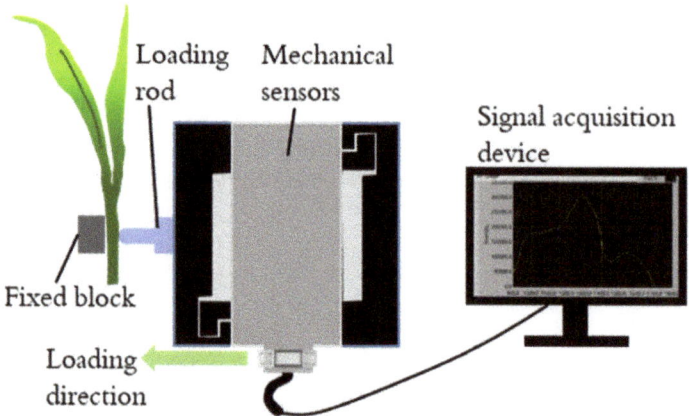

Figure 3. Setup of the mechanical test.

To determine the mechanical properties of the tea stalk, four loading modes were used at different locations, as shown in Figure 4 [17]. The mechanical properties of the finger engagement area from the time of contact to the wrapping of the tea stalk were determined using mode a. The extrusion properties at different positions in the vertical direction of the tea stalk were determined using mode b. The tensile properties of the tea stalks at different positions and under different bending angles were analyzed using mode c. Finally, the bending properties of the tea stalks at different positions were calculated using mode d. All experiments were loaded at a speed of 0.4 mm s^{-1}.

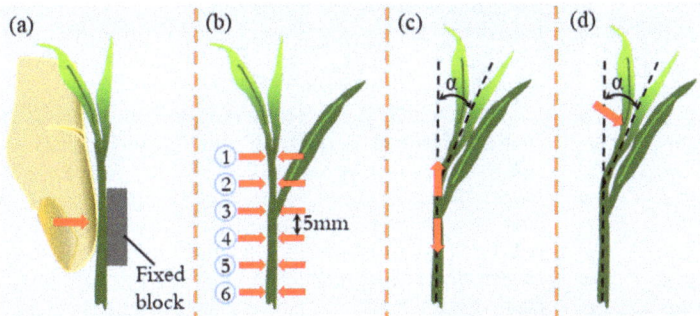

Figure 4. Loading modes used for the analysis of mechanical properties. (**a**) Flexible clamping force. (**b**) Damage forces in different locations. (**c**) Pull-off force. (**d**) Bending force. α is the stalk bending angle.

2.4. Stalk Microstructure Analysis

The correlation between the stalk structure and mechanical properties was analyzed. An optical microscope (MSD100-9, Meisidi Dongguan Technology Co., Ltd., Dongguan, China) was used to examine the transverse and longitudinal sections of the stalks at different positions. The maximum magnification of the microscope used was ×10,000. A five-megapixel high-definition (HD) electronic eyepiece enabled the display of the pictures on the computer. The working diagram of the microscope is shown in Figure 5. Stems at BIS, OTS, and STS were used as test samples. The stalk at BIS was selected for observation under a ×10 eyepiece and a ×10 objective lens. The stalks at OTS and STS were selected for observation under a ×10 eyepiece and a ×4 objective lens.

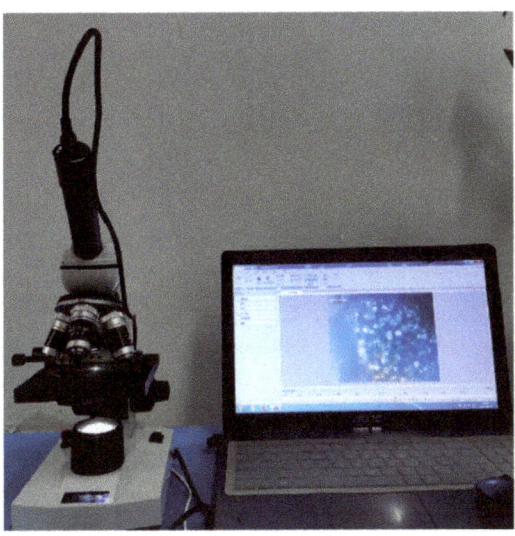

Figure 5. Microscopic view of the stalk cross-section.

3. Results and Discussion

During the picking process, the fingers exert compressive, frictional, bending, and pulling forces on the tea stalks. However, the breaking and bending forces required vary according to the location of the tea plantation. Therefore, the forces acting on the shoot tips, either individually or in combination, should be analyzed to explore the mechanisms underlying the breakage of tea buds upon hand-picking.

3.1. Microstructural Damage to Stalk Fracture

The wounds produced by blade-shear picking and hand-picking of tea stalks are shown in Figure 6. Under blade-shear picking, the blades squeezed the stalks, which resulted in an oval-shaped wound. The fracture interface was uneven and showed numerous burrs. The stalk tissue was torn at the point of fracture, and the interior of the fracture was also damaged through the crushing action, such that cavities were observed in the wood pith. After shear picking, the fractured sections and internally damaged tissues were extensively oxidized. Oxidation produces substances that darken the tea [18]. Blade-shear picking disrupts the tissues within the tea stalks, and such rupturing produces an excess tissue fluid that further increases the oxidation rate. In contrast, hand picking involves lifting off the buds by squeezing the stalks with the fingers, whereby the resulting fracture section is flat and burr-free. After equal oxidation periods, the oxidized area in a wound produced by hand picking was considerably smaller than that in a wound caused by blade-shear picking. The bud tissues showed a brownish-red color after the wound was oxidized by ambient air, particularly in the xylem and wood pith.

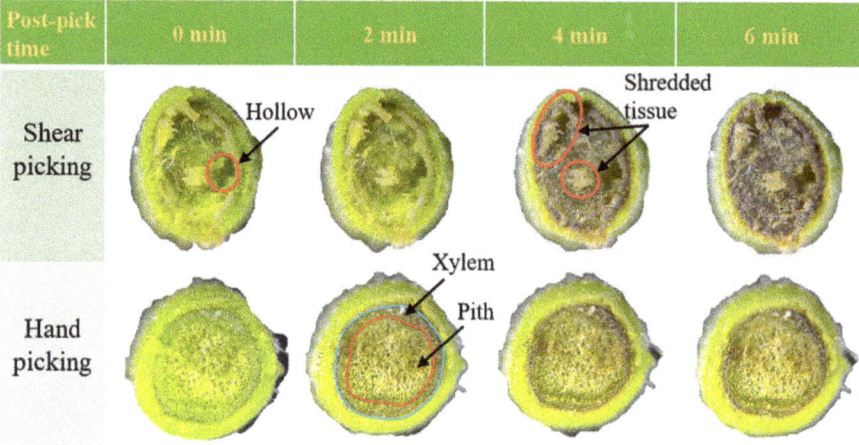

Figure 6. Appearance of the wound areas caused by hand and shear-blade picking of tea buds.

3.2. Analysis of Flexible Clamping Force

The structure of human fingers predominantly comprises skin, subcutaneous tissue, and phalanges [14]. When fingers engage the tea, the skin and subcutaneous tissue form indentations under the pressure exerted by the tea stalks. The depressed space formed by the thumb and forefinger then wraps around the tea stalk. The finger bones are considerably denser than the subcutaneous tissue. Therefore, when the fingers pinch the tea stalks, the flexible subcutaneous tissue creates a cushion, which prevents damage to the tea. Further, when fingers are wrapped around the tea stalk, the finger bones prevent the subcutaneous tissue from sinking. The grip of the fingers on the tea stalk then suddenly increases. The forces on the thumb and forefinger engagement area when in contact with the tea stalk are shown in Figure 7. The forces on the two intermeshing regions vary non-linearly with time. The contact force from the index finger slowly increased from 0 to 2.8 s, followed by a rapid increase in the contact force in the 2.8–5.6 s band. Meanwhile, the compression force from the thumb slowly increased from 0 to 6 s, with a rapid increase in the compression force in the 6–8.5 s band. These findings are consistent with those of Dzidek et al. [19]. However, Dzidek's study was conducted on the ventral region of the finger, where the pressure was

1.2 N when the ventral deformation was 1.46 mm. The previous work did not specify the force parameters of the thumb tip and the joint between the first and second joints of the index finger.

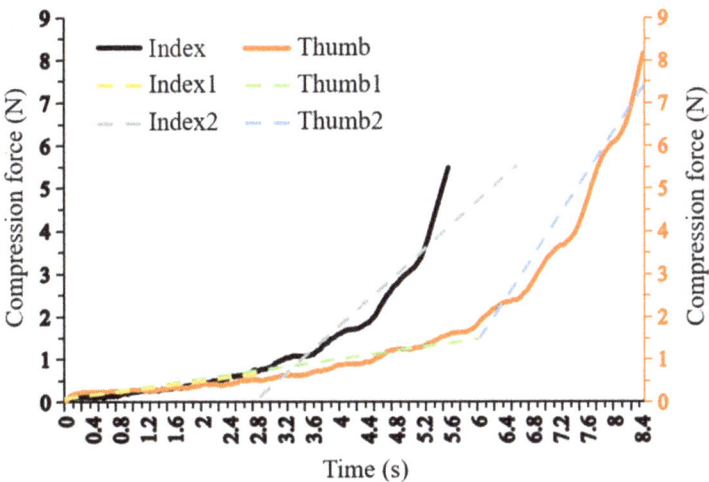

Figure 7. Forces on the engagement area.

When the index finger intermeshing region was deformed by approximately 1.6 mm, the contact force was approximately 1.5 N. At this point, the contact force from the thumb was approximately 0.8 N, which was lower because the subcutaneous tissue in the intermeshing region from the thumb is thicker than that of the index finger. Specifically, when the rod is loaded and the thumb intermeshing region is squeezed, the buffer zone of the thumb is larger than that of the index finger. Based on the mechanical variation trend, the intermeshing of the thumb and the index finger can be simplified as two separate linear elastic variations of flexible materials. As shown in Figure 7, the fitted curves for the anterior and posterior segments of the thumb were named thumb1 and thumb2, respectively. The thumb deformation was within 0–2.4 mm, and its elasticity coefficient was 783 N m^{-1} for thumb1 and the deformation interval was within 2.4–3.4 mm, with an elasticity coefficient of 6632 N m^{-1} for thumb2. The fitted curves for the anterior and posterior segments of the index finger were named index1 and index2, respectively. The index finger had an elasticity coefficient of 658 N m^{-1} in the deformation interval 0–1.1 mm. The deformation interval was within 1.1–2.2 mm when the elasticity coefficient was 3729 N m^{-1}. The area of the engagement zone was 143 mm^2.

3.3. Extrusion Properties at Different Positions of the Stalk Level

During tea picking, the clamping force is always applied to the tea stalk. The intensity of the clamping force directly affects the extent of the possible damage to the tea [20]. In mode b, the tea stalks were placed on the side of the fixing block. The probe was loaded to squeeze the stalk from the other side at an even speed. The data from 20 experiments were considered for each group, and the average value was used to represent the experimental results. Seven experimental points on the tea stalks were selected for these measurements, starting at the middle of the BIS, with other points 5 mm apart along the stem and down the stalk. The loading forces required to produce plastic deformation at different positions in the horizontal length of the tea stalk are shown in Figure 8. The width and length of the loading block was 1 and 10 mm, respectively, and the indentation area formed on the stalk was 1 ± 0.2 mm^2.

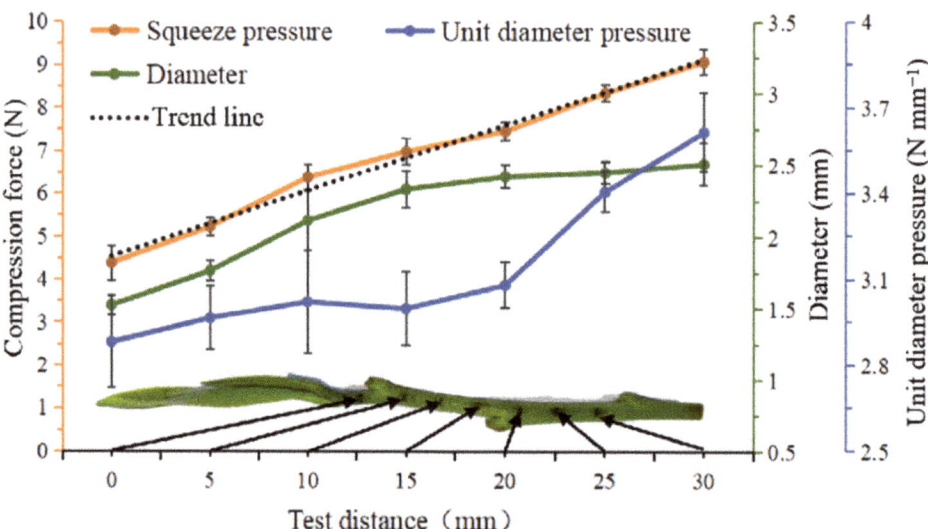

Figure 8. Maximum force on different points on the measured tea stalks.

As Figure 8 shows, the diameter of the tea stalk gradually increased from the tip of the bud downwards. As the diameter increased, the forces producing deformation in the stalk gradually increased and the loading force tended to be linearly distributed. The average maximum stalk deformation force was 4.38 N for BIS, 6.2 N for OTS, and 8.3 N for STS. Owing to the different diameters for the same parts of tea stalks during growth, the deformation forces per unit diameter at different positions along the stalk were investigated. As the diameter increased, the maximum deformation force per unit diameter tended to slowly increase, then level off, and then rapidly increase. Further, the tea stalk diameter underwent substantial mutation from BIS to OTS but not from OTS to STS.

The increase in the stalk deformation force with increasing diameter was attributed to the changes in the structure of the stalk tissue. This was in line with the findings of Cao et al. [21]. Previously, Cao's study showed a linear correlation between the stalk cross-sectional area and shear force. The shear force was 0.6 N when the cross-sectional area of the tea stalk was 1.8 mm^2. The results of this study showed a linear correlation between the stalk cross-sectional area and squeezing pressure. The squeezing pressure was 4.4 N for a tea stalk cross-sectional area of 1.8 mm^2. However, the previous research studied the shear force of the stalk and did not analyze the squeezing force between the fingers and the stalk. As shown in Figure 9, the stalk cross-section comprises the stalk bark, bast, xylem, and wood pith. The cross-sectional organization of the stalks was relatively similar at the stalk lengths of 0, 5, 10, and 15 mm. In contrast, the bast and medullary fibers of the stalk became more transparent, and the xylem diameter increased considerably at 20, 25, and 30 mm. The xylem in the tea stalks increased with increasing diameter. The cells of the stalk bast and wood pith showed progressive fibrillation from position 0 to 30 on the stalk. The xylem is the main structure responsible for maintaining the stalk in an upright position. As the stalk diameter increased, the bast of the stalk became progressively fibrous. This change was consistent with the trend of the deformation forces generated by the stalk. Therefore, the intensity of the deformation force generated by the stalk is directly related to the degree of fibrillation of the bast.

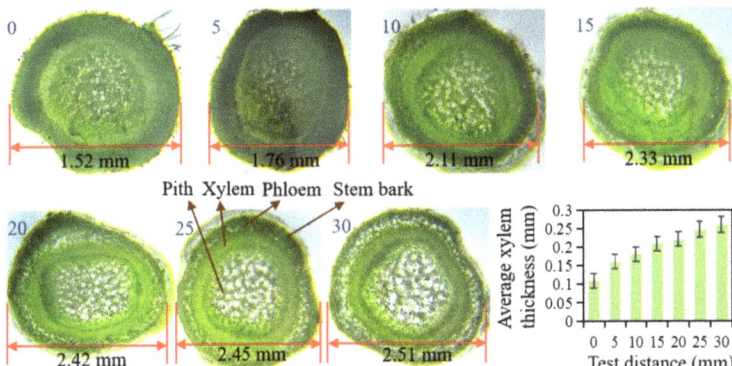

Figure 9. Microscopic cross-sectional view of different parts of tea stalks. Here, 0, 5, 10, 15, 20, 25, and 30 are distances (mm) along the stalks and indicate the positions on the stalk at which measurements were carried out.

3.4. Pull-off Force at Different Positions on the Stalk

When picking tea buds by hand, the fingers first bend the shoots at a certain angle and then the fingers lift off the buds. It is crucial to identify the difference in the pull-off forces between the bud break point and the rest of the stalk under bending to develop efficient bionic harvesting. The tea stalk diameter varies in size, whereby the pull-off force cannot be directly compared. Therefore, the pull-off force per unit diameter was adopted as a measurement. The pull-off force per unit diameter was evaluated separately for the BIS, OTS, and STS of the stalk, and the results are shown in Figure 10. For stalk bending angles between 0° and 90° in the BIS range, the stalk pull-off force per unit diameter ranged within 2.2–2.4 N. In turn, the pull-off force per unit diameter of the stalk at OTS ranged from 2.2 to 3.1 N, and that at STS ranged from 1.6 to 4.1 N. In all three cases, the stalk pull-off force per unit diameter increased and then decreased under the action of different bending angles. Specifically, as the bending angle increased from 0° to 30°, the partial force required to pull off the stalk increased, resulting in a larger combined force. On the other hand, the hardness of the stalk decreased when the bending angle exceeded 30°. The stalk xylem vessels became brittle and broke under the bending action and, consequently, the pull-off force was reduced.

When the stalk was subjected to axial tension, the breaking point occurred at the end of clamping. The cross-section of the point of fracture at BIS was smooth and burr-free, whereas that at OTS showed few filamentous fibers, and that at STS showed abundant filamentous fibers. The breakage of all tea stalks was a brittle break. This was attributed to the high water content of the stalks and the fact that they were not yet fully lignified. The axial cross-sectional organization of tea stalks is shown in Figure 11. The fibrous tissue in the stalk gradually increased with increasing diameter. The small variation range in the pull-off force at different stalk angles at BIS was attributed to the similarity of the organization of the various regions of the stalk in that section. The bending angle showed a lower effect on the pull-off force of the stalk at BIS. Furthermore, owing to its smaller xylem and diameter, BIS presented a lower pull-off force. The stalk bark, bast, xylem, and wood pith were clearly distinguished in the axial cross-sectional view of the stalk at OTS. However, the cellular tissue at this point was not yet mature compared with the STS stem tissue. Therefore, the mechanical trend of OTS was in line with that of STS. These findings were consistent with those of Huang et al. [22]. Previous studies by Hang showed that the average values of shear force at BIS and OTS were 0.97 and 1.2 N, respectively. The results of this study showed that the mean values of the pull-off forces at BIS and OTS were 2.2 and 2.6 N, respectively, at 0 deg. In this paper, the bending force, pull-off forces, and stalk structure were analyzed simultaneously. At OTS and STS, the stalks showed a gradual reduction in the stalk pull-off force at 30–90°. Because of the increase in diameter and xylem tissue, the stalk was more likely to break under bending action, thereby reducing the pull-off force.

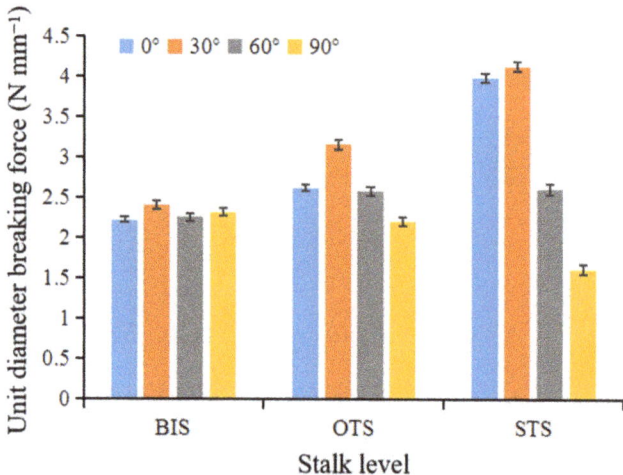

Figure 10. Tensile force on tea stalks under different bending actions. BIS: stalks between buds and leaves; OTS: one and two leaves interstitial stalks; STS: stalks between the second and third leaves.

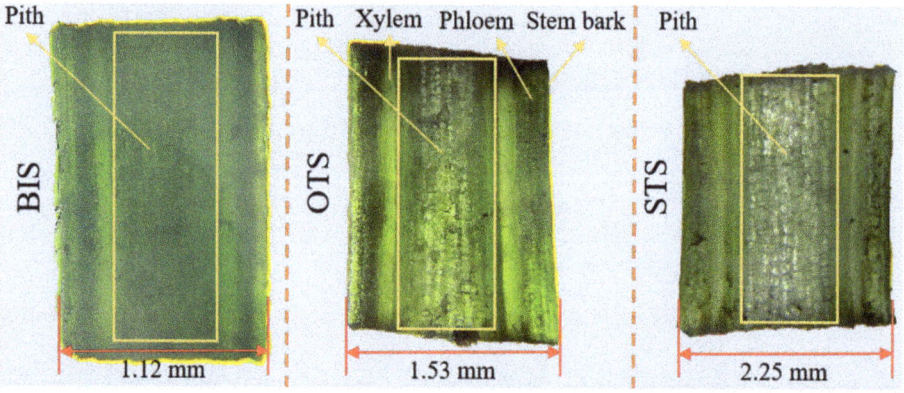

Figure 11. Longitudinal micro-sectional view of different parts of tea stalks. BIS: stalks between buds and leaves; OTS: one and two leaves interstitial stalks; STS: stalks between second and third leaves.

3.5. Forces Required for Bending at Different Stalk Positions

At the final stage during tea-bud picking, stalks should be bent at an angle that allows tea buds to be quickly picked [23]. Stalks should be bent at the BIS during picking, while remaining upright at other positions. There are diameter differences for the same stalk position, whereby the bending forces cannot be directly compared. Therefore, we selected tea samples with the largest diameter at BIS and the smallest diameter at OTS and STS for the experiments. To analyze the forces required to bend the different parts of the tea stalk, the experiments were conducted at different positions along the tea stalks, as shown in Figure 12.

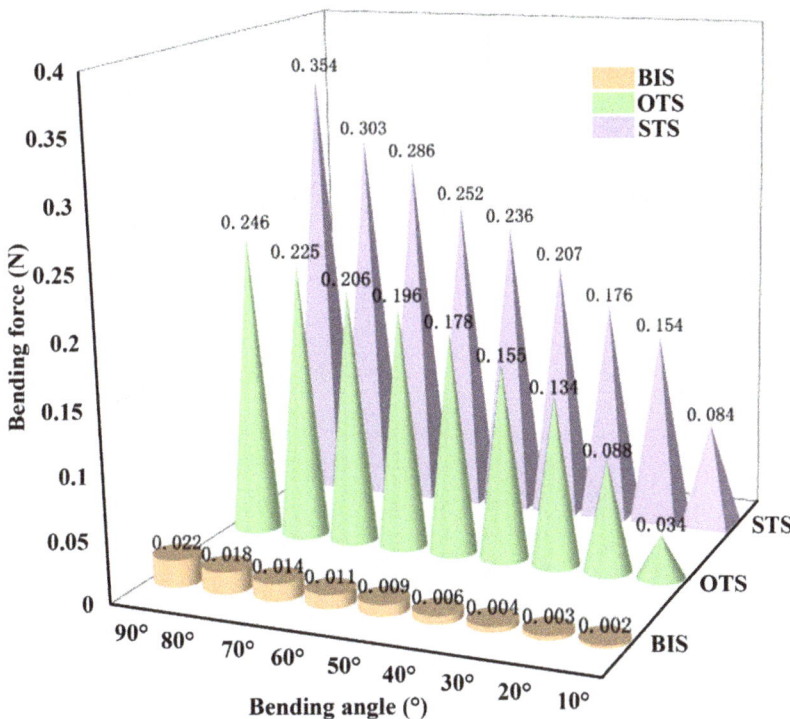

Figure 12. Stalk bending force. BIS: stalks between buds and leaves; OTS: one and two leaves interstitial stalks; STS: stalks between the second and third leaves.

Consistent with findings reported by Wu et al. [24], the bending force required by the tea stalk gradually increased as the bending angle increased, in the experiments described herein. Previously, Wu's study showed decreasing values of the stem stiffness from the bottom to the top. In this paper, the bending force of the stalk was measured at different positions. The test results show that the stiffness of the stalk decreases slowly from the bottom to the top and then decreases rapidly. Further, the bending resistance of the stalks was most pronounced at STS, and, because STS showed the largest xylem vessels, its potential for the stalk was the greatest and increased with an increasing angle. Conversely, the stalk showed the least bending resistance at BIS, which indicated a greater toughness. The tissue structure of the stalk at BIS can remain intact even under the effects of large angular bending. Indeed, bending forces of 0.022, 0.246, and 0.354 N were required at 90° for BIS, OTS, and STS, respectively. Furthermore, the bending force of BIS was considerably lower than those of OTS or STS owing to the small diameter of BIS and greater hardness of the stalk tissue in this case.

3.6. Picking Mechanics Program

The pinching, upward pulling, and picking of bionic harvesting was determined based on the characteristics of manual picking. Multiple forces act on tea stalks during tea bud harvesting, and the main ones are clamping force, tension, and bending force. A flow diagram of the load applied to the stalk during the three stages of manual picking is shown in Figure 13. The engagement gap is the distance between the contact surfaces of the index finger and the thumb. Contact without extrusion is represented by a positive value, whereas deformation extrusion is represented a negative value. The fingers guide the stalk into the engagement zone at the pinching stage, during which a clamping force is primarily used. The range of pressure action at STS was obtained from the finger engagement zone pressures, which have been previously measured as $0 < p < 417.5$ kPa. When engaged, old leaves fill the engagement gap and fluctuate at 1–5 mm in the engagement gap.

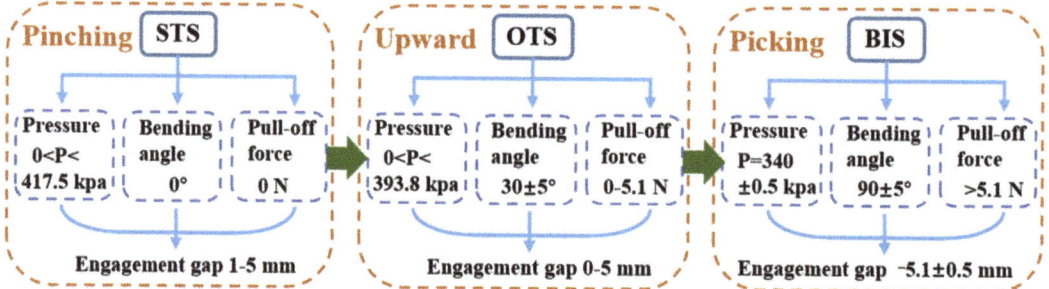

Figure 13. Force path of artificial shoot picking. BIS: stalks between buds and leaves; OTS: one and two leaves interstitial stalks; STS: stalks between the second and third leaves.

The fingers move upwards while bending to guide the stalk behind them into the bend. The range of pressure on the stalk at this point was $0 < p < 393.8$ kPa, and the stalks were bent at an angle of $30 \pm 5°$. The finger tension was less than the breaking tension of the stalk; thus, it was <5.1 N. During the picking stage, the fingers pinch the stalk, and at BIS, the stalk can act on a range of pressures of 340 ± 0.5 kPa. A higher bending angle of the stalk improved the picking. However, the bending angle of the wrist is limited; therefore, the bending angle at BIS was $90 \pm 5°$. At this point, the tension acting on the stalk is greater than the breaking tension of the stalk (i.e., tension is greater than 4.38 N). At this point, the fingers must squeeze the stalk to create a greater frictional force to pull it off. The engagement gap was measured as -5.1 ± 0.5 mm.

During manual picking, the fingers can be used to sense the gripping force and the shape of the stalks in real time. The strength and direction are adjusted in real time depending on the stalk position. As bionic picking simulates manual picking, a flow chart of tea bud bionic harvesting mechanics (Figure 14) based on the manual harvesting process was drawn. Bionic picking starts by clamping the tea plant on the lower part of the stalk and then moving upwards through the STS, OTS, and then BIS. To ensure that the stalks are not damaged by clamping, the maximum pressure that tea stalks can withstand was determined based on the maximum pressure at the most vulnerable point. This maximum clamping pressure was determined as 340 kPa throughout the picking process.

Tea buds should be picked at BIS, and OTS and STS should remain intact. Greater bending angles of BIS led to better picking, which is consistent with the principle of manual picking. The OTS and STS bending angles showed the highest pull-off force at 30°; therefore, a BIS-bend angle of 90° and OTS- and STS-bend angles of 30° were considered the most suitable for tea picking. Based on the bending force experiment (Figure 12), a bending force of 0.134 N was determined.

During the picking process, greater pulling forces loaded on the tea buds can lead to more efficient bud harvest. However, excessive tension can cause the tea stalks to break at STS or OTS. Therefore, it is important to ensure that the buds are pulled off without breaking other points of the stalk. The critical value of the tensile force should be less than that required to break the stalk at OTS. Based on the tensile tests, a pull-off force of 5.1 N was determined.

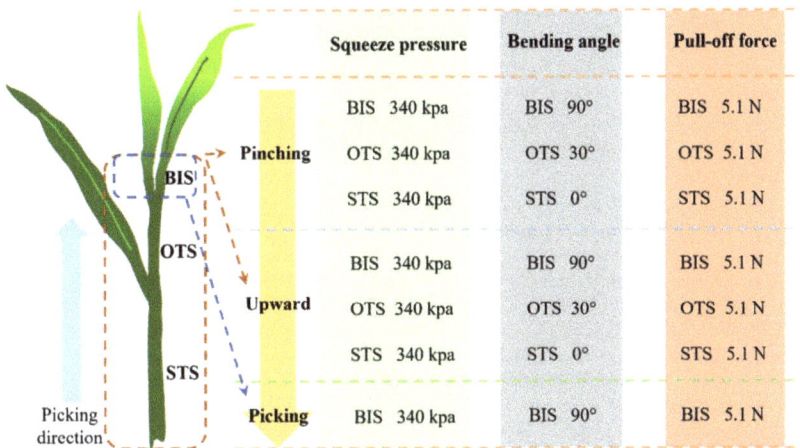

Figure 14. The path of the bionic shoot-picking force. BIS: stalks between buds and leaves; OTS: one and two leaves interstitial stalks; STS: stalks between the second and third leaves.

4. Conclusions

This study analyzed the process of manual picking of tea buds and investigated the mechanical functioning and mechanic paths for bionic tea-bud picking. The bionic picking mechanics paths obtained herein can be used to determine the structural design of a low-damage, fast-picking mechanism to use for tea shoots. The main findings of this study are as follows:

(1) Tea stalk breakage is brittle fracture. Finger engagement with the tea stalk is soft contact. Bionic picking of tea consists of three processes, namely: pinching, pulling upward, and picking. Finger engagement is simplified by the combination of the two moduli of elasticity materials that can change the clamping force as the position of the stalk changes. Pinching and upward lifting ensure that the stalks are bent at a specified angle in the specified position. Flexible clamping and picking effectively protect the stalk interior and wound structure.

(2) Tea stalks gradually lignify in a basipetal progression, and BIS shows low lignification and greater toughness. Fracture at BIS occurs mainly through bending forces and normal tension at the bending point. The OTS and STS stalks break easily under large-angle bending action, and later break easily under tension.

(3) A precise application of bending forces at different positions on the stalk during harvesting is crucial for appropriate bionic harvesting. The maximum clamping pressure of 340 kpa, bending force of 0.134 N, and pulling force of 5.1 N were determined for the bionic picking of tea leaves.

Author Contributions: Conceptualization, K.L., Z.W., C.C. and X.Z.; methodology, K.L., Z.W., C.C. and K.Q.; software, K.L. and M.A.; validation, K.L., X.Z. and Z.W.; formal analysis, K.L.; investigation, K.L.; data curation, K.L.; writing—original draft preparation, K.L.; writing—review and editing, K.L., Z.W., C.C. and K.Q.; supervision, K.L. and M.A.; funding acquisition, Z.W. and K.Q. All authors have read and agreed to the published version of the manuscript.

Funding: This research was funded by the National Key R&D Program of China [grant number 2021YFD1601102] and by the National Natural Science Foundation of China [grant number 52105239].

Institutional Review Board Statement: Not applicable.

Informed Consent Statement: Not applicable.

Data Availability Statement: Not applicable.

Acknowledgments: The authors would like to thank Zhengmin Wu from State Key Laboratory of Tea Plant Biology and Utilization for providing equipment and technical support during the experiments. We also thank other colleagues in the laboratory such as Kuan Qin, Xuenchen Zheng, and Minhui An for their help in the experiments.

Conflicts of Interest: The authors declare no conflict of interest.

References

1. Zhu, Y.P.; Wu, C.Y.; Tong, J.H.; Chen, J.N.; He, L.Y.; Wang, R.Y.; Jia, J.M. Deviation tolerance performance evaluation and experiment of picking end effector for famous tea. *Agriculture* **2021**, *11*, 128. [CrossRef]
2. Wu, X.L. Analysis of the World Tea Production and Trade Pattern and its Inspiration. *Tea Fujian* **2019**, *41*, 41–42.
3. Han, Y.; Xiao, R.H.; Song, Y.Z.; Ding, Q.W. Design and Evaluation of Tea-Plucking Machine for Improving Quality of Tea. *Appl. Eng. Agric.* **2019**, *35*, 979–986. [CrossRef]
4. Li, X.; Lin, Y.; Zhao, S.; Zhao, X.; Geng, Z.; Yuan, Z. Transcriptome changes and its effect on physiological and metabolic processes in tea plant during mechanical damage. *For. Pathol.* **2018**, *48*, e12432. [CrossRef]
5. Lin, Y.P.; Jin, X.Y.; Hao, Z.L.; Ye, N.X.; Huang, Y.B.; Tang, H.Y.; Chen, X.H.; Zhou, X.Y. Experiment on mechanical properties and crude fiber of tea leaf. *J. Tea Sci.* **2013**, *33*, 364–369.
6. Liu, Q.T.; Ou, Y.G.; Qing, S.L.; Wang, W.Z. Study progress on mechanics properties of crop stalks. *Trans. Chin. Soc. Agric. Mach.* **2007**, *38*, 172–176.
7. Du, Z.; Hu, Y.G.; Buttar, N.A. Analysis of mechanical properties for tea stem using grey relational analysis coupled with multiple linear regression. *Sci. Hort.* **2020**, *260*, 108886. [CrossRef]
8. Jia, J.M.; Ye, Y.Z.; Cheng, P.L.; Zhu, Y.P.; Fu, X.P.; Chen, J.N. Design and experimental optimization of hand-held manipulator for picking famous tea shoot. *Trans. Chin. Soc. Agric. Mach.* **2022**, *53*, 86–92.
9. Hao, M. Researches on the Identification of Tender Leaves and Bionic Plucking Fingers for High-Quality Green Tea. Master's Thesis, Nanjing Forestry University, Nanjing, China, 2019.
10. Du, Z.; Hu, Y.G.; Mahmood, A.; Wang, S. Determination of shearing force by measuring NDF and ADF in tea stems with hyperspectral imaging technique. *IFAC PapersOnLine* **2018**, *51*, 849–854. [CrossRef]
11. Wang, S. Research Design and Experimental Study on Portable Electric Tea Plucking Machine. Master's Thesis, Jiangsu University, Zhenjiang, China, 2018.
12. Miao, Y.B.; Zheng, J.F. Optimization design of compliant constant-force mechanism for apple picking actuator. *Comput. Electron. Agric.* **2020**, *170*, 105232. [CrossRef]
13. Zou, L.L.; Yuan, J.; Liu, X.M.; Li, J.G.; Zhang, P.; Niu, Z.R. Burgers viscoelastic model-based variable stiffness design of compliant clamping mechanism for leafy greens harvesting. *Biosyst. Eng.* **2021**, *208*, 1–15. [CrossRef]
14. Hou, Z.L.; Li, Z.G.; Fadiji, T.; Fu, J. Soft grasping mechanism of human fingers for tomato-picking bionic robots. *Comput. Electron. Agric.* **2021**, *182*, 106010. [CrossRef]
15. Wang, N.; Liu, W.; Lai, J. An attempt to model the influence of gradual transition between cell wall layers on cell wall hygroelastic properties. *J. Mater. Sci.* **2014**, *49*, 1984–1993. [CrossRef]
16. Du, Z.; Hu, Y.G.; Wu, W.Y.; Lu, Y.Z.; Buttar, N.A. Structural analysis on cutting notch of tea stalk by X-ray micro-computed tomography. *Inf. Process. Agric.* **2020**, *7*, 242–248. [CrossRef]
17. Lu, W.; Li, X.C.; Zhang, G.C.; Tang, J.H.; Ni, S.; Zhang, H.B.; Zhang, Q.; Zhai, Y.L.; Mu, G. Research on Biomechanical Properties of Laver (Porphyra yezoensis Ueda) for Mechanical Harvesting and Postharvest Transportation. *AgriEngineering* **2022**, *4*, 48–66. [CrossRef]
18. Liu, K. Research on the Enzymological Characteristics of Polyphenol Oxidase from Tea and the Effect of Infrared on Its Activity and Conformation. Master's Thesis, Jiangnan University, Wuxi, China, 2013.
19. Dzidek, B.M.; Adams, M.J.; Andrews, J.W.; Zhang, Z.; Johnson, S.A. Contact mechanics of the human finger pad under compressive loads. *J. R. Soc. Interface* **2017**, *14*, 20160935. [CrossRef]
20. Zhu, H.; Zhao, H.; Bai, L.; Ma, S.; Zhang, X.; Li, H. Mechanical Characteristics of Rice Root–Soil Complex in Rice–Wheat Rotation Area. *Agriculture* **2022**, *12*, 1045. [CrossRef]
21. Cao, W.C.; Xue, Y.F.; Zhou, J.G. Study on shearing properties of tea shoot. *J. Zhejiang Agric. Univ.* **1995**, *21*, 11–16.
22. Huang, Y.; Wei, K.; Wang, L.Y.; Cheng, H.; He, W.; Zhou, J. Study of developmental pattern of tea shoot tenderness on the base of texture analyser. *J. Tea Sci.* **2012**, *32*, 173–178.
23. Xue, Y.F.; Cao, W.C. Mechanical properties of tea young shoot under bending. *J. Zhejiang Agric. Univ.* **1994**, *20*, 43–48.
24. Wu, W.C.; Hu, Y.G.; Jiang, Z.H. Investigation on the bending behavior of tea stalks based on non-prismatic beam with virtual internodes. *Agriculture* **2022**, *12*, 370. [CrossRef]

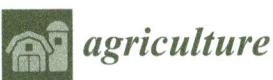

Article

Construction and Verification of Spherical Thin Shell Model for Revealing Walnut Shell Crack Initiation and Expansion Mechanism

Xiulan Bao [1,2], Biyu Chen [1,2], Peng Dai [1,2], Yishu Li [1,2] and Jincheng Mao [3,*]

1. College of Engineering, Huazhong Agricultural University, Wuhan 430070, China
2. Key Laboratory of Agricultural Equipment in Mid-Lower Yangtze River, Wuhan 430070, China
3. School of Mechanical and Electrical Engineering, Wuhan Institute of Technology, Wuhan 430073, China
* Correspondence: jun–lan@163.com; Tel.: +86-138-7122-9154

Abstract: Walnut shell breaking is the first step of deep walnut processing. This study aims to investigate the mechanical properties and fracture state of the Qingxiang walnut shell under unidirectional load and guide the complete separation of the walnut shell and kernel. The spherical thin shell model of the walnut (the fitting error is less than 5%) was established and verified. The process from the initiation to the expansion of walnut cracks was analyzed. The crack expansion rate was estimated in terms of the crack fracture regularity on the shell's surface. Based on the momentless theory and finite element simulation analysis, we found that the stress on the shell surface in the concentrated force action region was gradient distributed from inside to outside and that the internal forces were equal in all directions in the peripheral force action region. The unidirectional impact shell-breaking experiments confirmed the reliability of our spherical thin shell model and verified our hypothesis of walnut shell fracture along the longitudinal grain. Our results can provide a theoretical basis for the development and structural optimization of shell-breaking machinery.

Keywords: walnut; physical properties; crack; broken shell experiment

1. Introduction

Walnut is a plant of the genus Juglans, and walnut, cashew, almond, and hazelnut are known as the world's four dried fruit. Walnut kernels are rich in nutrients such as protein, vitamins, and cellulose. It contains high contents of unsaturated fatty acids and multiple proteins, which is very beneficial for health and can strengthen the brain [1–3]. The shell weight of dried fruits such as walnuts is relatively large in proportion to their total weight, but their edible part is little. Moreover, the hard shell poses a serious obstacle to the extraction of effective components (pulp) in processing. Walnut shell, mainly composed of lignin and hemicellulose, is hard with an irregular appearance, and thus it is difficult to peel [4]. Moreover, there is a large difference in size between different walnuts and a complex diaphragm connection between the shell and kernel with a small shell–kernel gap. These factors make it difficult for the walnut shell to be completely separated from the kernel, and thus it is also difficult to achieve a high complete kernel rate.

At present, the manual shell breaking method with a high cost and low efficiency is gradually being replaced by high-efficiency mechanical shell breaking. In order to realize the mechanization of walnut shell breaking, a large number of studies have been conducted [5]. Appropriate moisture content and force loading direction have been reported to greatly improve the processing efficiency and quality of walnuts [6–9]. A large number of tests have revealed that two pairs of normal concentrated forces can better achieve uniform shell rupture [10]. The research on the mechanical properties of walnut shell breaking from the perspective of finite elements provides a theoretical basis for the development of walnut shell breaking machinery [11,12]. Ojolo et al. designed a rotary sheller, but the shelling effect was far from satisfactory due to the large individual difference in walnut shells [13]. Li et al. developed a cone-basket walnut shell breaking device with a desirable processing effect but relatively low shelling efficiency [14]. Liu et al. designed a flexible belt-shearing extrusion shell-breaking device that improved the shelling rate and reduced the kernel breaking rate [15]. Ding et al. proposed a bionic knocking shell breaking method and developed a bionic knocking walnut shell breaking machine, which exhibited high shell breaking efficiency but a low complete kernel rate [16].

In order to improve the shell breaking efficiency and shell kernel separation rate, this study explored the shell breaking state and mechanical properties of walnut shells under unidirectional load based on the physical characteristics of the walnut shell. The walnut shell is a spherical shell composed of two hemispherical shells that are combined at the suture line (ridge line). It has been reported that when the walnut suture line (ridge line) is loaded with forces, the walnut shell and kernel will be divided into two parts directly from the ridge line. Therefore, this study selected the shell surface except for the ridge line for modeling and investigated the related characteristics of the continuous shell surface to provide a theoretical basis for the development of shell-breaking machinery.

2. Analysis and Verification of Walnut Characteristics

2.1. Materials and Instruments

This study used Qingxiang thin-skinned walnuts as experiment materials. Three sizes of walnuts with a diameter of 35 ± 2 mm for large, 33 ± 2 mm for medium, and 27 ± 2 mm for small were selected as the walnut samples. The test instruments mainly include a texture meter, a digital vernier caliper (with an accuracy of 0.02 mm), and a digital thickness measuring instrument (with an accuracy of 0.02 mm).

2.2. Tests and Analysis

2.2.1. Sphericity Measurement

The measurement direction of the triaxial size of a walnut is shown in Figure 1. The walnut was fixed with a plane fixture, and the maximum measurement value in each direction was used as the measurement result. The three-axis dimensions of three sizes (large, medium, and small) of walnuts were measured by a digital vernier caliper. The measurement results were recorded, and the sphericity was calculated according to Equation (1).

$$S = \frac{\sqrt[3]{abc}}{d} (d = \max\{abc\}) \tag{1}$$

where S is the sphericity, a is the edge diameter (mm), b is the transverse diameter (mm), and c is the longitudinal diameter (mm).

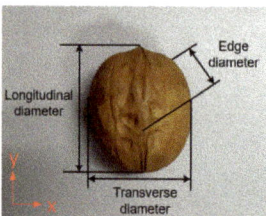

Figure 1. Schematic diagram of walnut diameter.

2.2.2. Sphericity Analysis

The average sphericity of large, medium, and small walnuts was 0.889, 0.883, and 0.904, with the standard deviations of 0.028, 0.012, and 0.019, respectively. Since the sphericity of the walnuts in all three sizes was above 88%, with a very small standard deviation, the selected walnuts were appropriate for approximate spherical modeling.

2.2.3. Shell Thickness Measurement

Since the walnut shell is symmetrically distributed, seven points were selected from half of the shell surface to measure the shell thickness, as shown in Figure 2. The thickness of each sampling point was measured by a digital thickness measuring instrument. Walnuts were divided into three groups (large, medium, and small sizes), with seven walnuts per group and seven thickness measurement points per walnut. The multiple measurement results were averaged.

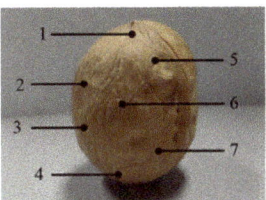

Figure 2. Schematic diagram thickness measurement points of the walnut shell. 1–7 are seven thickness measurement points.

2.2.4. Shell Thickness Analysis

The measurement results of walnut shell thickness at different measurement points are shown in Figure 3. Figure 3 shows that the shell thickness was correlated with the size and measurement point of the walnut. Therefore, these two factors affecting the shell thickness were selected as factor A (walnut size) and factor B (measurement point). Two-Way ANOVA was performed to reveal the difference in shell thickness between different groups (Table 1). The results showed that the p (test value) of the two factors was above 0.01, indicating that the shell thickness at any point on the selected shell surface was uniform between different size groups.

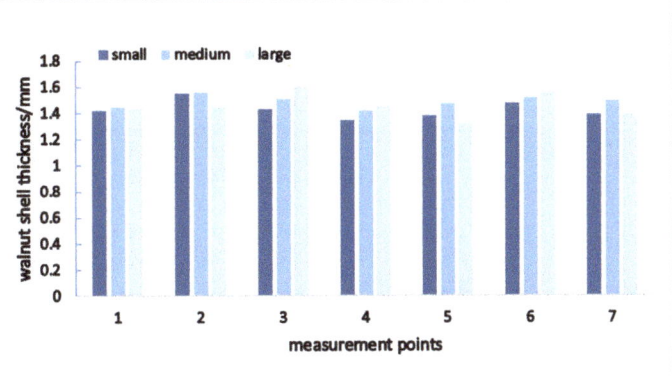

Figure 3. Walnut shell thickness at different measurement points.

Table 1. Two-way ANOVA of shell thickness.

Factors	Sum of Squares	Degree of Freedom	Mean Square	F	p
Factor A	0.01384	2	0.00692	3.89	0.15
Factor B	0.05885	6	0.00981	2.99	0.04
Error	0.03710	12	0.00309		
Sum	0.10978	20			

The above measurement results showed that the walnut shell was approximately spherical and that the shell thickness was uniform. Therefore, the walnut shell was simplified as a spherical thin shell model in this study, and the shell analysis was carried out by establishing the spherical thin shell model.

2.3. Fit Verification of Spherical Thin Shell Model

The previous study has shown that when the load is applied to the walnut, the stress is the largest at the load point, and the deformation area is concentrated near the load point. In addition, the shell thickness and compression stiffness vary with different positions, suggesting the mechanical properties are different at different positions of the walnut shell. When an external load is increased to a certain value, the walnut shell will be unstable or even break. According to elastic mechanics, the critical buckling pressure P_{cr} of thin spherical shells is calculated according to Equation (2):

$$P_{cr} = \frac{2E}{\sqrt{3(1-\mu^2)}}\left(\frac{h}{r}\right)^2 \qquad (2)$$

where P_{cr} is the critical pressure (GPa), E is the elastic modulus (GPa), μ is Poisson's ratio, h is the shell thickness (mm), and r is the radius (mm).

Experimental measurements were performed using a texture analyzer. The results were as follows: walnut elastic modulus E = 0.18 GPa and Poisson's ratio μ = 0.38. The shell thickness, the radius measurement value (r = min {a, b, c}/2), the elastic modulus, and the Poisson's ratio were substituted into the above formula to calculate the critical stress for breaking the shell, and then the shell breaking force was calculated according to the formula $F = P_{cr} \times S$, where F is the shell breaking force, P_{cr} is the critical pressure, S is the compressed area (S = 100 mm^2), and the corresponding theoretical calculation values are presented in Table 2.

Table 2. Shell breaking force comparison.

Shell-Breaking Force	Sizes	Small (27 ± 2 mm)	Medium (33 ± 2 mm)	Large (35 ± 2 mm)
Calculated Value/N		317.3	303.7	312.7
Observed Value/N		329.6	316.1	329.2
Deviation/%		3.7	3.9	5.0

The average shell breaking force of walnut actually measured by the texture analyzer was used as the observed value. The deviation value was calculated by the observed value and the calculated value, with the results presented in Table 2.

As shown in Table 2, there was a certain deviation between the calculated values from the spherical thin-shell model and the actually observed values in this study, indicating that the actual shell shape, shell thickness distribution, and other factors had a certain influence on the force characteristics of walnuts. Since the deviation values in the three groups were less than 5%, a high approximation level and a good model fitting degree were indicated.

3. Crack Analysis

During the experiment, under unidirectional (Y-direction) load, the force was increased with the increase in the downward loading displacement. After reaching the strength limit, the walnut was unstable and fractured. In this process, the fracture first occurred at the maximum stress (the load point). When the downward load displacement continued to increase, the walnut shell continued to bend downward in the load direction. At the same time, the crack expanded outward from the load point and ended when the crack length reached the maximum (Figure 4).

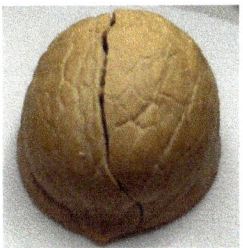

Figure 4. Walnut crack.

3.1. Crack Type

According to the characteristics of force and displacement, cracks fall into three basic types, namely, type I, type II, and type III. In the load concentration area, the load is the normal stress σ, and the direction is perpendicular to the surface of the walnut shell. When it is pressed downward, the walnut will eventually rupture to form a crack, and the relative slippage of a crack occurs between the two surfaces, which is a type II crack. Outside the concentrated action domain, the crack mainly extends outward under the action of the partial force pointing to each side of the walnut, and the crack characterized by tearing from the middle is a type I crack.

3.2. Crack Initiation

According to material mechanics, the brittle material will fail when the maximum principal normal stress reaches the unidirectional strength limit of the material under tensile or compressive load, which is the maximum normal stress yield criterion. The maximum normal stress yield criterion can be specified by the function as follows:

$$\sigma_M = MAX(|\sigma_x|, |\sigma_y|, |\sigma_z|) \qquad (3)$$

where σ_M is the ultimate strength, and σ_x, σ_y, and σ_z are the stresses in the three principal axis directions.

When $\sigma_M < \sigma_u$, the material will not break, and when $\sigma_M \geq \sigma_M$, the material will break. In our walnut shell breaking model, $\sigma_x = 0$, $\sigma_y = P_{cr}$, and $\sigma_z = 0$, and thus the limit pressure strength $\sigma_u = |\sigma_y| = P_{cr}$. Under load P_{cr}, $\sigma_1 = 0$, $\sigma_2 = -p$ (negative sign indicates pressure stress), $\sigma_3 = 0$, as a result, $\sigma_M = |\sigma_2| = p$. When $p \geq P_{cr}$, that is, $\sigma_M \geq \sigma_u$, according to the maximum normal stress yield criterion, the failure fracture of the walnut shell occurred, and the initial crack was generated, which was the crack initiation process.

3.3. Crack Expansion

Generally, two parameters in linear elastic fracture mechanics are employed to measure the crack generation ability, namely energy release rate G and stress intensity factor K. When the energy release rate G or the stress intensity factor K exceeds their critical value ($G \geq G_C$ or $K \geq K_C$), it is considered that fracture occurs, which is the fracture criterion. According to fracture mechanics, stress intensity factor K is a measure of crack severity, which is related to crack size, stress, and geometric shape. This study assumes that the mechanical behavior of a walnut shell is linear elastic, and thus we analyzed the crack characteristics of a walnut shell based on the knowledge of linear elastic fracture mechanics.

One previous study has shown that cracks generated on a certain material tend to expand to the positions where toughness was increasingly lowered. For wood, the toughness along the grain direction is lower than that in other directions, and thus wood tends to fracture in the grain direction [17]. The walnut shells in this study also exhibited a similar breaking pattern, namely, walnut shells fracture in the longitudinal direction (Y-axis direction), which was defined as the "along-grain direction", and the transverse direction (X-axis direction) is the "horizontal direction".

Based on this, we hypothesized that walnut shells might fracture "along the longitudinal grain". To test our hypothesis, the material critical strength K_C was calculated. The stress intensity factor K is related to the applied stress and the crack length. Based on linear elastic fracture mechanics, K is usually calculated by Equation (4) [18]:

$$K = FS\sqrt{\pi a} \qquad (4)$$

where parameter F is a function of the ratio a/b, which is related to the geometry; S is the load stress, and a is the crack length.

In the case of the ratio of $\alpha = a/b < 0.4$, F is calculated according to Equation (5):

$$F = 1.12S\sqrt{\pi a} \qquad (5)$$

In other cases, where $\alpha = a/b$, F is calculated according to Equation (6):

$$F = \sqrt{\frac{2}{\pi\alpha}\tan\frac{\pi\alpha}{2}}\left[\frac{0.923 + 0.199(1-\sin\frac{\pi\alpha}{2})^2}{\cos\frac{\pi\alpha}{2}}\right] \qquad (6)$$

3.3.1. Longitudinal (Along Grain) Direction

The crack length measurement in the longitudinal direction is shown in Figure 5. When the longitudinal ratio $\alpha = a/b = 0.51$ is substituted into Equation (6), longitudinal $F_Z = 1.48$ (Figure 5). Our results also showed that the average crack length of the longitudinal shell breaking of a walnut shell is $a = 34.3$ mm, and the shell breaking force is $S_Z = 310$ N. When these data were substituted into Equation (4), the fracture toughness along the grain direction of a walnut shell is $K_{ZC} = 1.51$ MPa·m$^{1/2}$.

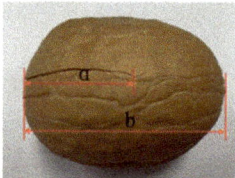

Figure 5. Crack length measurement in the longitudinal direction, a is the crack length, b is the longitudinal diameter.

3.3.2. Horizontal (X-Axis) Direction

The crack length measurement in the transverse direction is shown in Figure 6. When the transverse ratio $\alpha = a/b = 0.50$ was substituted into Equation (6), longitudinal $F_X = 1.47$. In addition, our results showed that the average crack length of a walnut shell is $a = 20.1$ mm, and the shell breaking force is $S_X = 468$ N. When the above data were substituted into Equation (4), we obtained the transverse fracture toughness of a walnut shell as $K_{ZC} = 1.72$ MPa·m$^{1/2}$.

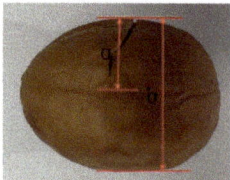

Figure 6. Crack length measurement in the horizontal direction, a is the crack length, b is the transverse diameter.

Our calculation results showed that the transverse fracture toughness was greater than the longitudinal fracture toughness, indicating that the longitudinal intensity is smaller than the transverse intensity, thus confirming our hypothesis that walnut shells might fracture "along longitudinal grain".

The actual observation also showed that most of the cracks were also longitudinal cracks. Therefore, it can be concluded that no matter whether the initial cracks of walnuts are along the longitudinal direction, they are always affected by the fracture properties along the longitudinal grain during the crack extension process, and under this influence, the cracks would be longitudinally shifted.

3.4. Crack Expansion Rate

In the experiments, the cracking time of a walnut shell under load pressure is so short that the process cannot be observed by eyes. The cracking time of a walnut shell can be estimated according to the relevant formula. According to brittle solid fracture mechanics, the crack expansion rate is calculated by Equation (7) [19]:

$$v(c) = v_T f(c/c_0, \alpha) \tag{7}$$

where v_T is the limit speed, and f is the function of scale one, which is calculated as:

$$f(c/c_0, 0) = 1 - c_0/c \tag{8}$$

where c_0 is the initial crack length, and c is the crack extension length.

The estimation of the limit speed is as follows:

$$v_T \approx 0.38 v_1 \tag{9}$$

where $v_1 = (E/\rho)^{1/2}$ is the longitudinal sound rate.

The initial conditions for calculating the crack expansion rate of walnuts are shown in Table 3, and the calculation results are shown in Table 4. The average shell cracking time was calculated as $t = a/v(c) = 4.75$ µs. The calculation results of the crack expansion rate showed that the crack formation time was very short. Based on it, we proposed that it is not necessary to consider the crack formation time. Instead, only the force loading time on the walnut shell surface should be taken into account in practical applications.

Table 3. The initial conditions for calculating the crack expansion rate of walnuts.

Initial Conditions	Elastic Modulus E	Density ρ	Initial Crack Length c_0	Average Length of Cracks a
Initial Value	0.18 GPa	0.5 kg/m^3	0	34.3 mm

Table 4. The calculation results of the walnut crack expansion rate.

Type	The Longitudinal Sound Rate v_1	The Limit Speed v_T	f	The Crack Expansion Rate $v(c)$
Results	19 km/s	7.22 km/s	1	34.3 mm

4. Shell Mechanics Analysis

4.1. Shell Deformation Process

The walnut shell breaking tests under unidirectional load were performed using a texture meter. The force-displacement curve during walnut shell breaking is shown in Figure 7. The force-displacement curve showed that the walnut shell breaking process under force load was summarized as follows: the AB section curve had a small slope with small fluctuations, which might be mainly due to the texture meter cylindrical indenter getting close contact with the irregular surface of the walnut; the BC section was a straight line with a fixed slope *k*. According to engineering mechanics, $\sigma = E\varepsilon$. The elastic deformation stage is characterized by a linear relationship between the load and the strain. Therefore, the walnut produces elastic deformation under a load of this section, and thus the BC section was the elastic compression stage. The slope of the CD section was decreased with the increase in the force-displacement in the transverse coordinate compared with that of the BC section. According to material mechanics, the CD section produces not only elastic deformation but also partial plastic deformation, and thus the CD section was a mixed deformation stage of elastic deformation and plastic deformation. When the load was increased to σ_D, the load stress reached the intensity limit of the walnut shell, and thus brittle fracture, as one type of fracture failure, occurred. The EF section showed the stage when the indenter continued to compress the walnut downward. Due to the brittle fracture of the walnut, the toughness of the walnut was reduced to a low value, and thus the load increase under unit displacement was small, eventually resulting in a small slope *k*. After point F, the texture meter indenter moved back to the initial position, and the load gradually decreased to zero.

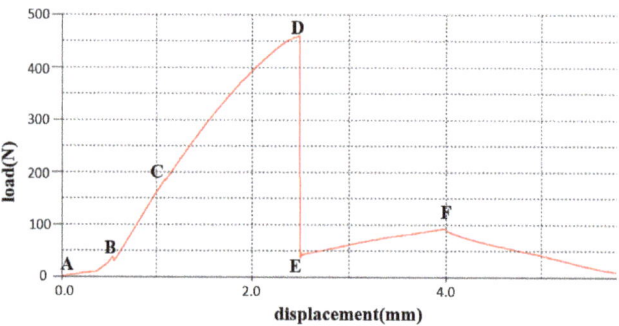

Figure 7. Force—displacement curve of the walnut shell breaking under load.

4.2. Internal Force Analysis

The small thickness and bending moment of the thin shell cause great stress and deformation, which has an important influence on the establishment of the mechanical model. Therefore, this study took the bending moment into full consideration in the analysis of the thin-shell model. In this study, the walnut shell was divided into the concentrated force region and peripheral force region. The concentrated force region was the region undertaking the unidirectional load. The presence of the normal external load resulted in a large bending moment in this region, which could not be ignored. Excluding the concentrated force region, the remaining region far from the concentrated force was defined as the peripheral force region with a negligible small bending moment.

4.2.1. Peripheral Force Region

Since the bending moment in the peripheral force region was negligible, the thin film theory (namely, the momentless theory) could be used for analysis. In a momentless state (Figure 8), only the stresses T_θ, T_φ, and $T_{\theta\varphi}$ were examined, while torques M_θ, M_φ, and $M_{\theta\varphi}$ were ignored. In equilibrium state:

$$M_\theta = M_\varphi = M_{\theta\varphi} = N_\theta = N_\varphi = 0 \tag{10}$$

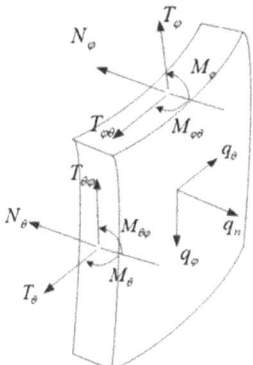

Figure 8. Section diagram of force.

Under static balance conditions:

$$T_\varphi r_0 \sin\varphi = -\int_0^\varphi r_0 R(q_\varphi \sin\varphi - q_n \cos\varphi) d\varphi \tag{11}$$

In any cross-section of the walnut shell (Figure 9), $q_\varphi = 0$, $q_n = -p$, $R = r$, $r_0 = r\sin\varphi$.

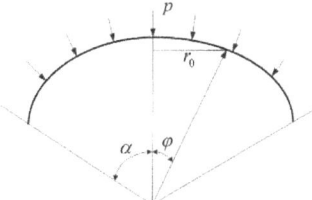

Figure 9. Cross-section diagram of force.

Thus:

$$T_\varphi r \sin^2\varphi = -\int_0^\varphi r^2 \sin\varphi p \cos\varphi \, d\varphi \tag{12}$$

Thus:

$$T_\varphi = -\frac{pr}{2} \tag{13}$$

Then, by the formula:

$$\frac{T_\varphi}{R_1} + \frac{T_\varphi}{R_2} - q_n = 0 \tag{14}$$

where R_1 and R_2 are the radiuses of the primary curvature, $R_1 = R_2 = r$, thus:

$$T_\theta = -\frac{pr}{2} \tag{15}$$

The results showed that T_θ was equal to T_φ, and thus the internal force was equal in any cross-section of the walnut shell surface within the peripheral force region, indicating that the peripheral force region of the walnut shell had an isotropic property.

4.2.2. Concentrated Force Action Region

The external load in the concentrated force action region resulted in a large unignorable bending moment. Therefore, this region cannot be simply analyzed by the momentless theory, and we resorted to the corresponding moment theory for mechanical analysis. In this study, the finite element analysis method was employed to simulate the concentrated force action area of the walnut shell to obtain an intuitive and specific shell stress distribution pattern. To this end, the walnut model was constructed, and the concentrated force was analyzed as follows.

Modeling: A 3D walnut model was constructed using a 3D scanner, and then the obtained 3D model was introduced into the finite element software ANSYS (Figure 10).

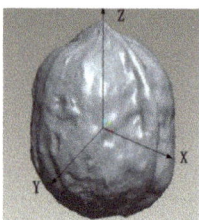

Figure 10. Walnut 3D scanned model.

Parameter setting: The elastic modulus of the walnut model was set as 0.18 GPa, the Poisson ratio as 0.3, and the walnut shell density as 0.5 kg/m^3.

Meshing: The grid properties were set, and the grid was endowed with material properties. The model was meshed with a mesh quality of >0.3, indicating a suitable meshing (Figure 11).

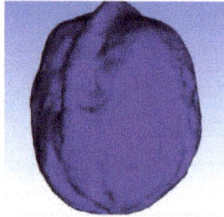

Figure 11. Meshing of the walnut model.

Force analysis: The 100 N contact load was added to the model, and then the simulation analysis of the loaded model was performed. The stress cloud diagram was obtained from the simulation analysis (Figure 12). The stress cloud diagram intuitively reflected the stress distribution in the concentrated force region. The results showed that under the load, the shell stress was gradient-distributed along the walnut shell, reaching the maximum at the load point, and it gradually decreased with the increasing distance from the load point.

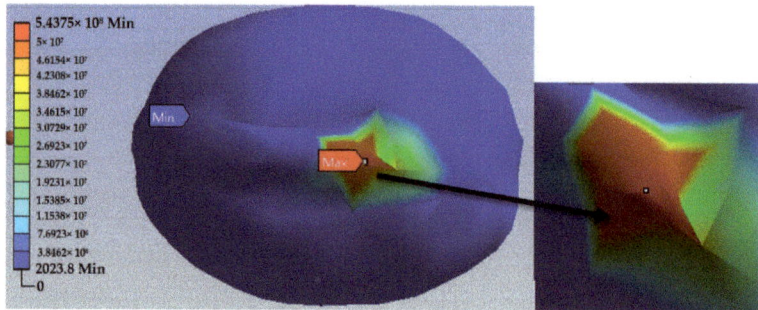

Figure 12. Stress cloud map of the walnut under unidirectional load.

5. Walnut Shell Breaking Experiments under Unidirectional Load

According to the requirements of walnut shell breaking under unidirectional load, this study designed a mechanical claw shell-breaking test bench (Figure 13) to carry out the walnut shell breaking tests under unidirectional load.

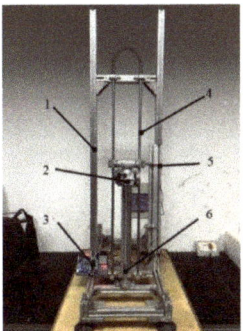

Figure 13. Mechanical claw shell breaking test bench. (1) Frame; (2) Three-fingered mechanical claws; (3) Microcontroller; (4) Sliding rail; (5) Proximity switch; (6) Impact table.

5.1. Test Procedure

On the test bench, a large walnut sample was grabbed by a three-fingered mechanical claw with the walnut ridge parallel to the impact table and the midpoint of the walnut shell surface touching the impact table when impacting, and then the mechanical claw was lifted to different heights to enable it to fall freely along the sliding rail until the walnut fell on the impact table to implement unidirectional load.

According to the momentum theorem, the force the walnut undertook was calculated by Equation (16).

$$F \cdot t = mv_2 - mv_1 \qquad (16)$$

where F is the force, which is unknown; t is the action time, which was set as 0.01 s; m is the mass; v_1 is the initial velocity; v_2 is the final velocity; both v_1 and v_2 are vectors.

The overall mass of the mechanical claws was 1.6 kg. In the experiment, walnuts and the impact table collided with almost no rebound, and thus $v_2 = 0$, and v_1 was measured as follows. Two proximity switches were installed on the test bench framework, the spacing of which was the calibration value X_0. The first proximity switch position was set as the starting position, and the second was set as the termination position. After the mechanical claw was placed at the starting position, the microcontroller was turned on. Then the mechanical claw was released to fall freely along the sliding rail. At this time, the timing program of the microcontroller was triggered to start timing. When the mechanical claw reached the termination position, the proximity switch was triggered again. Subsequently, the microcontroller stopped timing immediately after receiving the signal from the proximity switch, and t_0 (the time when the mechanical claw moved from the initial position to the termination position) was output and displayed. Then, according to the displacement formula $x = 1/2\, at^2$, the acceleration (a) of the mechanical claw to fall freely along the sliding rail was calculated as 9.8 m/s². Finally, the base of the impact table in the test bench was taken as the zero point, and X_0 (the spacing between the two proximity switches) was calibrated with 10 cm as the unit distance along the sliding rail. From different heights (h), the mechanical claw was released to fall freely along the sliding rail until the walnuts collided with the impact table and the shell broke. The velocity v during the impact was calculated by the formula $v^2 = 2\, ax$. a and x (namely, h) were substituted into the formula, and the v value (the initial velocity v_1 in Equation (16)) was obtained.

5.2. Test Results

The shell load force was calculated as follows. Based on multiple tests, the critical height for walnut shell breaking (h) was determined as 20 cm. When the height was above 20 cm, the walnut would be seriously broken. When the height was below 20 cm, the walnut failed to break. According to $v^2 = 2\ ax$, the initial velocity is $v_1 = 1.98$ m/s. In addition, when $t = 0.01$ s, $m = 1.6$ kg, $v_1 = 1.98$ m/s were substituted into the Equation (16), the load force F was calculated as 316.8 N in the process of collision, which was consistent with the results obtained by the equation in Section 2.3.

After the shell-breaking tests, the walnut cracks were analyzed (Figure 14). The crack expansion direction was consistent with our hypothesis of fracture along the longitudinal texture. The shell and kernel were separated from the walnut kernel intact; therefore, the shell-breaking effect was desirable.

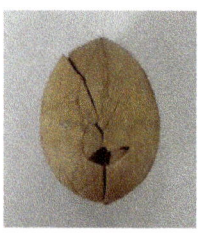 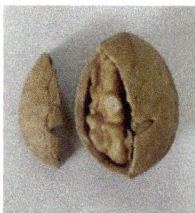

Figure 14. Walnut shell crack and complete kernel after shell-kernel separation.

6. Discussion and Conclusions

In this study, the spherical thin-shell model was established for walnut shell breaking tests, and the model fitting degree was tested by the elastic mechanical calculation based on the spherical thin-shell theory. The model deviation was found to be within 5%, indicating a good fitting degree of the model. Based on theoretical analysis of this model and walnut shell breaking experiments, the following conclusions were drawn:

(1) The walnut shell was divided into the concentrated force region and peripheral force region. In the peripheral force domain, the internal forces of the shell surface in all directions were calculated to be equal based on the momentless theory. In the concentrated force region, the finite element analysis method was used to intuitively exhibit the gradient distribution of the internal force on the shell from inside to outside. Based on these results, we suggested that the unidirectional force during shell breaking should be loaded on the middle of the walnut shell surface so as to make the shell surface force load uniform, thus improving the shell breaking effect and efficiency.

(2) Walnut cracks included type I and type II cracks. According to the maximum stress yield criterion, crack initiation occurred at the position where the load was applied, and the crack expansion direction was determined according to the fracture criterion and the stress intensity factor. Finally, the crack expansion rate could be used to determine the walnut shell breaking position and force loading time so as to obtain the complete kernel and improve the shell-kernel separation rate.

(3) The actually measured walnut shell breaking force under unidirectional load was in line with the theoretical value, and the observed crack extension direction was consistent with our hypothesis of fracture along the longitudinal texture. These results jointly verified the reliability of the theoretical model proposed in this study. Our results can provide a theoretical basis for the development and structural optimization of shell-breaking machinery.

Author Contributions: Conceptualization, X.B. and J.M.; methodology, X.B. and J.M.; software, P.D.; validation, B.C.; resources, X.B.; data curation, P.D. and Y.L.; writing—original draft preparation, B.C.; writing—review and editing, X.B. and J.M.; project administration, X.B. All authors have read and agreed to the published version of the manuscript.

Funding: This research was funded by the Nature Science Foundation of Hubei Province, China (No. 2021CFB 471), and the Nation Key Research and Development Program of China (No. 2018YFD0700804), and the National Natural Science Foundation of China (No. 51605181).

Institutional Review Board Statement: Not applicable.

Informed Consent Statement: Not applicable.

Data Availability Statement: Not applicable.

Conflicts of Interest: The authors declare no conflict of interest.

References

1. Song, Y.; Wang, X.H.; Zhang, R.; Liu, C.H.; Yu, S.Q.; Gao, S.; Zhang, R.L. Comparison of Quality Differences Among Varieties of Walnut from Xinjiang. *J. Chin. Cereals Oils Assoc.* **2019**, *34*, 91–97.
2. Lu, J.; Zhao, A.Q.; Cheng, C. Nutritional composition and physiological activity of walnut and its development and utilization. *Food Mach.* **2014**, *30*, 238–242.
3. Sütyemez, M.; Bükücü, Ş.B.; Özcan, A. 'Helete Güneşi:' A New Walnut Cultivar with Late Leafing, Early Harvest Date, and Superior Nut Traits. *Agriculture* **2021**, *11*, 991. [CrossRef]
4. Aleksandra, V.C.; Marie-Christine, R.; Jacqueline, V.; Sara, K.; Arijana, M.; Draženka, K.; Estelle, B. Valorisation of walnut shell and pea pod as novel sources for the production of xylooligosaccharides. *Carbohydr. Polym.* **2021**, *263*, 117932.
5. Liu, M.Z.; Li, C.H.; Cao, C.M. Research progress of key technology and device for size-grading shell-breaking and shell-kernel separation of walnut. *Trans. Chin. Soc. Agric. Eng.* **2020**, *36*, 294–310.
6. Wang, J.; Liu, M.; Wu, H.; Peng, J.; Peng, B.; Yang, Y.; Cao, M.; Wei, H.; Xie, H. Design and Key Parameter Optimization of Conic Roller Shelling Device Based on Walnut Moisture-Regulating Treatments. *Agriculture* **2022**, *12*, 561. [CrossRef]
7. Khir, R.; Pan, Z.; Atungulu, G.G.; Thompson, J.F.; Shao, D. Size and moisture distribution characteristics of walnut and their components. *Food Bioprocess Technol* **2013**, *6*, 771–782. [CrossRef]
8. Froogh, S.; Mohammadali, H.D. Mechanical behavior of walnut under cracking conditions. *J. Appl. Sci.* **2008**, *8*, 886–890.
9. Kocturk, B.O.; Gurhan, R. Determination of mechanical properties of various walnut according to different moisture levels. *J. Agric. Sci.* **2007**, *13*, 69–74.
10. Wu, Z.Y. Mechanical analysis of walnut shelling. *J. Nanjing Agric. Univ.* **1995**, *18*, 116–123.
11. Tu, C.; Yang, W.; Yin, Q.J. Optimization of technical parameters of breaking macadamia nut shell and finite element analysis of compression characteristics. *Trans. Chin. Soc. Agric. Eng.* **2015**, *31*, 272–277.
12. Yan, R.; Gao, J.; Zheng, J.H. Analysis of mechanical properties of walnut shell breaking based on workbench. *Agric. Mech. Res.* **2014**, *36*, 38–41.
13. Ojolo, S.J.; Damisa, O.; Orisaleye, J.I. Design and development of cashew nut shelling machine. *J. Engineering. Des. Technol.* **2010**, *8*, 146–157. [CrossRef]
14. Li, Z.X.; Liu, K.; Yang, L.L. Design and experiment of cone basket walnut shell breaking device. *J. Agric. Mach.* **2012**, *43*, 146–152.
15. Liu, M.Z.; Li, C.H.; Zhang, Y.B. Shell Crushing Mechanism Analysis and Performance Test of Flexible-belt Shearing Extrusion for Walnut. *Trans. Chin. Soc. Agric. Mach.* **2016**, *47*, 266–273.
16. Ding, R.; Cao, C.M.; Zhan, C. Design and experiment of bionic-impact type pecan shell breaker. *Trans. Chin. Soc. Agric. Eng.* **2017**, *33*, 257–264.
17. Xu, B.H.; Wang, Y.X.; Zhao, Y.H. Advances in the study of the toughness of wood-striped fractures. *Mech. Pract.* **2016**, *38*, 493–500.
18. Norman, E.D.; Jiang, S.Y.; Zhang, Y.Q. *Mechanical Behavior of Engineering Materials*; China Machine Press: Beijing, China, 2015.
19. Law, B.; Gong, J.H. *Fracture Mechanics of Brittle Solids*; Higher Education Press: Beijing, China, 2010.

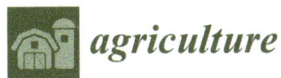

Article

Design and Performance Evaluation of a Multi-Point Extrusion Walnut Cracking Device

Hong Zhang [1,2], Hualong Liu [1,2], Yong Zeng [1,2,*], Yurong Tang [1,2], Zhaoguo Zhang [3] and Ji Che [4]

1. College of Mechanical and Electronic Engineering, Tarim University, Alar 843300, China
2. Agricultural Engineering Key Laboratory, Ministry of Higher Education of Xinjiang Uygur Autonomous Region, Tarim University, Alar 843300, China
3. Faculty of Modern Agricultural Engineering, Kunming University of Science and Technology, Kunming 650000, China
4. Xinjiang Jiangning Light Industry Mechanical Engineering Technology Co., Ltd., Urumqi 830011, China
* Correspondence: 120190040@taru.edu.cn; Tel.: +86-155-0457-7650

Abstract: The practical problems of existing methods of walnut cracking under compression loading, including incomplete walnut-shell crushing, broken walnut kernels, and so on, are widespread in walnut processing and are constraints that hinder mechanized walnut processing. Therefore, attempts have been made to design and optimize a multi-point extrusion walnut cracking device. For this, walnuts were fed manually into a cracking unit through the hopper. The tangential force of the grading roller graded the walnuts and dropped them into the gap between the rotating cracking roller and extrusion plate, causing them to crack. The developed machine was tested and the parameters were optimized using a central composite design (CCD). The objective functions involving the cracking angle (CA: 0.17, 0.27, 0.52, 0.76, 0.86°) and roller speed (RS: 63, 75, 105, 135, 147 r/min) were calculated. The shell cracking rate (*SCR*), whole kernel rate (*WKR*), and specific energy consumption (Es) regression models were established using the quadratic regression orthogonal combination test and the parameters were optimized using MATLAB software. The results showed that the most significant factors for the RS were the linear terms of the *SCR* and *WKR*, whereas for the CA the most significant factor was the linear term of the Es. The interaction term of the two factors had a significant effect on the three indicators. The optimal parameter combination was determined to be 0.47° for the CA and 108 r/min for the RS. On this basis, the adaptability test showed that the cracking device had a better cracking effect on walnuts with a gap between the walnut shell and kernel greater than 1.6 mm and a shell thickness less than 1.2 mm. The results have practical significance for the design of walnut cracking devices.

Keywords: walnut; multi-point extrusion; central composite design (CCD); parameter optimization

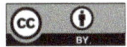

1. Introduction

The Walnut (*Juglans regia* L.) is one of the oldest cultivated fruit species in the world [1]. The kernels have excellent nutritional and therapeutic value due to their high content of unsaturated fatty acids [2] and abundant amino acids and minerals [3,4]. In post-harvest and processing, compared to other operations (e.g., cleaning, drying, storing, etc.), walnut-shell cracking to extract the kernel from the internal nut is not only the most important operation but also the fundamental goal, which can be attributed to the fact that the usable part of tree nuts is not the walnut itself but the kernel, especially the whole kernel because consumers prefer whole kernels [5]. However, during the process of walnut cracking, unexpected phenomena (e.g., incomplete nutshell cracking and broken nut kernels) occur with existing cracking devices, which are the key factors that affect the quality of the final kernel and limit the development of the initial processing [6]. The cracking performance is strongly related to the intrinsic properties of the walnut (e.g., shell thickness and moisture content), cracking device configurations (e.g., roll and hammer), and operational conditions (e.g., shaft rotation speed). Hence, several researchers have proposed a series of effective methods to improve cracking performance in terms of the three aspects mentioned above [7–9], particularly the latter two factors.

Li [10] studied the effects of the gap between the two rotating cracking rollers and roller speed on walnut cracking. It was found that increasing the rotational speed and decreasing the pitch increased the fracture force, thereby resulting in an increase in the specific deformation of the walnut shell [11]. Shi et al. [12] evaluated a cam rocker bidirectional extrusion walnut cracking device using squeeze clearance, camshaft speed, and walnut circumference as the test factors. Bernik et al. [5] investigated the cracking quality of three types of walnuts at different speeds under a modified centrifugal cracking machine. By analyzing the above-mentioned research, it was found that the contact type between the walnut and the cracking device was mostly a single point or line load. However, it was also found that the contact types mentioned above would result in uneven forces on the shell, poor crack extension, and easy damage to the inner kernel [13]. Additionally, studies have also suggested that different contact types have a significant effect on walnut cracking. For example, Zhang et al. [14] reported that spherical compression was the best process for walnut cracking. In addition, Shen [15] discovered that adding spikes to the surface of the V-indenter for shell cracking was substantially more successful. According to the above analyses, increasing the stress concentration areas contributes to the generation and expansion of cracks while reducing the inner shell force and deformation value of walnut kernels, thus further minimizing mechanical damage to the kernels.

Unfortunately, there are few practical applications for walnut cracking devices based on multiple load contact. For instance, Cao et al. [13] observed superior walnut-cracking outcomes using a hammer head with seven grooves. Furthermore, He et al. [16] improved cracking device performance by adding rectangular or trapezoidal grooves to the surfaces of the cracking rollers. Nonetheless, the quality of cracking still needs to be improved. Therefore, by integrating the results of previous research, a multi-point extrusion walnut cracking device was designed and its operating parameters were optimized using the RSM in this work. The influence of each factor on the evaluation index and the interaction between the factors were analyzed, respectively. The best combinations of parameters were determined using the regression analysis method with the help of MATLAB software, which was used to verify the practical suitability of several walnut varieties.

2. Materials and Methods

2.1. Materials

'Wen 185', which is the typical walnut cultivar in the local market, was selected and used as the experimental sample. In the harvest season of 2021, fresh-harvested walnuts (*Juglans regia* L.) were collected from the Wensu Walnut Experimental Station (latitude: 41°27′67″ N, longitude: 80°24′17″ E, and at a 1056 m altitude), Xinjiang, China. A moderate walnut moisture content is known to improve the quality of cracking [17]. Thus, according to our previous study [18], walnut shells with a moisture content range of 7–9% and kernels with a moisture content range of 10–13% were used in the walnut cracking experiments.

2.2. Principles of a Walnut Cracking Device

A walnut cracking machine, including the frame, control panel, speed-regulating motor, feed hopper, grading cylinder, deflector, and cracking device (Figure 1a), was designed and manufactured. A control panel was used to adjust the speed of the grading cylinder and rotating cracking roller to meet the requirements of different working conditions. After feeding, the walnuts were rolled with the cylinder and were moved forward by the driving of the helical steel ribs. Different walnut sizes fell off the corresponding spaces of the cylinder and the walnuts were graded according to their size. Walnuts fell through the guide chute into the cracking device, which was composed of a rotating cracking roller and extrusion plate with 'V' grooves. The wedge-shaped space formed by the extrusion plate and rotating cracking roller was the part where the walnuts were cracked by the squeezing-type device. The space could be adjusted by the retainer bolt and the position-limit mechanism as a means of adapting to the different walnut dimensions. The shells were cracked by the squeezing, rolling, and grinding of the extrusion plate and rotating cracking roller and then ejected. In order to ensure the appropriate extrusion shearing forces on the walnut, several spikes were added to the surface of the rotating cracking roller and extrusion plate (Figure 1b) to increase the stress concentration areas. Thus, this designed cracking machine was able to simultaneously carry out walnut grading and cracking. The main technical parameters of the walnut cracking device are listed in Table 1.

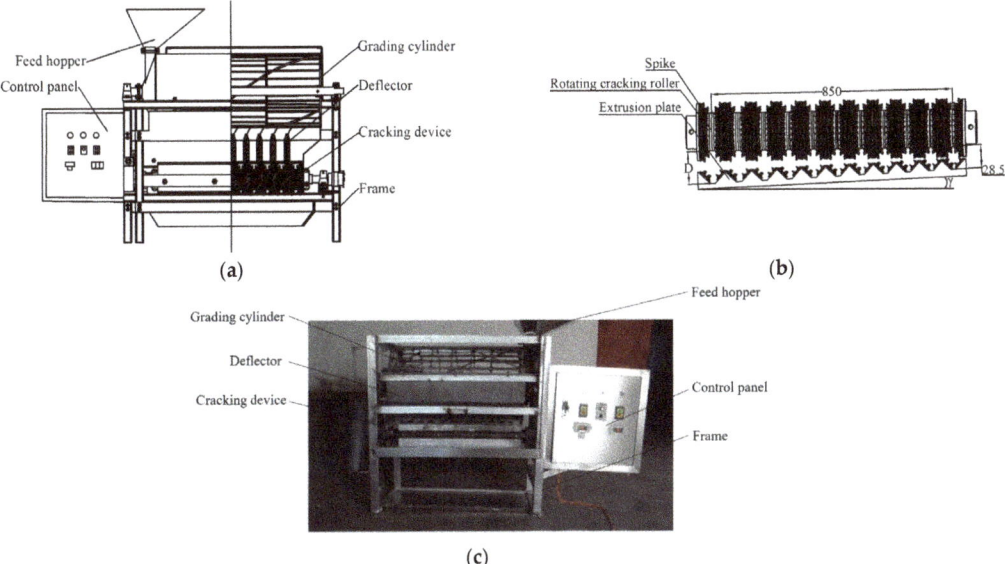

Figure 1. Overall structural schematic diagram of the walnut cracking device: (**a**) final assembly drawing, (**b**) the gap between rotating cracking roller and extrusion plate, (**c**) structural schematic photo of the prototype.

Table 1. Parameters of the cracking device.

Parameters	Size
Length × width × height/(mm × mm × mm)	1200 × 800 × 1200
Overall weight/kg	165
Inlet size/(mm × mm)	90 × 45
Productivity/(kg/h)	1080
Power of cracker/kw	0.75
Grading accuracy/(%)	≥96
Cracking angle/(°)	0–1
Roller speed/(r/min)	0–210

2.3. Design of Grading Cylinder

The length (L), width (W), and thickness (T) [17] of 200 randomly selected walnuts were measured (Figure 2) using a DELI DL91150 digital caliper (DELI Group Co., Ltd., Ningbo, China) with an accuracy of 0.01 mm. To classify the walnuts more accurately, the equivalent diameter of walnut samples was calculated based on Equation (1) mentioned in Zeng et al. [19] and the statistical results are shown in Figure 3. The measurements showed that the measured diameters conformed to a normal distribution and were mainly in the range of 32–42 mm ($p < 0.05$). The proportion of walnuts sized 32–37 mm was 34.74%, sized

37–39 mm was 35.26%, and sized 39–42 mm was 30%, respectively. Thus, based on these size distributions, the rotary fence cylinder of the walnut grader with three stages was designed as shown in Figure 4, namely, the gaps between the fences were 37 mm, 39 mm, and 42 mm, respectively.

$$D_P = \left[\frac{(W+T)^2}{4}L\right]^{(\frac{1}{3})} \quad (1)$$

where D_P is the walnut equivalent diameter (mm); L is the length (mm); W is the width (mm); T is the thickness (mm).

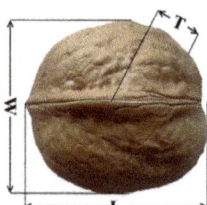

Figure 2. Characteristic parameter analysis of walnuts.

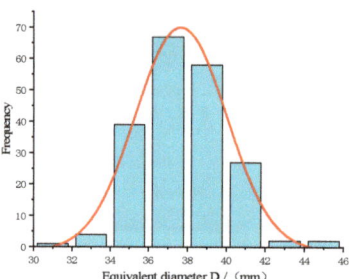

Figure 3. Equivalent diameter distribution of walnuts.

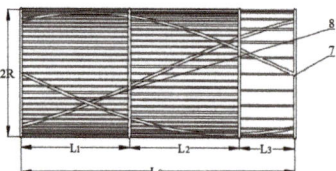

Figure 4. Schematic diagram of grading cylinder.

The grading cylinder diameter was calculated, as per Jeffrey et al. [20] where the grading cylinder speed is equal to 50% of the critical speed.

$$R = \frac{1}{2}\left(\frac{0.19Q_m}{F_i K_v d_b g^{0.5} \tan \alpha}\right)^{0.4} \quad (2)$$

of which,

$$K_v = \begin{cases} 1.35 & (\alpha = 3°) \\ 1.85 & (\alpha = 5°) \end{cases} \quad (3)$$

where Q_m is the feeding capacity (kg/h); α is the angle of inclination of the grading cylinder (°); K_v is the velocity correction factor; d_b is the material bulk density (kg/m³); g is the acceleration due to gravity (m/s²); F_i is the filling degree, taken as 0.25–0.33. Substituting

Q_m = 1080 kg/h, F_i = 0.25, α = 5°, K_v = 1.85, d_b = 470 kg/m³ [13], and g = 9.8 m/s² into Equation (2) gives a grading roller radius of R = 0.16 m.

The length of the grading cylinder is related to the tumbling time of the walnuts in the grading cylinder. As the length increases, the grading time also increases, and the grading accuracy increases. However, the length should not be too long. After the length exceeds a certain value, it does not significantly increase the grading efficiency but increases the cost of the grading cylinder. Thus, the length of the grading cylinder is generally taken to be 2–6 times its diameter [21].

The length of the grading cylinder was calculated as follows where the classifying cylinder speed is equal to 50% of the critical speed.

$$L_0 = 15\sqrt{2}K_v(2R)^{0.5}g^{0.5}\pi^{-1}t_i \tan \alpha \tag{4}$$

where t_i is the residence time (min); L_0 is the grading cylinder length (m).

Substituting K_v = 1.85, R = 0.18 m, t_i = 0.5 min, and α = 5° into Equation (4), we obtain L_0 = 0.97 m, taking L_0 = 1 m. To ensure the accuracy and efficiency of grading, the grading roller is divided into 3 grades according to the proportions of the different sizes of walnuts (L_1 = L_2 = 0.35 m, L_3 = 0.3 m), as shown in Figure 4.

2.4. Design of Rotating Cracking Roller, Extrusion Plate, and Cracking Angle

For extrusion-style devices, the gap between the rotating cracking roller and extrusion plate and the speed of the rotating cracking roller are both principal factors. The gap significantly influences the deformation degree of the walnut shells, whereas the speed has an important impact on the efficiency of the walnut cracking [22]. The conditions under which walnuts can enter the gap between the rotating cracking roller and extrusion plate are as follows (Figure 5).

$$mg + \mu F_N + \mu F_R \cos \varepsilon > F_R \sin \varepsilon \tag{5}$$

Because of $\sum F_x$ = 0, bring $F_N = F_R \cos \varepsilon + \mu F_R \sin \varepsilon$ into Equation (5) then,

$$mg + \mu F_R \cos \varepsilon + \mu^2 F_R \sin \varepsilon + \mu F_R \cos \varepsilon > F_R \sin \varepsilon \tag{6}$$

Bring $\mu = \tan \beta$ into Equation (6), then,

$$\varepsilon < \sin^{-1}\left(\frac{mg\cos^2\beta}{F_R}\right) + 2\beta \tag{7}$$

where F_R is the positive pressure of the rotating cracking roller on the walnut (N); F_N is the positive pressure of the extrusion plate on the walnut (N); ε is the angle between the positive pressure F_R and the horizontal line (°); β is the friction angle between the rotating cracking roller and extrusion plate and the walnut (°); μ is the friction coefficient between the rotating cracking roller, extrusion plate, and walnut, $\mu = \tan \beta$.

A cross-sectional view of the walnut along the thickness direction is shown in Figure 6. The walnut is squeezed into the gap in the direction of its thickness under the following conditions:

$$t < e \leqslant t + 2h \tag{8}$$

Or,

$$t < e \leqslant T - d \tag{9}$$

where e is the gap between the rotating cracking roller and extrusion plate (mm); h is the walnut shell thickness (mm); t is the wide diameter of the kernel (mm); d is the space between the kernel and the inner wall of the shell (mm), i.e., the gap between the walnut shell and kernel.

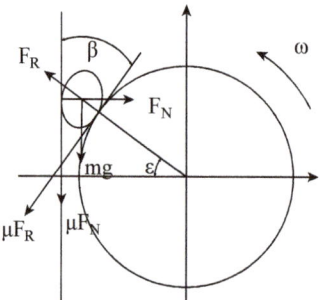

Figure 5. Forces of walnut in extrusion cracking device.

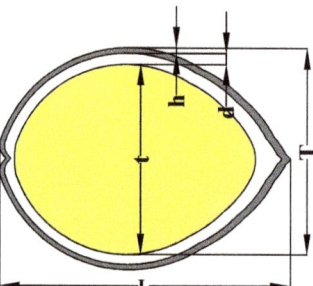

Figure 6. Transverse sectional view of a walnut.

The gap between the rotating cracking roller and extrusion plate was the largest when $e = t + 2h$ or $e = T - d$. At this point, the shell was subjected to a squeezing pressure, whereas the squeezing pressure on the kernels was zero. This is the ideal state for walnut cracking so the kernels are not damaged. When $t < e \leq t + 2h$ or $t < e \leq T - d$ was met, the external shell was just crushed but the internal kernel was not broken. The gap (d) between the walnut shell and kernel was generally 1.85 mm and the shell thickness (h) was 0.86 mm for the 'Wen 185' [23]. Thus, the minimum gap (e) was designed to be 28.5 mm.

The small end of the gap between the rotating cracking roller and the extrusion plate (right end in Figure 1b) was used as an example for the analysis. The walnut shape is assumed to be ellipsoidal [20], and then we have

$$\cos \varepsilon = \frac{r + e}{r + W} \tag{10}$$

Simplifying Equation (10), the radius of the rotating cracking roller is given by

$$r = \frac{e - W \cos \varepsilon}{\cos \varepsilon - 1} \tag{11}$$

In summary, the radius the of rotating cracking roller was 75 mm. If the gap (e) became smaller and the rotating cracking roller diameter remained the same so that $\varepsilon \geq \sin^{-1} ((mg\cos^2 \beta)/F_R) + 2\beta$, the cracking device did not work properly. In this paper, the gap (e) was replaced by the angle between the rotating cracking roller and extrusion plate, which was treated as a studied factor, as shown in Figure 1b. Note that the angle could be adjusted by the bolt (GB/T 5782M12 × 80) and a DELI DL305300 full-circle protractor (DELI Group Co., Ltd., Ningbo, China) with an accuracy of 0.3°. According to the above analysis and Equation (12), the cracking angle (γ) was selected in the range of 0 to 1°.

$$\tan \gamma = \frac{(D - 28.5)}{850} \tag{12}$$

where D is the big end of the gap between the rotating cracking roller and extrusion plate (mm); γ is the angle of the rotating cracking roller and extrusion plate (°).

2.5. Cracking Quality Index Measurement Method

2.5.1. Shell-Cracking Rate

To evaluate the performance of walnut cracking under different working parameters, the shell cracking rate was treated as the evaluation index, as per Zhang et al. [14], as shown in Equation (13):

$$SCR = \left(1 - \frac{M_1}{M_0}\right) \times 100\% \qquad (13)$$

where SCR is expressed as the shell-cracking rate achieved in one pass through the machine (%); M_0 is the total weight of the walnuts (kg); M_1 is the mass of unbroken walnuts (kg). As shown in Figure 7, a degree of walnut breakage greater than one-half the size of a walnut was identified as a broken walnut. Among them, one-quarter walnuts and one-half walnuts were identified as shell-wrapped kernels.

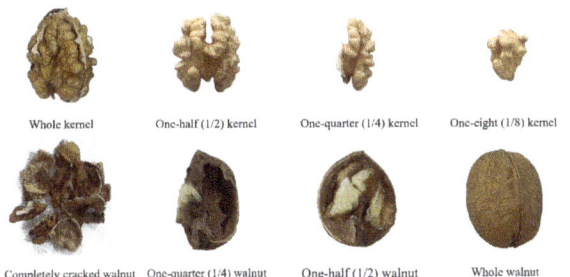

Figure 7. The different particle sizes of cracked walnuts and walnut kernels.

2.5.2. Whole Kernel Rate

Following walnut cracking, each kernel was visually evaluated to determine the state of the kernel. Each kernel was visually classified into four types, as shown in Figure 7. Kernels with greater than a 1/4 volume were defined as a "complete kernel" [17]. The *WKR* can be calculated by using:

$$WKR = \frac{M_3}{M_2} \times 100\% \qquad (14)$$

where M_2 is the total mass of kernels obtained after cracking (kg); M_3 is the mass of kernels identified as greater than 1/4 kernels after cracking (kg).

2.5.3. Specific Energy Consumption

The energy consumption of cracking was measured using a power meter (DL333502, Deli Group Co., Ltd., Ningbo, China). The power meter was connected to a power source and the cracking device was connected to the power meter. The energy required for operating the machine without load was first recorded and then subtracted from the energy data collected when the machine was running under load. The real-time power and cracking duration were recorded during the running periods. The *Es* was calculated using the method of Meng et al. [24]:

$$Es = \frac{\int_0^t (P_t - P_0)dt}{M} \qquad (15)$$

where P_t is the real-time power during the cracking process (W); P_0 is the operating power without walnuts in the hopper (W); t is the cracking duration (s).

2.6. Experimental Design and Statistical Analysis

Each experiment with 5 kg of 'Wen-185' walnuts (electronic balance, precision 0.01 g) was conducted and then repeated three times. The results were averaged and the data were recorded as shown in Table 2. A central composite design (CCD) of two variables (CA, RS) with five levels was adopted using the Design Expert software program (V8.0.6, Stat-Ease Co., Minneapolis, MN, USA). The range of values for the single factors was selected according to the preliminary experiments (not shown). The variables and their levels are given in Table 2. A multiple regression analysis was carried out to obtain an empirical model for each response variable, namely, the SCR, WKR, and Es. The second-order polynomial of the following forms was fitted to the data of the response.

$$Y = \beta_0 + \sum_{i=1}^{2} \beta_i X_i + \sum_{i=1}^{2} \beta_{ii} X_i^2 + \beta_{ij} X_i X_j \tag{16}$$

where Y represents the dependent responses; β_i, β_{ii}, and β_{ij} represent the regression coefficients of the process variables; X_i and X_j are coded as independent variables. Analysis of variance (ANOVA) was used to test the adequacy of the acquired model. The validity of the model was confirmed by the equation analysis, lack of fit (p = 0.05) tests, and R^2 (the ratio of the explained variation to the total variation) analysis. The variable level combinations and responses of the experiments are shown in Table 2. A numerical optimization module in the software was used to obtain the optimal operating parameters.

Table 2. Design and results of the experiments.

Test NO.	X_1 (°)	X_2 (r/min)	SCR/(%)	WKR/(%)	Es/(kJ/kg)
1	0.27 (−1)	75 (−1)	93.66	81.62	2.26
2	0.76 (1)	75 (−1)	93.52	82.36	1.92
3	0.27 (−1)	135 (1)	99.54	88.23	3.41
4	0.76 (1)	135 (1)	94.82	81.36	1.84
5	0.17 (−1.414)	105 (0)	99.42	87.98	2.62
6	0.86 (1.414)	105 (0)	95.14	83.64	2.26
7	0.52 (0)	63 (−1.414)	92.66	81.46	1.89
8	0.52 (0)	147 (1.414)	93.81	87.28	2.84
9	0.52 (0)	105 (0)	97.62	91.02	1.64
10	0.52 (0)	105 (0)	98.65	92.15	1.72
11	0.52 (0)	105 (0)	97.85	93.89	1.35
12	0.52 (0)	105 (0)	97.35	91.78	1.92
13	0.52 (0)	105 (0)	98.84	94.26	1.82

Note: X_1 cracking angle, X_2 roller speed, SCR shell-cracking rate, WKR whole kernel rate, Es specific energy consumption.

The degree of influence of every factor in the model can be reflected by the magnitude of the contribution ratio K, which is proportional to the magnitude of the influence [25]. Its calculation is shown in Equations (17) and (18):

$$\delta = \begin{cases} 0 & F \leq 1 \\ 1 - \frac{1}{F} & F > 1 \end{cases} \tag{17}$$

$$K_j = \delta_j + \frac{1}{2} \sum_{\substack{i=1 \\ i \neq j}}^{m} \delta_{ij} + \delta_{jj} \quad j = 1, 2, \cdots, m \tag{18}$$

where K_j is the contribution ratio (%); δ is the assessment values for the F-values; F represents the F-values in the ANOVA table; δ_j is the primary item contribution rate (%); δ_{jj} is the secondary item contribution (%); δ_{ij} is the contribution of the interaction items (%).

3. Results and Discussion

3.1. Effects of Single Factors on Responses

The dimension reduction method was carried out to study the effects of the single factors on the experimental responses. For the model of the percentage of the SCR, the coded independent variables were in turn set at −1.414, −1, 0, 1, and 1.414, whereas the other independent variables were fixed at 0. As shown in Figure 8a$_1$, the SCR first increased and then decreased as the coded values of the rotating cracking roller speed (X_2) ascended, and the SCR increased with the decreasing cracking angle (X_1), which showed that the appropriate values of X_1 and X_2 could improve the quality of the walnut cracking. The WKR increased and then decreased with the increase in X_1 and X_2 in the range of −1.414 to 1.414 (Figure 8b$_1$), which indicated that the WKR could be improved with a suitable parameter combination of X_1 and X_2. As shown in Figure 8c$_1$, the Es decreased and then increased with the increase in X_1 and X_2 in the range of −1.414 to 1.414, which indicated that the Es could be reduced with a suitable parameter combination of X_1 and X_2.

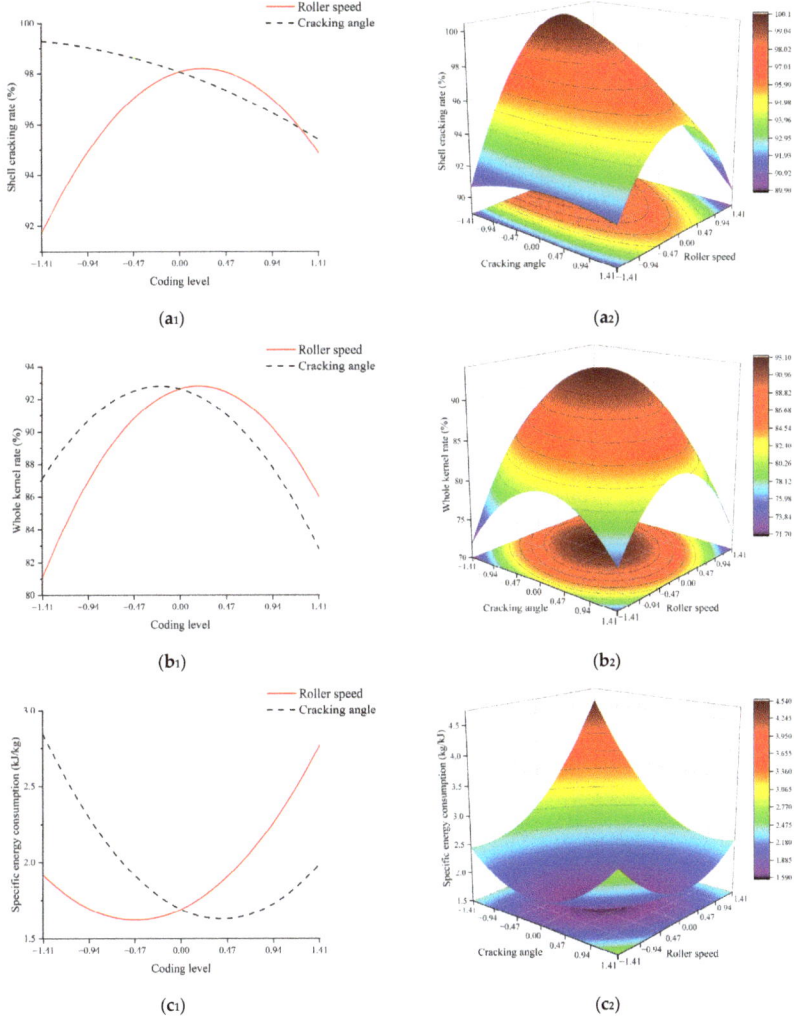

Figure 8. Influence of experimental factors on SCR (**a$_1$,a$_2$**), WKR (**b$_1$,b$_2$**), Es (**c$_1$,c$_2$**).

3.2. Optimization and Verification of Regression Models

3.2.1. Effect of Variables on SCR

The measured values of the *SCR* are presented in Table 2. The *SCR* varied between 92.66% and 99.54% with the combinations of the variables studied. According to the ANOVA results shown in Table 3, a second-order polynomial equation was extremely conspicuous ($p < 0.01$) for the responses. There was no significant lack of fit and the high R^2 (0.9232) values showed that most of the variability could be explained by the variables tested. The contributions of each factor affecting the *SCR* were calculated by Equations (17) and (18). The results showed that the RS was the most important factor, followed by the CA. Their contribution ratios were 2.276 and 1.337, respectively. The results in Table 3 indicated that, in this case, the linear term of the CA was extremely significantly different ($p < 0.01$), and the RS was significantly different ($p < 0.05$). The interaction terms of the CA and RS were significantly different ($p < 0.05$). The predicted model for the *SCR* can be described by the following equation in terms of the actual factors under the tested conditions.

$$SCR = 98.06 - 1.36X_1 + 1.10X_2 - 1.15X_1X_2 - 0.36X_1^2 - 2.38X_2^2 \qquad (19)$$

Table 3. Analysis of variance (ANOVA) applying response surface quadratic model.

Variation Source	Squares	df	SCR F	p	Squares	df	WKR F	p	Squares	df	Es F	p
β_0	69.3	5	13.86	0.0009 **	275.32	5	26.75	0.0002 **	3.31	5	10.35	0.0039 **
β_1	14.89	1	14.89	0.0038 **	18.81	1	9.14	0.0193 *	0.73	1	11.44	0.0117 *
β_2	9.69	1	9.69	0.0110 *	23.95	1	11.63	0.0113 *	0.73	1	11.39	0.0118 *
$\beta_1\beta_2$	5.24	1	5.24	0.0396 *	14.48	1	7.03	0.0328 *	0.38	1	5.92	0.0453 *
β_{11}	0.9	1	0.9	0.3313	102.01	1	49.55	0.0002 **	0.92	1	14.4	0.0068 **
β_{22}	39.46	1	39.46	0.0002 **	143.98	1	69.94	<0.0001 **	0.74	1	11.58	0.0114 *
R^2			0.9232				0.9503				0.8809	
Lack of fit	4.07	3	1.36	0.1458	6.62	3	1.13	0.436	0.26	3	1.83	0.2823

Note: "**" means extremely significant ($p < 0.01$), "*" means significant ($p < 0.05$).

The representation of the response surface is given in Figure 8a$_2$. The model's expression permits the evaluation of the effects of the factors. As shown in Figure 8a$_1$, the RS was at a level of 0, the CA increased from 0.17° to 0.86°, and the *SCR* dropped from 99.27% to 95.42%. With the increase in the CA, the *SCR* showed a slow decrease. The reason for this behavior was that as the CA increased, the walnuts were subjected to reduced positive pressure and friction between the rotating cracking roller and extrusion plate. When the gap was larger than the size of the walnut, the amount of extrusion deformation decreased, which was not helpful for the expansion of the crack. Some of the walnuts were not completely cracked (lower kernel exposure rate), leading to a decrease in the *SCR*. When the CA was at a level of 0, the *SCR* increased from 91.74% to 98.19% as the RS increased from 63 r/min to 111.89 r/min. The reason was that when the RS was low, the walnuts had enough frictional squeeze to achieve cracking within the gap between the cracking roller and the extrusion plate. When the RS exceeded 111.89 r/min, the *SCR* dropped to 94.86%. There were two possible reasons for this. On the one hand, walnuts were quickly thrown out of the gap between the cracking roller and the extrusion plate, which reduced the friction extrusion enacted upon the walnuts. On the other hand, as the loading speed increased, the amount of shell deformation (walnut shell flexibility) used to break the walnut shells [26] increased, which led to incomplete cracking for a portion of the walnuts. Kilickan and Guner [27] reported that the specific deformation of the olive fruit and pit increased as the compression speed increased. Also, the flexible shell prevented the walnut from cracking [11], which led to a reduced *SCR*.

3.2.2. Effect of Variables on WKR

The WKR varied from 81.36% to 94.26% with the combinations of the variables (Table 2). The ANOVA results are shown in Table 3 and the model was extremely conspicuous ($p < 0.01$) for the responses. There was no significant lack of fit and the high R^2 (0.9503) values showed that most of the variability could be explained by the variables tested. According to Equations (17) and (18), the factors affecting the WKR were the RS (K = 2.329) and the CA (K = 2.299). The results in Table 3 indicate that, in this case, the linear terms of the CA and RS were significantly different ($p < 0.05$). The interaction terms of the CA and RS were significantly different ($p < 0.05$). The predicted model for the WKR can be described by the following equation in terms of the actual factors.

$$WKR = 92.62 - 1.53X_1 + 1.73X_2 - 1.90X_1X_2 - 3.83X_1^2 - 4.55X_2^2 \tag{20}$$

The representation of the response surface is given in Figure 8b$_2$. The model's expression permits the evaluation of the effects of the factors. As shown in Figure 8b$_1$, when the CA was at a level of 0, the increase in the RS from 63 r/min to 110.53 r/min led to the WKR increasing dramatically from 81.08% to 92.78%. Then, the WKR declined to 85.97% when the RS increased from 110.53 r/min to 147 r/min. The reason was that the increase in the RS led to a decrease in the fracture force [26], which protected the fragile kernels and increased the WKR. When the RS exceeded 105 r/min, the WKR dropped sharply. The increase in the specific deformations of the walnut led to damage to the kernel. The kernel had a much smaller fracture force than its shell [28]. Similarly, when the RS was at a level of 0, the CA increased from 0.17° to 0.86° and the WKR increased from 87.13% to a maximum of 92.77% (CA = 0.46°) before decreasing to 82.79%. A possible reason for this was that the walnut was subjected to the ideal squeezing pressure for cracking the shell when the gap increased to the thickness of the walnut.

3.2.3. Effect of Variables on Es

The values of the Es varied from 1.35 kJ/kg to 3.41 kJ/kg as shown in Table 2. Table 3 shows a high correlation coefficient (R^2 = 0.8809) and no significant lack of fit for the responses, indicating that the polynomial fitted well for predicting the Es. The CA was the most important factor, followed by the RS, which was obtained by calculating the contribution ratio of the Es using Equations (17) and (18). Their contribution ratios were 2.259 and 2.241, respectively. The results in Table 3 indicate that, in this case, the linear terms of the CA and RS were significantly different ($p < 0.05$). The quadratic terms of the CA and RS were significantly different ($p < 0.05$). The predicted model for the Es can be described by the following equation in terms of the actual factors.

$$Es = 1.69 - 0.30X_1 + 0.30X_2 - 0.31X_1X_2 + 0.36X_1^2 + 0.33X_2^2 \tag{21}$$

The representation of the response surface is given in Figure 8c$_2$. The model's expression permits the evaluation of the effects of the factors. As shown in Figure 8c$_1$, as the CA increased from 0.17° to 0.61°, the Es decreased from 2.84 kJ/kg to 1.63 kJ/kg. This is because as the gap between the rotating cracking roller and extrusion plate increased, the walnuts were subjected to less squeezing friction, which lowered the resistance to the roller rotation. As the CA exceeded 0.61°, the Es increased with the CA to 1.99 kJ/kg. This was attributed to the fact that the movement of the walnuts in the gap was disordered, which led to increased energy consumption. The Es decreased slightly with the increasing RS and then gradually increased. It first decreased from 1.92 kJ/kg to 1.62 kJ/kg and then increased to 2.77 kJ/kg. This was due to the increase in the RS, which increased the power consumption and fracture energy required by the walnuts [29]. The possible reason for the decrease in the Es when the RS was less than 90.16 r/min is that at a lower RS, it took longer to complete the cracking of the walnuts. The working time of the cracking device increased, thus the Es of the cracking device increased. As the RS increased, the working efficiency also increased, which resulted in a slight decrease in the Es.

3.3. Determination and Validation of the Optimal Parameters

In the cracking process, the selection of the CA for the SCR and WKR was contradictory. Reducing the CA improved the SCR, but when the CA was too small, it reduced the WKR. Increasing the CA ensured the quality of the walnut kernels but seriously reduced the SCR. To enhance the walnut processing yield, the WKR was maximized while retaining a lower Es and an appropriate SCR. The mathematical models of the SCR, WKR and Es multi-objective functions were constructed, with weights of 0.3, 0.4, and 0.3, respectively. The weights of the WKR in the optimization solution equation were set larger than those of the SCR and Es. Because the magnitudes of the objective functions varied, the linear effectiveness coefficient approach was deployed to turn each objective function into a dimensionless function before applying the respective objective regression equation for comprehensive optimization. The nonlinear programming mathematical model in the following was established by analyzing Equations (19)–(21):

$$\begin{cases} F(X) \begin{cases} Y_1 = \max(SCR) \\ Y_2 = \max(WKR) \\ Y_3 = \min(Es) \end{cases} \\ s.t. \begin{cases} P = \eta_1 Y_1 + \eta_2 Y_2 + \eta_3 Y_3 \\ 0.17° \leq X_1 \leq 0.86° \\ 63 \text{ r/min} \leq X_2 \leq 147 \text{ r/min} \end{cases} \end{cases} \quad (22)$$

Based on the mathematical model and the regression equations for the SCR, WKR, and Es, the regression equations were optimally solved using MATLAB R2020a (Math-works, Inc. MA, USA) software [30]. The optimum parameters for working were as follows: the CA was 0.47° and the RS was 108.16 r/min. The optimum results were an SCR of 98.40%, WKR of 92.94%, and Es of 1.80 kJ/kg.

The before and after tests of the cracking device optimization are shown in Figure 9 and Table 4. The performance of the walnut cracking using the tip point roller press was superior, and the cracking effect of the walnut cracking device was significantly improved after optimization. Before optimization, the mixture of shells and kernels contained fewer shell-wrapped kernels, relatively intact shells (>1/4 shell), and broken kernels (<1/4 kernel). After optimization, the mixture did not include shell-wrapped kernels but contained many broken shells (<1/8 shell) and relatively intact kernels (>1/4 kernel). Validation experiments were carried out based on the optimal parameters. The measured values of the SCR, WKR, and Es were 97.24%, 92.03%, and 1.88 kJ/kg, respectively, which were close to the predicted values within the acceptable limits of the error percentage (0.98–4.44%). This demonstrates that the regression equations could predict the experimental results from the response surface.

Table 4. Comparison of parameters of cracking device before and after optimization.

Program	CA/(°)	RS/(r/min)	SCR/(%)	WKR/(%)	Es/(kJ/kg)
Before optimization	0.35	150	94.18	56.23	2.12
After optimization	0.47	108	97.24	92.03	1.88

3.4. Variety Adaptability Test

Mixed intercrop planting of multiple species of walnuts is a common phenomenon in Xinjiang, especially in the Hotan and Kashgar regions. Generally, different varieties of walnuts have irregular shapes, large size differences, varying shell thicknesses, and different gaps between the walnut shell and kernel. Previous devices have failed in achieving ideal adaption and cracking performance due to significant differences in the physical properties of the walnut varieties [28,31]. To do this, five common walnut varieties (i.e., 'Wen-185', 'Xinwen-179', 'Xinxin2', 'Zha-343', and 'Xinfeng') were used as test samples to confirm the cracking device's adaptability to the different varieties [23]. In the harvest season of

2021, fresh-harvested walnuts were collected from the Wensu Walnut Experimental Station, Xinjiang, China.

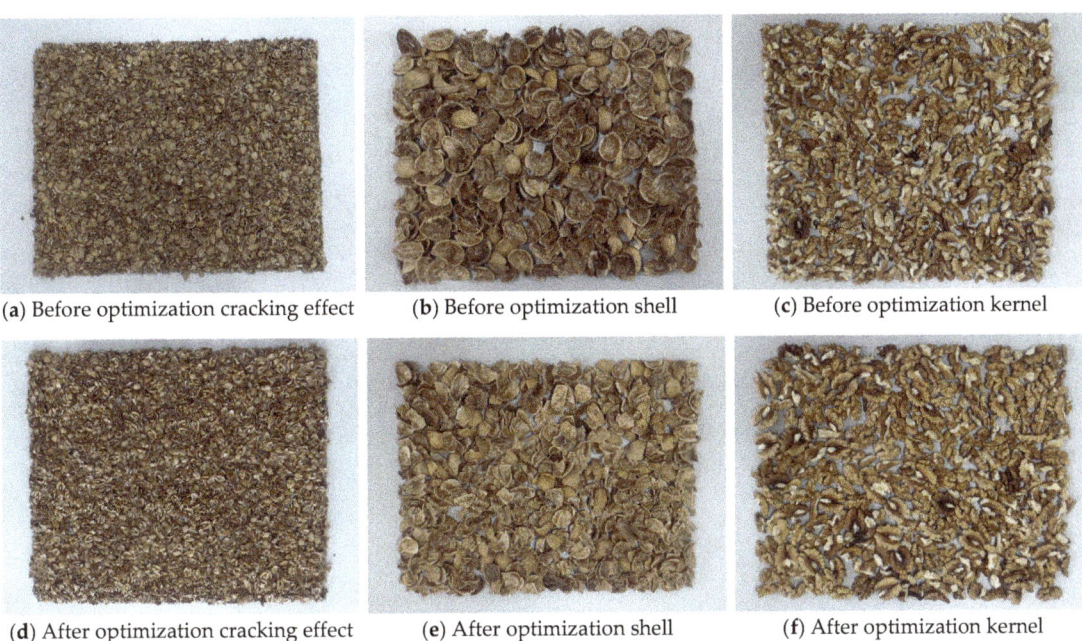

Figure 9. Prototype experimental conditions, (**a**–**c**) show plots of experimental results before device optimization, and (**d**–**f**) show plots of experimental results after device optimization.

The *t*-test in the IBM SPSS 25.0 (Armonk, NY, USA: IBM Corp) software was used to analyze the significance of the evaluation indicators of the cracking effects of the different varieties of walnuts obtained from the acclimatization trials (Table 5). There were significant differences in the cracking characteristics of the different walnut varieties [5,23]. For the SCR, the cracking unit was well-adapted to the 'Wen-185', 'Xinwen-179', 'Zha-343', and 'Xinxin2' varieties, with an *SCR* greater than 95%. Koyuncu et al. [32] showed that the shell thickness is inversely related to the shell cracking and kernel extraction quality. For the *WKR*, the cracking unit was highly adaptable to the 'Wen-185', 'Xinwen-179', 'Zha-343', and 'Xinfeng' varieties, with a *WKR* greater than 90%. When the walnuts were the same size, the smaller the value of the kernel diameter (t) and the larger the gap between the walnut shell and kernel (d), the greater the deformation allowed by the shell without damaging the kernel, which is conducive to maintaining the integrity of the kernel. For the Es, the cracking unit was highly adaptable to the 'Wen-185', 'Xinwen-179', and 'Zha-343' varieties, with an *Es* of less than 2 kJ/kg. With an increase in the *Es* with increasing shell thickness, similar results were reported by Kacal and Koyuncu et al. (linear relationship) [9,32,33]. In summary, at the same moisture content and size, the cracking device had excellent shelling results for walnuts with a shell thickness (h) < 1.2 mm and a gap between the walnut shell and kernel (d) $\geq$ 1.6 mm.

Table 5. Results of variety adaptability test.

Varieties	Thickness (mm)	Gap between Walnut Shell and Kernel (mm)	SCR (%)	WKR (%)	Es (kJ/kg)
Wen-185	0.86 ± 0.03 a	1.85 ± 0.24 a	97.24 ± 0.41 a	92.03 ± 0.36 a	1.88 ± 0.07 a
Xinwen-179	0.86 ± 0.03 a	1.84 ± 0.24 a	96.54 ± 0.39 a	92.87 ± 0.33 a	1.91 ± 0.08 a
Zha-343	1.16 ± 0.34 a	1.59 ± 0.25 a	96.26 ± 0.54 a	90.07 ± 0.86 a	1.96 ± 0.06 a
Xinxin-2	1.20 ± 0.11 a	1.57 ± 0.11 b	95.99 ± 0.42 a	84.83 ± 1.29 b	2.41 ± 0.12 b
Xinfeng	1.48 ± 0.15 b	1.67 ± 0.26 a	84.62 ± 0.40 b	92.11 ± 0.39 a	3.24 ± 0.11 b

Note: Data in the table are "mean ± standard deviation" of samples, different letters in the same column indicate significant differences ($p < 0.05$).

Wang et al. [17] conducted walnut cracking experiments and discovered that walnut moisture content had a significant impact on the cracking quality. Zheng et al. [23] reported that the shell thickness and geometric mean diameter affected the quality of kernel extraction from cracked walnuts. In this paper, we also found a significant effect of the gap between the walnut shell and kernel on the cracking effect of walnuts. There was a relationship between the shell thickness and the energy consumption of the cracking quality, which is shown in Table 5. Therefore, the material properties (shell thickness, moisture content, gap between walnut shell and kernel, etc.), walnut cracking characteristics (cracking force, cracking energy, power of walnut cracking, etc.) and the correlation between them for the different walnut varieties still need to be studied in depth.

4. Discussion

The different types of walnut cracking devices were compared and the results are listed in Table 6 [9,10,12,17,34–36]. It is clear that compared to other types, the extrusion type had a higher working efficiency [22,36]. In addition, the load with multiple contact points was significantly better than a pair of forces and two pairs of forces, showing a larger SCR and WKR. Studies have suggested that single point or line loads cause uneven forces on the shell, poor crack extension, and damage to the kernels [13]. However, multi-point walnut cracking not only contributes to crack generation and expansion but also reduces the stress value and deformation used to break walnut shells on the condition that the kernel stays whole [8]. Additionally, it is worth pointing out that many walnut cracking devices only focused on the improvement of the SCR but ignored the WKR. Fortunately, the walnut cracking device designed in this work considered simultaneously a larger SCR and WKR. Nonetheless, the following two points of the multi-point extrusion type walnut cracking device need to be further enhanced.

(1) The multi-point extrusion walnut cracking device is integrated with walnut grading and walnut cracking, where the accuracy of the grading affects the cracking performance. The mixed grade of the walnuts causes a mismatch between the size of the walnuts and the cracking angle, which indirectly affects the cracking performance of the walnut cracking device [36]. The accuracy of grading needs to be further improved.
(2) The posture of the walnut falling into the gap between the rotating cracking roller and extrusion plate after grading is generally random. Therefore, it is necessary to seek a directional cracking device that can realize the breakage of the walnut shell, which is beneficial for improving walnut cracking.

Table 6. Comparison of different types of walnut cracking devices.

Principle	Name	Loading Style	Results of Cracking
Shear type	Walnut shearing extrusion flexible shell-crushing device [9]	Two pairs of forces	WKR = 75%, SCR = 98%
	6HP-400 cone basket walnut shelling device [34]	Two pairs of forces	WKR = 90.3%, SCR = 97.3%
Impact type	Conic roller shelling device based on walnut moisture-regulating treatments [17]	A pair of forces	WKR = 84.54%, SCR = 99.15%
	Secondary shell-breaking machine for pecans [35]	A pair of forces	WKR = 83.86%, SCR = 87.58%, Ph = 500 kg/h
	Clearance walnut sheller [10]	A pair of forces	WKR = 83.6%, SCR = 94%
Extrusion type	Cam rocker bidirectional extrusion walnut shell-breaking device [12]	Two pairs of forces	WKR = 61.39%, SCR = 92.36%
	Squeezed walnut shell-breaking machine with self-grading and multi-station [36]	Two pairs of forces	WKR = 84.72%, SCR = 91.5%
	Multi-point extrusion walnut cracking device	Multiple pairs of forces	WKR = 92.03%, SCR = 97.24%, Es = 1.88 kJ/kg, Ph = 850 kg/h

Note: Ph walnut cracking efficiency.

5. Conclusions

The present work described an engineering solution to the walnut cracking problem. A machine for cracking walnuts was designed and manufactured and also evaluated for performance. The response surface test results showed that all the parameters had a significant influence on the three indicators, whereas only the CA had an extremely significant effect on the SCR. The obtained regression equation could be used to quantitatively predict the cracking quality under different operating parameters. Taking all the indices into comprehensive consideration, the machine performance was found to be optimum at a CA of 0.47° and an RS of 108 r/min. For the 'Wen-185' walnut, the SCR, WKR, and Es were 97.24% against the predicted 98.40%, 92.03% against the predicted 92.94%, and 1.88 kJ/kg against the predicted 1.80 kJ/kg, respectively. The variety adaptability tests showed that the cracking device was well-adapted to the 'Wen185', 'Xinwen-179', and 'Zha-343' varieties. The cracking device had excellent cracking results for walnuts with a shell thickness (h) < 1.2 mm and a gap between the walnut shell and kernel (d) $\geq$ 1.6 mm, for example, the 'Wen-185', 'Xinwen-179', 'Zha-343' varieties, as well as other walnut varieties with thin shells and a larger gap between the walnut shell and kernel. This paper provides a theoretical reference for improving and optimizing walnut cracking devices' processing parameters.

Author Contributions: Conceptualization, H.Z. and Y.Z.; methodology, H.L.; software, H.L.; validation, Y.T.; formal analysis, J.C.; investigation, H.L.; resources, H.Z.; data curation, H.L.; writing—original draft preparation, H.L.; writing—review and editing, H.Z. and Y.Z.; visualization, H.L. and Z.Z.; supervision, H.Z. and Y.Z.; project administration, Y.T.; funding acquisition, H.Z. All authors have read and agreed to the published version of the manuscript.

Funding: This research was financially supported by the Chinese Natural Science Foundation (12002229, 31160196), the President's Foundation of Tarim University (TDZKBS202001), the Open Project of the Modern Agricultural Engineering Key Laboratory (TDNG2022101, TDNG2021104), and the Shishi Science and Technology Program (Grant No. 2021ZB01).

Institutional Review Board Statement: Not applicable.

Informed Consent Statement: Not applicable.

Data Availability Statement: The data presented in this study are available on request from the corresponding author.

Acknowledgments: The authors express their thanks to the Chinese Natural Science Foundation (12002229, 31160196), the President's Foundation of Tarim University (TDZKBS202001), the Open Project of the Modern Agricultural Engineering Key Laboratory (TDNG2022101, TDNG2021104), and the Shishi Science and Technology Program (Grant No. 2021ZB01) for their financial support and to all of the people who assisted with the writing of this paper. The authors are grateful to the anonymous reviewers for their comments.

Conflicts of Interest: The authors declare no conflict of interest.

Abbreviations

CA	Cracking Angle
RS	Roller Speed
SCR	Shell-Cracking Rate
WKR	Whole Kernel Rate
Es	Specific Energy Consumption
CCD	Central Composite Design
RSM	Response Surface Methodology
ANOVA	Analysis of Variance

References

1. Ghafari, A.; Chegini, G.R.; Khazaei, J.; Vahdati, K. Design, construction and performance evaluation of the walnut cracking machine. *Int. J. Nuts Relat. Sci.* **2011**, *1*, 70–74.
2. Geng, S.; Ning, L.; Ma, T.; Chen, H.; Zhang, Y.; Sun, X. Comprehensive analysis of the components of walnut kernel (*Juglans regia* L.) in China. *J. Food Qual.* **2021**, *95*, 825–834. [CrossRef]
3. Sütyemez, M.; Bükücü, Ş.B.; Özcan, A. 'Helete Güneşi', a New Walnut Cultivar with Late Leafing, Early Harvest Date, and Superior Nut Traits. *Agriculture* **2021**, *11*, 991. [CrossRef]
4. Brunner-Parra, C.F.; Croquevielle-Rendic, L.A.; Monardes-Concha, C.A.; Urra-Calfuñir, B.A.; Avanzini, E.L.; Correa-Vial, T. Web-Based Integer Programming Decision Support System for Walnut Processing Planning: The MeliFen Case. *Agriculture* **2022**, *12*, 430. [CrossRef]
5. Bernik, R.; Stajnko, D.; Demsar, I. Comparison of the kernel quality of different walnuts (*Juglans regia* L.) varieties shelled with modified centrifugal sheller. *Erwerbs-Obstbau* **2020**, *62*, 213–220. [CrossRef]
6. Liu, M.; Li, C.; Zhang, Y.; Wang, L. Advances and recent patents about cracking walnut and fetching kernel device. *Recent Pat. Mech. Eng.* **2015**, *8*, 44–58. [CrossRef]
7. Wang, W.; Wang, Y.; Wang, P.; Lu, J.; Tian, Z. Structure improvement design and test of cone basket walnut shelling. *J. Agric. Mech. Res.* **2022**, *44*, 124–129.
8. Ding, R.; Cao, C.; Zhan, C.; Lou, S.; Sun, S. Design and experiment of bionic-impact type pecan shell breaker. *Trans. Chin. Soc. Agric. Eng. Trans. CSAE* **2017**, *33*, 257–264.
9. Liu, M.; Li, C.; Zhang, Y.; Yang, M.; Hou, Y.; Gao, L. Shell crushing mechanism analysis and performance test of flexible-belt shearing extrusion for walnut. *Trans. Chin. Soc. Agric. Mach.* **2016**, *47*, 266–273.
10. Li, X. *Parameters Optimization of Clearance Walnut Sheller*; Sichuan Agricultural University: Ya'an, China, 2018.
11. Sharifian, F.; Derafshi, M.H. Mechanical behavior of walnut under cracking conditions. *J. Appl. Sci.* **2008**, *8*, 886–890. [CrossRef]
12. Shi, M.; Liu, M.; Li, C.; Cao, C.; Li, X. Design and Experiment of Cam Rocker Bidirectional Extrusion Walnut Shell Breaking Device. *Trans. Chin. Soc. Agric. Mach.* **2022**, *53*, 140–150.
13. Cao, C.; Jiang, L.; Wu, C.; Li, Z.; Wang, T.; Ding, R. Design and test on hammerhead of pecan shell-breaking machine. *Trans. Chin. Soc. Agric. Mach.* **2017**, *48*, 307–315.
14. Zhang, H.; Shen, L.; Lan, H.; Li, Y.; Liu, Y.; Tang, Y.; Li, W. Mechanical properties and finite element analysis of walnut under different cracking parts. *Trans. Chin. Soc. Agric. Eng. Trans. CSAE* **2018**, *11*, 81–88. [CrossRef]
15. Shen, L. *Design and Experimental Study on the Walnut Cracking Machine with Impact Extrusion Type*; Tarim University: Alar, China, 2017.
16. He, Y.; Wang, X.; Cao, S.; Wang, M.; Liu, H. Design and experimental study of a roller extrusion type walnut shell breaking device. *Jiangsu Agric. Sci.* **2012**, *40*, 350–352.
17. Wang, J.; Liu, M.; Wu, H.; Peng, J.; Peng, B.; Yang, Y.; Cao, M.; Wei, H.; Xie, H. Design and key parameter optimization of conic roller shelling device based on walnut moisture-regulating treatments. *Agriculture* **2022**, *12*, 561. [CrossRef]
18. Man, X. *Optimization of the Process Parameters of Hot-Air and Microwave-Vacuum Synergistic Drying for Walnut Shell Breaking*; Tarim University: Alar, China, 2021.
19. Zeng, Y.; Jia, F.; Meng, X.; Han, Y.; Xiao, Y. The effects of friction characteristic of particle on milling process in a horizontal rice mill. *Adv. Powder Technol.* **2018**, *29*, 1280–1291. [CrossRef]
20. Ashok, G.; Denis, Y. Chapter 6—Roll Crushers, Mineral Processing Design and Operation; Elsevier Science: 2016. Available online: https://www.elsevier.com/books/mineral-processing-design-and-operations/gupta/978-0-444-63589-1 (accessed on 8 August 2022).
21. Hu, Y.; Li, J.; Lu, H.; Xiao, H. Design and experiment of equant-diameter roller screening machine for fresh tea leaves. *Trans. Chin. Soc. Agric. Mach.* **2015**, *46*, 116–121.

22. Liu, M.; Li, C.; Cao, C.; Wang, L.; Li, X.; Che, J.; Yang, H.; Zhang, X.; Zhao, H.; He, G.; et al. Walnut fruit processing equipment: Academic insights and perspectives. *Food Eng. Rev.* **2021**, *13*, 822–857. [CrossRef]
23. Zheng, X.; Zhang, E.; Kan, Z.; Zhang, H.; Li, H.; Chou, W. Improving cracking characteristics and kernel percentage of walnut by optimal position of cutting on shell. *Trans. Chin. Soc. Agric. Eng. Trans. CSAE* **2018**, *34*, 300–308.
24. Meng, X.; Jia, F.; Xiao, Y.; Han, Y.; Zeng, Y.; Li, A. Effect of operating parameters on milling quality and energy consumption of brown rice. *J. Food Sci. Technol.* **2019**, *56*, 674–682. [CrossRef]
25. Shen, G.; Wang, G.; Hu, L.; Yuan, J.; Wang, Y.; Wu, T.; Chen, X. Development of harvesting mechanism for stem tips of sweet potatoes. *Trans. Chin. Soc. Agric. Eng. Trans. CSAE* **2019**, *35*, 46–55.
26. Altuntas, E.; Erkol, M. The effects of moisture content, compression speeds, and axes on mechanical properties of walnut cultivars. *Food Bioprocess Technol.* **2011**, *4*, 1288–1295. [CrossRef]
27. Kilickan, A.; Guner, M. Physical properties and mechanical behavior of olive fruits (*Olea europaea* L.) under compression loading. *J. Food Eng.* **2008**, *87*, 222–228. [CrossRef]
28. Gharibzahedi, S.M.T.; Mousavi, S.M.; Hamedi, M. Mechanical behavior of Persian walnut and its kernel under compression loading: An experimental and computational study. *J. Food Process. Preserv.* **2008**, *36*, 423–430. [CrossRef]
29. Khazaei, J.; Rasekh, M.; Borghei, A.M. *Physical and Mechanical Properties of Almond and Its Kernel Related to Cracking and Peeling*; Cambridge Universuty Press: Chicago, IL, USA, 2002.
30. Yang, R.; Chen, D.; Zha, X.; Pan, Z.; Shang, S. Optimization design and experiment of ear-picking and threshing devices of corn plot kernel harvester. *Agriculture* **2021**, *11*, 904. [CrossRef]
31. Ebubekir, A.; Yakup, O. Physical and mechanical properties of some walnut (*Juglans regia* L.) cultivars. *Int. J. Food Eng.* **2008**, *4*, 99–107.
32. Koyuncu, M.A.; Ekinci, K.; Gun, A. The effects of altitude on fruit quality and compression load for cracking of walnuts (*Juglans regia* L.). *J. Food Qual.* **2004**, *27*, 407–417. [CrossRef]
33. Kacal, M.; Koyuncu, M.A. Cracking characteristics and kernel extraction quality of hazelnuts: Effects of compression speed and positions. *Int. J. Food Prop.* **2017**, *20*, 233–240. [CrossRef]
34. Wang, W.; Tian, Z.; Wang, P.; Wang, Y. Design and experiment of 6HP-400 cone basket walnut shelling. *Packag. Food Mach.* **2021**, *39*, 84–88.
35. Cao, C.; Li, Z.; Luo, K.; Wang, T.; Wu, Z.; Xie, C. Design and experiment of secondary shell breaking machine for Pecan. *Trans. Chin. Soc. Agric. Mach.* **2019**, *50*, 128–135.
36. Liu, X. *Development and Test of a Squeezed Walnut Shell Breaking Machine with the Self-Grading and Multi-Station*; Southwest University: Chongqing, China, 2021.

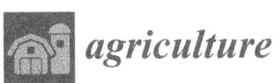

Article

Comparative Evaluation of Physicochemical Properties, Microstructure, and Antioxidant Activity of Jujube Polysaccharides Subjected to Hot Air, Infrared, Radio Frequency, and Freeze Drying

Bengang Wu [1,2], Chengcheng Qiu [1], Yiting Guo [1,2,*], Chunhong Zhang [3], Dan Li [3], Kun Gao [1], Yuanjin Ma [1] and Haile Ma [1,2]

[1] School of Food and Biological Engineering, Jiangsu University, 301 Xuefu Road, Zhenjiang 212013, China
[2] Institute of Food Physical Processing, Jiangsu University, 301 Xuefu Road, Zhenjiang 212013, China
[3] Naval Medical Center of PLA, Naval Medical University (Second Military Medical University), Shanghai 200433, China
* Correspondence: 1000005604@ujs.edu.cn

Abstract: In this study, we used four drying methods (hot air, freezing, infrared, and radio frequency) to dry fresh jujube and its polysaccharide extracts by a two-step drying method, and the effects of the drying methods on the physical and chemical properties, structural properties, and antioxidant activity of jujube polysaccharides were studied. The results showed significant differences in the yield, drying time, monosaccharide content, molecular weight, apparent viscosity, thermal stability, and microstructure of the polysaccharides treated under the different drying methods. In contrast, no significant differences in the monosaccharide composition and functional groups of the polysaccharide samples obtained from the different drying methods were observed. Among all the tested methods, the freeze-drying extraction rate was the highest, reaching 4.52 ± 0.19%, while its drying time was the longest. Although the extraction rate of radio frequency drying was only 3.55 ± 0.21%, the drying time was the shortest, compared with hot air drying, the drying time was reduced by 76.67–83.29%, and the obtained polysaccharides exerted good antioxidant activity. Therefore, radio frequency drying is a potential polysaccharide extraction and drying technique, and this study can provide a theoretical basis for its industrial production.

Keywords: jujube polysaccharide; drying methods; physicochemical property; structural characteristic; antioxidant activity

1. Introduction

Jujube is a fruit of the plant jujube tree, a plant of the family rhamnaceae. It is a specialty species native to China and has a long history [1]. Jujube has high nutritional and medicinal value, such as nourishing the yin and kidney, strengthening the body, softening blood vessels, and enhancing the physiological function of each viscus [2]. Jujube extracts have been proven to have many bioactive substances, among which polysaccharide is considered one of the most important bioactive components [3]. Modern medical research shows that jujube polysaccharides (JPSs) have antioxidant, antiviral, antitumor, and other functions, so the development prospect of jujube polysaccharides is extensive [4].

Fresh jujube has high water content, so it easily deteriorates, leading to the loss of its nutrients, which is not conducive to further extraction of bioactive components [5]. Traditional drying techniques, such as hot air drying (HAD) and freeze drying (FD), are easy to control. However, these traditional drying techniques have many problems, such as high energy consumption, low drying efficiency, a long drying time, low quality of the products after drying, and expensive freeze-drying equipment. Therefore, in this case, it is imperative for us to find a new drying technology with the attributes of a short drying

Citation: Wu, B.; Qiu, C.; Guo, Y.; Zhang, C.; Li, D.; Gao, K.; Ma, Y.; Ma, H. Comparative Evaluation of Physicochemical Properties, Microstructure, and Antioxidant Activity of Jujube Polysaccharides Subjected to Hot Air, Infrared, Radio Frequency, and Freeze Drying. *Agriculture* 2022, 12, 1606. https://doi.org/10.3390/agriculture12101606

Academic Editor: Jiangbo Li

Received: 29 August 2022
Accepted: 30 September 2022
Published: 4 October 2022

Publisher's Note: MDPI stays neutral with regard to jurisdictional claims in published maps and institutional affiliations.

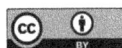

Copyright: © 2022 by the authors. Licensee MDPI, Basel, Switzerland. This article is an open access article distributed under the terms and conditions of the Creative Commons Attribution (CC BY) license (https://creativecommons.org/licenses/by/4.0/).

time, high drying efficiency, and good product quality. Radio frequency drying (RFD) is a new drying technique that generates heat inside food through ion conduction and dipole rotation, so that water can be evaporated [6]. Infrared drying (IRD) is a new method that radiates materials with the energy generated by an infrared emitter, and the infrared waves are absorbed and converted into heat energy by the materials [7]. These new drying methods have the advantages of a short drying time, high efficiency, and good product quality, which can be a complete or partial alternative to the traditional methods. A large number of studies have revealed that different drying techniques have significant effects on the structural characteristics and biological activities of polysaccharides derived from loquat leaves [8], dandelion [9], and mulberry leaves [10]. However, the effects of these different drying techniques on the structural characteristics and biological activities of the polysaccharides extracted from jujube are still unclear.

In this study, four drying methods (HAD, FD, IRD, and RFD) were used to perform a two-step drying treatment on fresh jujube to extract its polysaccharides (Figure 1). The effects of these drying methods on the physicochemical and structural properties of jujube polysaccharides in terms of thermogravimetric characteristics, rheological properties, and FT-IR spectroscopy were determined, and its antioxidant activity (DPPH and ABTS) was also studied. The detailed results can contribute to a better knowledge of jujube polysaccharide extraction and further provide more information for the practical industrial application of this two-step drying method.

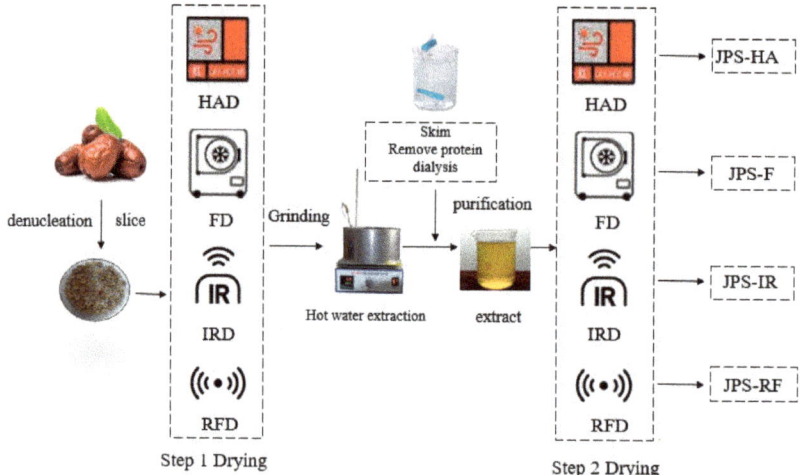

Figure 1. Schematic diagram of the two-step drying method of jujube polysaccharide extraction.

2. Materials and Methods

2.1. Materials and Chemicals

Fresh jujubes (*Ziziphus jujuba* Mill., Huizao) were collected from Xinjiang, China. Monosaccharides and uronic acids were purchased from Aladdin Biochemical Technology Co., Ltd. (Shanghai, China). Other chemicals used in this study were all analytical grade and purchased from Sinopharm (Shanghai, China).

2.2. Drying Procedures

Firstly, the jujubes were denucleated, sliced, and divided into four groups according to different drying processes, which were hot air drying (HAD), freeze drying (FD), infrared drying (IRD), and radio frequency drying (RFD). Briefly, in the FD process, jujube slices were placed in a glass Petri dish (5 mm diameter) and were freeze-dried for 48 h at −40 °C. In the HD process, jujube slices were placed into an oven at 70 °C. In the IRD process, the infrared device power was adjusted to 900 W, and the corresponding surface temperature of the jujube slices reached 70 °C. In the RFD process, well-calibrated radio frequency equipment (HGJL-6RFS, Hefei Hagong Jinlang Equipment Technology Co., Ltd., Hefei, China) was used to dry jujube slices at an anode voltage of 70%, and the distance of the sample tray to the heater was set to 6 cm. The endpoints of the four drying methods were chosen as when the jujube samples reached a constant weight. The used time and final moisture content of the samples for each method were recorded.

2.3. Extraction of Polysaccharides from Jujube

Hot water extraction of polysaccharides from jujube was carried out by the previously reported method, with slight modification [2]. Briefly, the dried jujube was ground and sifted through 60 mesh. An appropriate amount (50 g) of the sample was taken and treated with petroleum ether and 80% (v/v) ethanol for 2 h, respectively, to remove oil and small molecules. Then, the obtained sample was dried and extracted with 500 mL of deionized water at 90 °C for 4 h. The supernatant was collected after centrifuging and precipitated with four volumes of anhydrous ethanol at 4 °C overnight. Subsequently, the collected precipitates were redissolved in appropriate amount of deionized water and dialyzed with deionized water (molar mass cutoff: 3.5 kDa) for 4 h. Finally, the dialysate was subjected to HAD, FD, IRD, and RFD, to obtain the final polysaccharide powder, and the obtained products were labeled as JPS-H, JPS-F, JPS-IR, and JPS-RF.

2.4. Determination of Physicochemical Properties of Polysaccharides

2.4.1. Analysis of Chemical Components

The total sugar content of polysaccharides was determined by the phenol-sulfuric acid method, with D-glucose as a standard [11]. The protein content was identified by the Coomassie brilliant blue G-250 method. The carbazole sulfuric acid method was used to determine the uronic acid content of polysaccharides [12]. The polyphenol content in polysaccharides was determined by the Folin–Ciocalteu method [13]. All tests were performed in triplicate.

2.4.2. Monosaccharide Composition and Content of JPSs

The monosaccharide composition was determined by high-performance liquid chromatography (HPLC) (LC-20AT, Shimadzu Co., Ltd., Kyoto, Japan) with PMP precolumn derivatization [14]. Briefly, 2 mg of sample was accurately weighed into a 10 mL hydrolytic tube, and 2 mL of 2 M trifluoroacetic acid (TFA) was added, sealed with nitrogen, and hydrolyzed at 110 °C for 6 h. After hydrolysis, rotation evaporation was used to dry the obtained solution to remove TFA. After that, 3 mL of methanol was added to the tubes, and the step of evaporation–methanol washing was repeated 4 times to ensure that all TFA was removed. The hydrolysate was dissolved in 2 mL of distilled water, and 450 µL of 0.5 M PMP solution and 450 µL of 0.3 M NaOH were added into the hydrolysate sequentially. After mixing well, the mixture was incubated at 70 °C for 40 min, and then 450 µL of 0.3 M HCl was added to terminate the reaction. The hydrolyzed sample was filtered through a 0.45 µm aqueous membrane and analyzed by HPLC with an XDB-C18 column (4.6 × 50 mm, 25 cm). A mixture of maltose, rhamnose, arabinose, galactose, glucose, mannose, xylose, and glucuronic acid, at a series of concentrations, was selected as external standards for sugar identification and quantitation. Three replications were conducted for each test.

2.4.3. Molecular Weight of JPSs

The weight-average molecular weight (Mw), number-average molecular weight (Mn), molecular weight distribution (Mw/Mn), and root-mean-square rotation radius (Rg) of JPSs were determined by size-exclusion chromatography (HPSEC) equipped (G136A, Agilent Technologies, Santa Clara, CA, USA) with a MultiAngle Laser Light scattering (SEC-MALLS) detector and a differential refraction detector (RI) detector, according to the method of Gu et al. [15]. An accurate amount of sample (4 mg) was weighed and dissolved in 4 mL of 0.1 M NaCl solution containing 0.02% NaN$_3$ (w/v) (mobile phase). The solution was filtered through a 0.45 µm aqueous membrane and injected into the HPSEC for detection. Data were analyzed using Astra 6.1.7 software.

2.4.4. Thermogravimetric Analysis (TGA)

The thermogravimetric analysis (TGA) determination of JPSs followed the method of Liu et al. [16]. The TGA was conducted on a DTG-60 thermal analyzer (Shimadzu, Kyoto, Japan) to investigate the thermal properties of polysaccharides. Briefly, the samples (10 mg) were placed in a sealed aluminum pan and heated from 30 to 700 °C at a heating rate of 10 °C/min^{-1} under nitrogen. The empty, sealed aluminum pan was utilized as a control.

2.4.5. Determination of Rheological Properties

The rheological properties of JPSs were determined at room temperature (25 °C) using a DHR-1 rheometer (Discovery HR-1, TA Corporation, USA) equipped with a plate (40 mm diameter, 1 mm gap). Determination of apparent viscosity (η) of samples was performed in the shear rate range of 0.1–100 s^{-1} [17].

2.4.6. FT-IR Spectroscopy Analysis

The dried JPS samples were analyzed by an ATR-FTIR spectrometer (Semefi Technology Co., Ltd., Huludao, China). For all samples, 32 scans were performed at 4 cm^{-1} resolution in a scanning range of 4000–600 cm^{-1}. The obtained spectrograms were analyzed by OMNIC (Thermo Inc., Waltham, MA, USA).

2.5. Scanning Electron Microscopy (SEM)

Scanning electron micrographs of JPSs were conducted according to the modified method of Wang et al. [18]. The dried polysaccharide powders were mounted onto a specimen stub, with the assistance of conductive tape, and sputter-coated with gold. The well-prepared samples were photographed using a Hitachi S-3400N scanning electron microscope (Hitachi Inc., Tokyo, Japan), and the images were captured at a voltage of 15 kV.

2.6. Antioxidant Activities of JPS

2.6.1. Determination of DPPH Radical-Scavenging Assay

The DPPH radical-scavenging activity of dried JPS powders was determined based on the method of Wang et al. [19]. A series of concentrations of JPS solution (1 mL) was mixed with 3 mL of 0.2 mM DPPH ethanol solution. After shaking well, the mixture was incubated in dark at 37 °C for 30 min. The absorbance was measured at 517 nm with the absolute ethanol as the control. The DPPH radical-scavenging activity was calculated as follows:

$$DPPH\ radical\text{-}scavenging\ activity\ (\%) = \left(1 - \frac{A_1}{A_0}\right) \times 100\% \qquad (1)$$

where A_1 is the absorbance of JPS, and A_0 is the absorbance of the control.

2.6.2. Determination of ABTS Radical-Scavenging Activity

The ABTS radical-scavenging activity was basically measured as described by Chen et al. [20]. A stock solution of ABTS (7 mM) was prepared by dissolving ABTS in ethanol. Then, potassium persulfate was added to the prepared stock solution (final concentration was 2.45 mM), and the mixed solution was allowed to stand overnight at ambient temperature in darkness. The ABTS working solution was prepared by diluting the stock solution until the absorbance measured between 0.7 to 0.734. Subsequently, an aliquot of 2 mL of JPS solution was mixed with ABTS working solution in equal volume at room temperature in darkness for 10 min. Then, the absorbance was recorded at 734 nm, with ABTS working solution as the control. The ABTS radical-scavenging activity was calculated as follows:

$$ABTS\ radical\text{-}scavenging\ activity\ (\%) = \frac{A_0 - A_1}{A_0} \times 100\% \tag{2}$$

where A_1 is the absorbance of JPS, and A_0 is the absorbance of the control.

2.7. Statistical Analysis

All experiments were performed in three replicates, and the experimental results were expressed as the mean ± standard deviation (SD). Statistically significant differences in results were determined by one-way analysis of variance (ANOVA) with Duncan's multiple range test. SPSS 26.0 (IBM Corporation, Chicago, IL, USA) was used for all statistical analyses, at the significance level of $p = 0.05$.

3. Results and Discussion

3.1. Yields and Chemical Compositions of JPSs

As shown in Table 1, the extraction rate of JPS-F was the highest among all the tested methods, reaching 4.52%. Compared with HAD, the extraction rate of FD was increased by 53.2%, which was due to the fact that FD rendered porous structures into the jujube tissues; as a result, it was easier for water to penetrate the jujube tissues during the extraction process, though this method required the longest duration compared with the other methods [21]. Moreover, the lower processing temperature and less oxygen content in the environment were more conducive to extracting polysaccharides during the FD process [9]. As for extraction time, the longest duration of FD was used to dry fresh jujube to a constant weight, reaching 48 h. In contrast, the durations of IRD and RFD required to dry jujube to the same water content as FD decreased significantly ($p < 0.05$).

Table 1. Extraction rate, drying duration, and chemical composition of JPSs treated with different drying methods.

Sample	JPS-HA	JPS-F	JPS-IR	JPS-RF
Yield (%)	2.95 ± 0.08 a	4.52 ± 0.19 c	3.10 ± 0.19 a	3.55 ± 0.21 b
Step 1 drying time (h)	4.25 ± 0.35 b	48.00 ± 0.00 c	0.88 ± 0.06 a	0.71 ± 0.06 a
Step 2 drying time (h)	5.10 ± 0.14 b	48.00 ± 0.00 c	1.42 ± 0.12 a	1.19 ± 0.02 a
Total sugar content (%)	66.19 ± 0.81 a	76.06 ± 1.24 d	69.33 ± 0.93 b	74.26 ± 0.98 c
Total uronic acid content (%)	11.95 ± 0.004 a	15.65 ± 0.005 b	18.78 ± 0.002 c	19.18 ± 0.003 c
Total phenol content (%)	0.55 ± 0.07 a	1.17 ± 0.10 b	0.61 ± 0.07 a	1.04 ± 0.13 b
Protein content (%)	2.93 ± 0.13 b	1.41 ± 0.13 a	2.83 ± 0.54 a	1.69 ± 0.27 c

Note: Values are means ± standard deviation. Values followed by different letters in each column indicate significant differences ($p < 0.05$).

In general, the extracted crude polysaccharides contained many substances, such as proteins and polyphenols, which might combine with other components and show various activities. Therefore, it is necessary to measure the chemical composition of crude polysaccharides. As shown in Table 1, the total sugar contents were 66.19%–76.06%, indicating that polysaccharide was the dominant constituent in the extract. In addition, glucuronic acid was found in the extracts dried with these four methods, indicating the presence of pectin-like polysaccharides in jujube. Similar results were obtained in polysaccharides extracted from loquat and okra [22]. Although the samples were deproteinized and dialyzed, they still contained a small amount of protein and polyphenols, which may be due to the presence of protein–polysaccharide and polyphenol–polysaccharide complexes in the extracted polysaccharides. Such complexes can enhance the biological activity of polysaccharides to some extent [23].

3.2. Monosaccharide Compositions and Molecular Weights of JPSs

Monosaccharide is the natural basic unit that can determine the structures and characteristics of polysaccharides [24]. As shown in Table 2, the standard monosaccharides used were maltose (Mal), rhamnose (Rha), arabinose (Ara), galactose (Gal), glucose (Glu), glucuronic acid (GluA), mannose (Man), and xylose (Xyl). In general, the different drying methods had no effect on the monosaccharide composition of JPS. However, they had a significant effect on the monosaccharide content, which is consistent with the study of Chen et al. (2020), who investigated the effect of different drying methods on the structural characteristics of polysaccharides from bamboo shoots [25]. From Table 2, it can be seen that the seven tested monosaccharides and a uronic acid all can be detected in the polysaccharides that were extracted using the different drying methods. Among these monosaccharides, Mal was the predominant sugar, followed by Ara. The difference in monosaccharide content may be related to the oxygen content and environmental temperature. Compared with HAD, the Glu and Ara contents in the JPSs treated with FD, IRD, and RFD were significantly ($p < 0.05$) reduced, which is probably due to the hydroxyl oxidation and intermolecular hydrogen bond breakage of the polysaccharides in the environment, affecting the monosaccharide contents [26].

Table 2. Monosaccharide constituents and molecular weight of JPSs treated with different drying methods.

Sample	JPS-HA	JPS-F	JPS-IR	JPS-RF
Mw ($\times 10^5$ Da)	1.62 (±1.38%)	0.87 (±1.11%)	1.26 (±1.33%)	1.20 (±1.87%)
Mn ($\times 10^5$ Da)	1.20 (±6.09%);	0.77 (±4.93%)	0.93 (±6.02%)	0.92 (±1.85%)
Mw/Mn	1.34 (±6.24%)	1.13 (±5.05%)	1.36 (±6.17%)	1.30 (±2.63%)
Rg (nm)	38.7 (±0.1%)	27.9 (±0.2%)	38.0 (±0.1%)	30.1 (±0.1%)
Mal	40.81 ± 1.54 b	36.18 ± 0.00 ab	39.41 ± 0.65 ab	34.73 ± 3.51 a
Rha	3.89 ± 0.00 b	3.74 ± 0.06 b	3.39 ± 0.18 a	3.44 ± 0.06 a
Gal	6.81 ± 0.02 b	6.90 ± 0.02 b	5.87 ± 0.32 a	6.26 ± 0.03 a
Ara	10.33 ± 0.15 c	9.18 ± 0.36 b	8.35 ± 0.35 a	8.36 ± 0.11 a
Glu	5.03 ± 0.05 c	3.37 ± 0.03 a	4.09 ± 0.20 b	3.15 ± 0.06 a
GluA	3.52 ± 0.03 a	4.36 ± 0.35 a	2.31 ± 1.55 a	3.11 ± 1.57 a
Man	1.69 ± 0.00 b	1.75 ± 0.00 c	1.55 ± 0.04 a	1.70 ± 0.00 bc
Xyl	1.91 ± 0.04 a	1.95 ± 0.09 a	1.82 ± 0.02 a	1.90 ± 0.04 a

Note: Values are means ± standard deviation. Values followed by different letters in each column indicate significant differences ($p < 0.05$).

JPSs' molecular weight plays an important role in their functional properties and biological activity [24]. The molecular weight of polysaccharides obtained from the different drying methods was analyzed, and the data are shown in Table 2. The larger the Mw/Mn value of the polydispersion coefficient is, the wider the range of molecular weight distribution, which indicates that the polymer is in a mixed state and its purity is relatively low. The Mw/Mn value of JPS-F was the smallest, indicating that the range of its molecular weight distribution is the smallest among these four polysaccharides. The Mw values of JPS-HA, JPS-F, JPS-IR, and JPS-RF are 1.62×10^5, 0.87×10^5, 1.26×10^5, and 1.20×10^5 Da, respectively. Additionally, the smallest molecular weight of JPS-F also indicated that FD-extracted polysaccharides are loosely bound to other macromolecules within or between cells [27]. This is probably because the glycosidic bonds were broken under low temperature and low oxygen conditions, which further leads to the reduction of Mw.

3.3. Thermal Properties of JPSs

Figure 2A shows the thermal property of JPSs obtained under different drying conditions. The thermogravimetric analysis (TGA) curves of all JPSs were similar in shape over a defined temperature range (30 to 700 °C). In the first stage (below 250 °C), the free and bound water of the JPSs evaporated, and the weight loss was about 20%. The second stage of thermal degradation occurred at about 250~500 °C, which is mainly because of the decomposition of polysaccharide chains and the rupture of hydrogen bonds as well as the degradation of thermal unstable functional groups, resulting in a fast weight loss (about 40%). In the final stage, when the temperature exceeds 500 °C, the weight loss of the JPSs remains constant [16]. According to Figure 2A, JPS-F has the worst thermal stability among all the polysaccharides, which may be related to its flocculent porous structure.

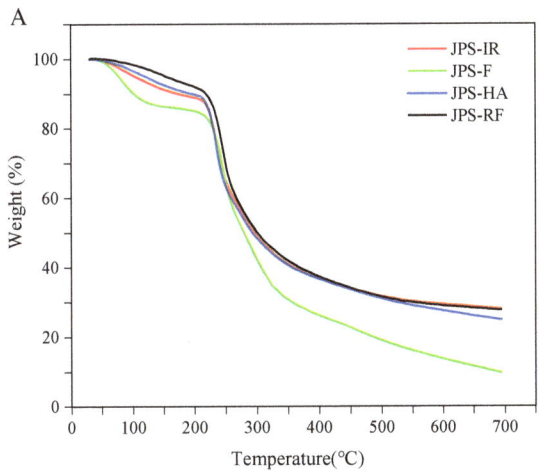

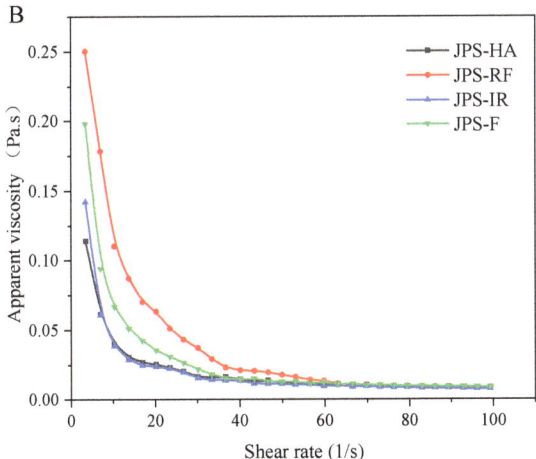

Figure 2. *Cont.*

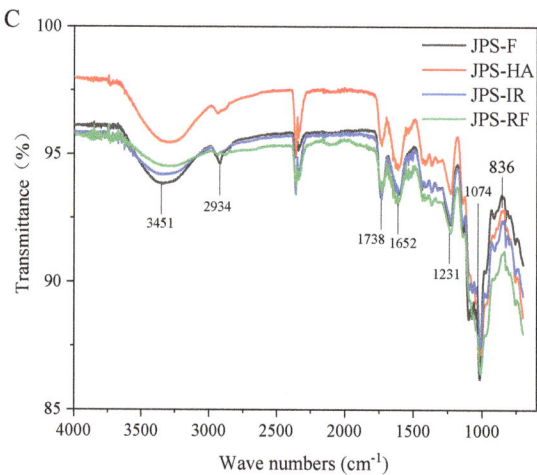

Figure 2. Thermogravimetric analysis (**A**), apparent viscosity (**B**), and FT-IR spectra (**C**) of JPSs dried under different methods.

3.4. Rheological Properties of JPSs

Viscosity is a vital property of polysaccharides that can influence their bioactivities. The flow behavior of the JPSs is displayed in Figure 2B, which shows that the apparent viscosity decreased with the shear rate increasing from 0.1 to 100 s^{-1}. Non-Newtonian shear-thinning behaviors could be found in JPS solutions at a low shear rate range (0.1–50 s^{-1}), while nearly Newtonian flow behavior was found at a high shear rate range (50–100 s^{-1}). The flow behavior alterations result from many reasons, and a large number of experimental studies have shown that the shear-thinning behavior of polysaccharides was related to the untangling of molecular chains in solution [28,29]. The results showed that the apparent viscosity of the JPSs was affected by the different drying methods. Among them, JPS-RF has the highest apparent viscosity, which is consistent with the results of Li et al. [9], who studied the effects of RF drying on dandelion polysaccharide. This result might be related to the molecular weight, monosaccharide composition, and uronic acid content of JPS-RF.

3.5. FT-IR Spectra of JPSs

FT-IR spectra can be used to efficiently and rapidly characterize the structural groups of polysaccharides. As presented in Figure 2C, the FT-IR spectra of JPS-HA, JPS-F, JPS-IR, and JPS-RF were similar, which indicates that the functional groups of these four JPSs had not changed during the different drying processes. It can be seen that these crude JPSs all exhibited a broadly stretched intense peak at 3451 cm^{-1}, for the hydroxyl stretching vibration, and a weak C-H stretching vibration at 2934 cm^{-1}. The absorption peak at 1738 cm^{-1} was the stretching vibration of the esterified carboxylic groups [30]. Moreover, the strong absorption peak at 1652 cm^{-1} was the C-O, demonstrating that the JPSs were acidic polysaccharides. Absorptions between 1000 and 1100 cm^{-1} showed the stretching vibrations of the pyranose ring. Moreover, the peak at 836 cm^{-1} in the JPSs indicated the existence of α-type glycosidic linkage [10].

3.6. Surface Morphology of JPSs

As a visual analytical technique, SEM can be directly used to observe the microscopic characteristics of polysaccharides [24]. SEM images of JPS-HA, JPS-F, JPS-IR, and JPS-RF are shown in Figure 3. The surface structures of the polysaccharides extracted by the different drying methods differed. Among them, JPS-HA, JPS-IR, and JPS-RF showed a flake structure, and JPS-HA also exhibited many pores, which may be caused by long-term exposure to a high-temperature environment. As the temperature rose, the water content in the jujube evaporated gradually, and the internal structure of the tissue was dislocated and irreversibly damaged. In the FD process, water was released by sublimation, which renders JPS-F a loose and porous structure.

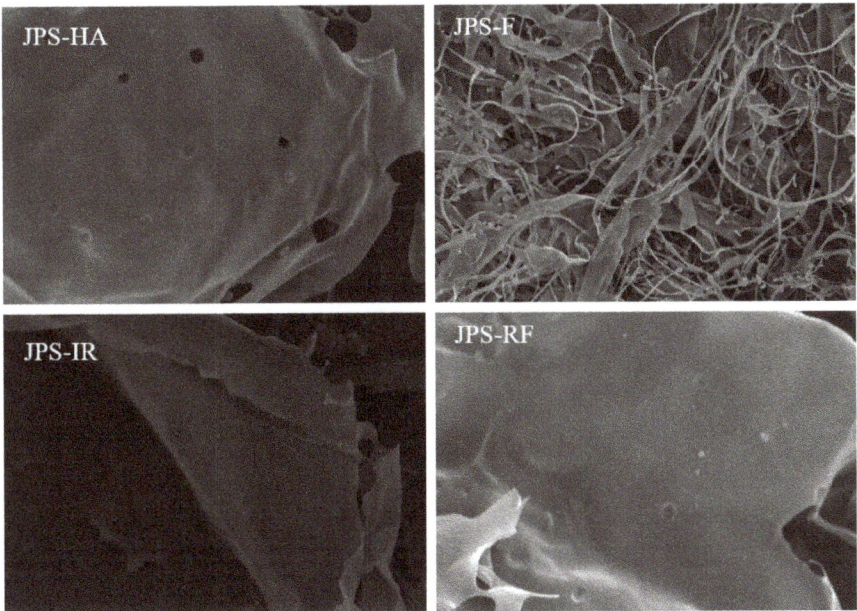

Figure 3. Scanning electron micrographs (500×) of four polysaccharides obtained from different drying methods.

3.7. Antioxidant Activity of JPSs

DPPH and ABTS radical scavenging methods were used to evaluate the antioxidant capacity of the JPSs extracted by the different drying methods [31]. As shown in Figure 4A, polysaccharides obtained from the four drying methods all showed good DPPH free radical-scavenging activity at different concentrations (0–1.0 mg/mL), and the antioxidant activity of JPSs increased with the increase in polysaccharide concentration during the entire process. When the concentration reaching 1 mg/mL, the four JPSs all showed their highest antioxidant activity, which was 59.42% (JPS-HA), 63.07% (JPS-F), 67.99% (JPS-IR), and 70.60% (JPS-RF). Since the DPPH scavenging activity is proportional to the JPS concentration, the IC_{50} value can be selected to compare the antioxidant activity of the polysaccharides treated with the different drying methods [19]. As can be seen in Figure 4B, among the four JPSs, the IC_{50} value of JPS-RF was the lowest, while that of the JPS-HA sample was the highest, indicating that JPS-RF could scavenge 50% of the free DPPH radicals at a lower concentration. Figure 4C shows the ABTS free radical scavenging capacity of JPS-HA, JPS-F, JPS-IR, and JPS-RF. The scavenging capacity of JPSs for ABTS radicals exhibited a similar tendency to the DPPH radical scavenging ability, which increased with the increase in the JPS concentration. The IC_{50} values are shown in Figure 4D. The IC_{50} value of the traditional drying method (HAD)-obtained JPSs showed no significant difference from the FD method, while the IC_{50} of JPS-RF was significantly lower than that of the other methods' treated samples. Similar to the DPPH scavenging ability, the lowest value of IC_{50} for the ABTS test was observed in the RF-dried jujube polysaccharides, which was 0.21 mg/mL.

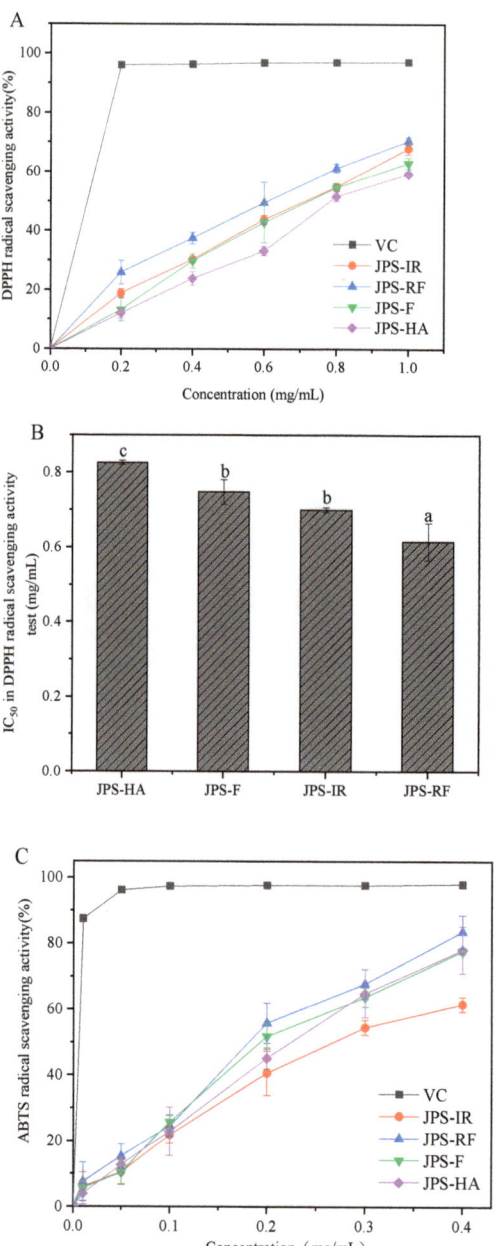

Figure 4. *Cont.*

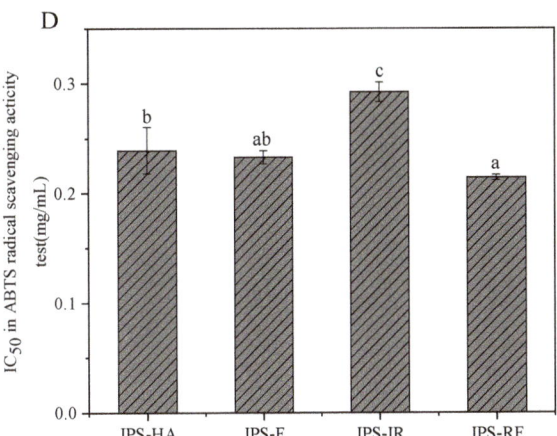

Figure 4. Effects of different drying methods on the antioxidant ability of JPSs. DPPH radical-scavenging activity (**A**) and its IC_{50} value (**B**); ABTS radical-scavenging ability (**C**) and its IC_{50} value (**D**). Bars with different letters differ significantly ($p < 0.05$).

By combining the results of the DPPH and ABTS tests, it was found that RFD technology is a promising drying method for extracting polysaccharides from jujube with high antioxidant activity, among the tested four methods. This result is consistent with the study of [9], who treated dandelion with different drying methods to study the structural activity of its polysaccharides. There are many factors affecting the antioxidant activity of jujube polysaccharides, such as the composition and proportion of monosaccharides, molecular weight, polyphenol content, and uronic acid content [10,32].

4. Conclusions

The effects of different drying techniques on the physical and chemical properties, functional structure, and antioxidant activity of JPSs were studied and compared. The results showed that different drying techniques not only affected the drying time of jujube and jujube polysaccharides but also significantly affected the physicochemical properties and antioxidant activity of jujube polysaccharides. The extraction time, molecular weight, monosaccharide composition, apparent viscosity, uronic acid content, and polyphenol content of the JPSs obtained from the different drying techniques were different. Compared with HAD, the polysaccharides obtained by RFD improved the drying efficiency and showed strong antioxidant activity. The current results can provide a theoretical basis for extracting and drying polysaccharides from jujube using this two-step drying method in industrial application.

Author Contributions: Conceptualization, B.W. and Y.G.; methodology, C.Q.; software, K.G.; formal analysis, Y.M.; data curation, C.Z.; writing—original draft preparation, C.Q. and B.W.; writing—review and editing, Y.G.; visualization, D.L.; supervision, Y.G.; project administration, H.M. All authors have read and agreed to the published version of the manuscript.

Funding: China Postdoctoral Science Foundation (Nos. 2021M700908 and 2022TQ0128) and the Key Laboratory of Storage of Agricultural Products, Ministry of Agriculture and Rural Affairs (No. kf2022002).

Institutional Review Board Statement: Not applicable.

Informed Consent Statement: Not applicable.

Data Availability Statement: Not applicable.

Conflicts of Interest: The authors declare that they have no conflict of interest.

References

1. Liu, X.M.; Liu, Y.; Shan, C.H.; Yang, X.Q.; Zhang, Q.; Xu, N.; Xu, L.Y.; Song, W. Effects of five extraction methods on total content, composition, and stability of flavonoids in jujube. *Food Chem. X* **2022**, *14*, 100287. [CrossRef] [PubMed]
2. Xu, D.; Xiao, J.; Jiang, D.; Liu, Y.; Gou, Z.; Li, J.; Shi, M.; Wang, X.; Guo, Y.; Ma, L.; et al. Inhibitory effects of a water-soluble jujube polysaccharide against biofilm-forming oral pathogenic bacteria. *Int. J. Biol. Macromol.* **2022**, *208*, 1046–1062. [CrossRef] [PubMed]
3. Liu, Y.; Liao, Y.; Guo, M.; Zhang, W.; Sang, Y.; Wang, H.; Cheng, S.; Chen, G. Comparative elucidation of bioactive and volatile components in dry mature jujube fruit (*Ziziphus jujuba* Mill.) subjected to different drying methods. *Food Chem. X* **2022**, *14*, 100311. [CrossRef] [PubMed]
4. Ruan, J.; Han, Y.; Kennedy, J.F.; Jiang, H.; Cao, H.; Zhang, Y.; Wang, T. A review on polysaccharides from jujube and their pharmacological activities. *Carbohydr. Polym. Technol. Appl.* **2022**, *3*, 100220. [CrossRef]
5. Chen, Q.; Bi, J.; Wu, X.; Yi, J.; Zhou, L.; Zhou, Y. Drying kinetics and quality attributes of jujube (*Zizyphus jujuba* Miller) slices dried by hot-air and short- and medium-wave infrared radiation. *LWT Food Sci. Technol.* **2015**, *64*, 759–766. [CrossRef]
6. Gong, C.; Zhao, Y.; Zhang, H.; Yue, J.; Miao, Y.; Jiao, S. Investigation of radio frequency heating as a dry-blanching method for carrot cubes. *J. Food Eng.* **2019**, *245*, 53–56. [CrossRef]
7. Chen, C.; Wongso, I.; Putnam, D.; Khir, R.; Pan, Z. Effect of hot air and infrared drying on the retention of cannabidiol and terpenes in industrial hemp (*Cannabis sativa* L.). *Ind. Crops Prod.* **2021**, *172*, 114051. [CrossRef]
8. Fu, Y.; Feng, K.L.; Wei, S.Y.; Xiang, X.R.; Ding, Y.; Li, H.Y.; Zhao, L.; Qin, W.; Gan, R.Y.; Wu, D.T. Comparison of structural characteristics and bioactivities of polysaccharides from loquat leaves prepared by different drying techniques. *Int. J. Biol. Macromol.* **2020**, *145*, 611–619. [CrossRef]
9. Li, F.; Feng, K.L.; Yang, J.C.; He, Y.S.; Guo, H.; Wang, S.P.; Gan, R.Y.; Wu, D.T. Polysaccharides from dandelion (*Taraxacum mongolicum*) leaves: Insights into innovative drying techniques on their structural characteristics and biological activities. *Int. J. Biol. Macromol.* **2021**, *167*, 995–1005. [CrossRef]
10. Ma, Q.; Santhanam, R.K.; Xue, Z.; Guo, Q.; Gao, X.; Chen, H. Effect of different drying methods on the physicochemical properties and antioxidant activities of mulberry leaves polysaccharides. *Int. J. Biol. Macromol.* **2018**, *119*, 1137–1143. [CrossRef]
11. Yang, B.; Wu, Q.; Luo, Y.; Yang, Q.; Wei, X.; Kan, J. High-pressure ultrasonic-assisted extraction of polysaccharides from Hovenia dulcis: Extraction, structure, antioxidant activity and hypoglycemic. *Int. J. Biol. Macromol.* **2019**, *137*, 676–687. [CrossRef]
12. Chen, S.; Qin, L.; Xie, L.; Yu, Q.; Chen, Y.; Chen, T.; Lu, H.; Xie, J. Physicochemical characterization, rheological and antioxidant properties of three alkali-extracted polysaccharides from mung bean skin. *Food Hydrocoll.* **2022**, *132*, 107867. [CrossRef]
13. Lester, G.E.; Lewers, K.S.; Medina, M.B.; Saftner, R.A. Comparative analysis of strawberry total phenolics via Fast Blue BB vs. Folin–Ciocalteu: Assay interference by ascorbic acid. *J. Food Compos. Anal.* **2012**, *27*, 102–107. [CrossRef]
14. Liu, X.-X.; Gu, L.-B.; Zhang, G.-J.; Liu, H.-M.; Zhang, Y.-T.; Zhang, K.-P. Structural characterization and antioxidant activity of polysaccharides extracted from Chinese yam by a cellulase-assisted method. *Process Biochem.* **2022**, *121*, 178–187. [CrossRef]
15. Gu, J.; Zhang, H.; Zhang, J.; Wen, C.; Zhou, J.; Yao, H.; He, Y.; Ma, H.; Duan, Y. Optimization, characterization, rheological study and immune activities of polysaccharide from *Sagittaria sagittifolia* L. *Carbohydr. Polym.* **2020**, *246*, 116595. [CrossRef] [PubMed]
16. Liu, X.-Y.; Yu, H.-Y.; Liu, Y.-Z.; Qin, Z.; Liu, H.-M.; Ma, Y.-X.; Wang, X.-D. Isolation and structural characterization of cell wall polysaccharides from sesame kernel. *LWT* **2022**, *163*, 113574. [CrossRef]
17. Du, Q.; Ji, X.; Lyu, F.; Liu, J.; Ding, Y. Heat stability and rheology of high-calorie whey protein emulsion: Effects of calcium ions. *Food Hydrocoll.* **2021**, *114*, 106583. [CrossRef]
18. Wang, Y.; Liu, Y.; Huo, J.; Zhaoa, X.; Zheng, J.; Wei, X. Effect of different drying methods on chemical composition and bioactivity of tea polysaccharides. *Int. J. Biol. Macromol.* **2013**, *62*, 714–719. [CrossRef]
19. Shang, H.; Cao, Z.; Zhang, H.; Guo, Y.; Zhao, J.; Wu, H. Physicochemical characterization and in vitro biological activities of polysaccharides from alfalfa (*Medicago sativa* L.) as affected by different drying methods. *Process Biochem.* **2021**, *103*, 39–49. [CrossRef]
20. Chen, X.M.; Ma, Z.; Kitts, D.D. Effects of processing method and age of leaves on phytochemical profiles and bioactivity of coffee leaves. *Food Chem.* **2018**, *249*, 143–153. [CrossRef]
21. Yan, J.K.; Wu, L.X.; Qiao, Z.R.; Cai, W.D.; Ma, H. Effect of different drying methods on the product quality and bioactive polysaccharides of bitter gourd (*Momordica charantia* L.) slices. *Food Chem.* **2019**, *271*, 588–596. [CrossRef] [PubMed]
22. Shi, H.; Wan, Y.; Li, O.; Zhang, X.; Xie, M.; Nie, S.; Yin, J. Two-step hydrolysis method for monosaccharide composition analysis of natural polysaccharides rich in uronic acids. *Food Hydrocoll.* **2020**, *101*, 105524. [CrossRef]
23. Liu, J.; Wang, X.; Yong, H.; Kan, J.; Jin, C. Recent advances in flavonoid-grafted polysaccharides: Synthesis, structural characterization, bioactivities and potential applications. *Int. J. Biol. Macromol.* **2018**, *116*, 1011–1025. [CrossRef] [PubMed]
24. Chen, Z.L.; Wang, C.; Ma, H.; Ma, Y.; Yan, J.K. Physicochemical and functional characteristics of polysaccharides from okra extracted by using ultrasound at different frequencies. *Food Chem.* **2021**, *361*, 130138. [CrossRef]
25. Chen, G.J.; Hong, Q.Y.; Ji, N.; Wu, W.N.; Ma, L.Z. Influences of different drying methods on the structural characteristics and prebiotic activity of polysaccharides from bamboo shoot (*Chimonobambusa quadrangularis*) residues. *Int. J. Biol. Macromol.* **2020**, *155*, 674–684. [CrossRef]
26. Zhang, M.; Wang, F.; Liu, R.; Tang, X.; Zhang, Q.; Zhang, Z. Effects of superfine grinding on physicochemical and antioxidant properties of *Lycium barbarum* polysaccharides. *LWT Food Sci. Technol.* **2014**, *58*, 594–601. [CrossRef]

27. Sila, D.; Doungla, E.; Smout, C.; Van Loey, A.; Hendrickx, M. Pectin Fraction Interconversions: Insight into Understanding Texture Evolution of Thermally Processed Carrots. *J. Agric. Food Chem.* **2006**, *54*, 8471–8479. [CrossRef]
28. Xu, Y.; Liu, N.; Fu, X.; Wang, L.; Yang, Y.; Ren, Y.; Liu, J.; Wang, L. Structural characteristics, biological, rheological and thermal properties of the polysaccharide and the degraded polysaccharide from raspberry fruits. *Int. J. Biol. Macromol.* **2019**, *132*, 109–118. [CrossRef]
29. Yuan, Q.; He, Y.; Xiang, P.-Y.; Huang, Y.-J.; Cao, Z.-W.; Shen, S.-W.; Zhao, L.; Zhang, Q.; Qin, W.; Wu, D.-T. Influences of different drying methods on the structural characteristics and multiple bioactivities of polysaccharides from okra (*Abelmoschus esculentus*). *Int. J. Biol. Macromol.* **2020**, *147*, 1053–1063. [CrossRef]
30. Lammers, K.; Arbuckle-Keil, G.; Dighton, J. FT-IR study of the changes in carbohydrate chemistry of three New Jersey pine barrens leaf litters during simulated control burning. *Soil Biol. Biochem.* **2009**, *41*, 340–347. [CrossRef]
31. Sridhar, K.; Charles, A.L. In vitro antioxidant activity of Kyoho grape extracts in DPPH and ABTS assays: Estimation methods for EC50 using advanced statistical programs. *Food Chem.* **2019**, *275*, 41–49. [CrossRef] [PubMed]
32. Fan, L.; Li, J.; Deng, K.; Ai, L. Effects of drying methods on the antioxidant activities of polysaccharides extracted from Ganoderma lucidum. *Carbohydr. Polym.* **2012**, *87*, 1849–1854. [CrossRef]

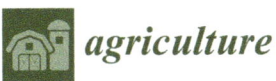

Article

Potato Slices Drying: Pretreatment Affects the Three-Dimensional Appearance and Quality Attributes

Jun-Wen Bai, Yi Dai, Yu-Chi Wang, Jian-Rong Cai, Lu Zhang and Xiao-Yu Tian *

School of Food and Biological Engineering, Jiangsu University, Zhenjiang 212013, China
* Correspondence: tianxy@ujs.edu.cn

Abstract: In the current study, the effects of steam blanching, saline immersion, and ultrasound pretreatment on the drying time, three-dimensional (3D) appearance, quality characteristics, and microstructure of potato slices were investigated. All the pretreatment methods enhanced the drying kinetics relative to the untreated potato slices. The 3D appearance was evaluated by reconstructed 3D images, shrinkage, and curling degree. The reconstructed images could well reproduce the appearance changes in the potato slices during drying. All the three pretreatment methods reduced the shrinkage during the drying process relative to the untreated potatoes. The curling degree was evaluated by the height standard deviation (HSD) of the material surface. The results showed that saline immersion inhibited the curling of the potato slices during the drying process, while ultrasound aggravated the curling of the potato slices. The potatoes treated by blanching obtained a lower total color difference (ΔE), higher total polyphenol content, and antioxidant capacity compared with the samples treated with saline immersion and ultrasound pretreatments. The observation of the microstructure by scanning electron microscope (SEM) verified the effects of the pretreatments on the drying time and appearance deformation. Therefore, it is of great significance to regulate the 3D appearance and quality characteristics of agricultural products during the drying process by an appropriate pretreatment.

Keywords: potato; pretreatment; drying; three-dimensional appearance; quality; microstructure

1. Introduction

Potato (*Solanum tuberosum* L.) is known as one of the world's five major crops along with corn, rice, wheat, and sorghum [1]. Potato is rich in nutrition, including starch, protein, vitamins, polyphenols, and trace elements, so it is used as a favorite composition of functional food [2,3]. Therefore, potato is getting higher and higher in the position of agricultural and sideline products, and the demand is also growing. However, potato, like other vegetables, has a high moisture content, so it is easy for it to rot and sprout during storage [4]. This has a great effect on the quality of potatoes [5]. Drying is an effective way to prolong the shelf life of fruits and vegetables.

There are many drying methods used in the processing of fruits and vegetables, including hot-air drying, infrared drying, freeze drying, microwave drying, and hybrid drying technology [6,7]. Each drying technique has its own advantages and disadvantages. However, the most commonly used drying method in potatoes is still hot-air drying [8]. Drying can effectively prevent the growth of microorganisms, reduce enzyme activity, and slow down some water-mediated chemical reactions [9,10]. However, the drying process always consumes a lot of energy and will have a significant impact on the shape, color, flavor, and nutrition of dried products [10]. Therefore, it is necessary to develop operations to minimize the adverse effects of the drying process, reduce the time and energy requirements, and maximize the retention of the original characteristics of the product [11].

Fruits and vegetables are usually subjected to physical or chemical pretreatment before drying to shorten the drying time, reduce the energy consumption, and preserve

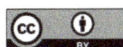

the quality of products [12]. It was found that blanching pretreatment can damage the structure of cell membranes and thus shorten the drying time [13]. Mehta et al. [14] reported that dried vegetables coupled with blanching as a pretreatment showed less degradation in terms of polyphenols and flavonoids. Liu et al. [15] observed that blanching pretreatment could not only shorten the drying time but also inhibit browning and maintain the anthocyanin level in purple-flesh sweet potato drying. It has also been reported that vacuum-dried potato chips pretreated with blanching have a better texture and a lower glycemic index [16]. Osmotic solution immersion pretreatment, such as sucrose or salt solution, has been widely used in drying pretreatments because of its ability to ensure the quality of dried products [17]. Zou et al. [18] reported that sucrose solution immersion pretreatment can improve the color and sensory quality of dried products. It was reported that osmotic solution pretreatment shortens the drying time and reduces the specific energy consumption in potato drying [19]. Moreover, Chinenye et al. [20] found that the volume of potato chips treated by saline immersion was higher by 6% than non-treated samples.

Ultrasound as a pretreatment method has attracted considerable interest in drying processes, since it can form microscopic channels in the tissue due to cavitation and sponge effects, which can promote the migration of water and accelerate the drying process [21,22]. For potato slices drying processes, it has been reported that ultrasound pretreatment can effectively shorten the drying time and reduce the specific energy consumption [23]. Zhang et al. found that ultrasound pretreatment can increased hardness of potato chips and reduce the destruction of the cellular structure [24]. The results of Xu et al. [25] showed that ultrasound pretreatment could improve the content of flavonoids and polyphenols in dried products. Rashid et al. [26] also reported that appropriate ultrasound pretreatment can well maintain phytochemical compounds. Generally speaking, suitable pretreatment before a drying process can improve the drying efficiency and enhance the product quality, but few people have paid attention to the influence of pretreatment on the appearance changes in dried products.

Appearance (especially for 3D appearance) is one of the most important indicators for people when evaluating dried products, and it has a great impact on subsequent further processing, packaging, and transportation [27]. For consumers, products with a uniform and regular appearance generally have a better degree of acceptability. At present, the main method for studying the appearance changes in dried samples is through two-dimensional images. For example, Khazaei et al. [28] applied an analog camera collect images to monitor shrinkage during dehydration in grape drying. However, a single camera can only obtain the data of a projected area of a sample's surface, and the thickness change in the material cannot be measured effectively. Therefore, Sampson et al. [29] used top and side cameras to obtain the thickness and projected area of materials so as to measure the volume changes in apple slices during the drying process. However, a side camera cannot fully reflect the thickness change during the drying process of the material. In addition, a two-dimensional image cannot perfectly simulate the morphological change in the drying process that occurs in a 3D space. Therefore, it is necessary to use 3D image technology to evaluate the shape change in materials during drying. Cai et al. [30] used a Kinect V2 sensor to build an image acquisition platform, and the morphological changes in potato slices under different drying temperatures were studied. However, the detection accuracy of a Kinect sensor is relatively low [31], which makes the quantification and analysis of 3D information rough. Therefore, there has been less information about the 3D appearance changes in fruits and vegetables during drying by pretreatment methods.

The objective of this study was to investigate the effects of blanching, saline immersion, and ultrasound pretreatments on the drying time, internal quality, and external quality characteristics of dried potato slices, including the 3D appearance, color, total polyphenol content, antioxidant properties, and microstructure.

2. Materials and Methods

2.1. Material

Fresh potatoes of the same variety "Holland fifteen" were purchased from a supermarket near Jiangsu University (Zhenjiang, China). All the potato samples were transported to the laboratory and stored at room temperature (about 20 °C) before experimentation. The average initial moisture content of potatoes was 84.23 ± 2.36% (wet basis). Before drying, the potatoes were washed, peeled, and sliced to a thickness of 2 mm using an electric slicer (MS-305C, Foshan Komle Electric Appliance Co., Ltd., Foshan, China). Then, the samples were subjected to pretreatment.

2.2. Pretreatment Methods

In this study, potato slices were subjected to three kinds of pretreatments. (1) For steam-blanching pretreatment, potato slices were processed by steam cooker (total volume 4 L) at atmospheric pressure. The power of the steam cooker was 1000 W to ensure the continuous boiling of the water. The blanching times were 30, 60, and 90 s, respectively. (2) Saline immersion pretreatment was referred to as the method of Chinenye et al. [20] with some modifications. Potato slices were soaked in a salt solution for 60 min. The concentrations of the salt solutions were 5%, 10%, and 20%, respectively. (3) For ultrasound pretreatment, the potato slices were immersed in distilled water and then subjected to an ultrasound bath. The parameters set to 240 W and 40 °C according to the relevant studies. The treatment times were 10 min, 30 min, and 60 min, respectively.

2.3. Hot-Air Drying Experiment

The potato slice samples were dried in hot-air drier, which was described in previous study [30]. The drying process was carried out at 65 °C with an air velocity of 3 m/s and a relative humidity of 10% (RH). A quantity of 100 ± 5 g samples was used for all drying runs in the experiment. The weight loss was periodically recorded by taking out the rotating glass and weighing it on an electronic balance within an accuracy of ±0.01 g during drying. Drying was stopped when the moisture content of the samples reached the desired final moisture content of 6.00% (wet basis). All the drying experiments were conducted in triplicate.

2.4. Moisture Ratio (MR)

The moisture ratio was calculated using Equations (1) and (2).

$$\mathrm{MR} = \frac{M_t - M_e}{M_0 - M_e} \quad (1)$$

where M_0 is the initial dry basis moisture content; M_t is the dry basis moisture content at the drying time t; MR is the moisture ratio; and M_e is the equilibrium moisture content. The equilibrium moisture content, M_e, was much smaller than M_0 and M_t and could generally be ignored [32]. Therefore, the calculation of MR can be simplified as:

$$\mathrm{MR} = \frac{M_t}{M_0} \quad (2)$$

2.5. Three-Dimensional Appearance Evaluation Index

The 3D image acquisition platform used in this experiment was independently built by the team [33]. Using binocular snapshot sensor (Gocator3210, LMI technologies Inc., Vancouver, BC, Canada), the measurement range was −50~50 mm in the horizontal direction, −77~77 mm in the vertical direction, −55~55 mm in the depth direction, and the detection accuracy was ±0.035 mm. The 3D point cloud images were periodically collected at an interval of 10 min during drying. The collected images were processed by the software Cloud Compare (version 2.1), including background removal, noise removal, point cloud filtering, and surface reconstruction.

The time-varying appearance images of one potato slice during drying is shown in Figure 1. The three images from top to bottom in each column represent a color physical image, 3D reconstructed image and height distributed image, respectively. The 3D reconstructed image obtained from the point cloud data was fairly close to the physical image of the potato slice, which benefitted from good measurement accuracy due to laser scanning [34,35]. Therefore, the reconstructed 3D images could well reproduce the appearance changes in the potato slices during drying. The height distribution of the potato slice in Figure 1 is represented by pseudo-color images, and the color from blue to red indicates that the height value of the pixels on the material changed from small to large. It was found that potato slice obviously curled with the process of drying, especially after a drying time of 40 min.

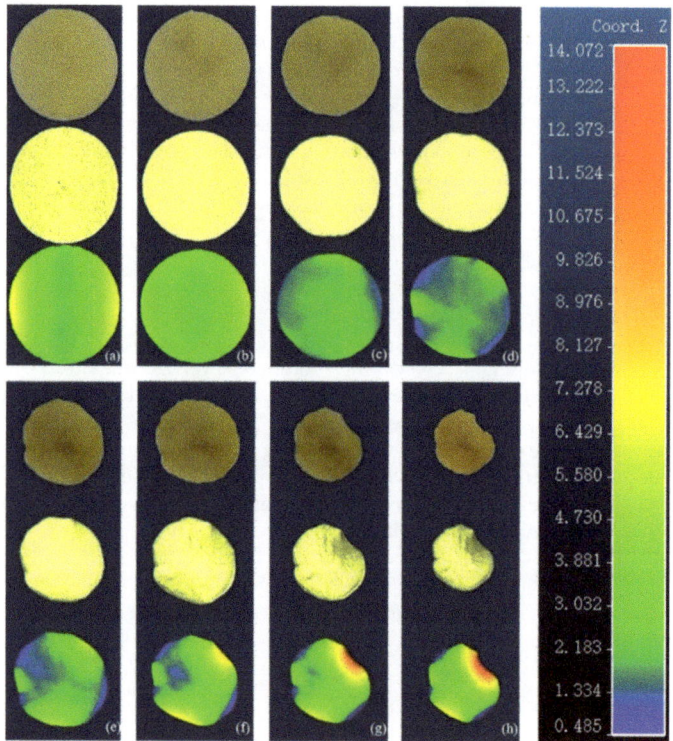

Figure 1. Time-varying appearance images of one potato slice during drying. (**a–h**) represent potato slices dried at 65 °C, 10% RH, 3 m/s for 0, 10, 20, 30, 40, 50, 60, and 70 min, respectively. The three images from top to bottom in each column represent color physical image, 3D reconstructed image, and height distributed image, respectively.

2.5.1. Shrinkage

The surface model was composed of tens of thousands of triangles. First, the distance between two points was calculated by Euclid's formula, and the three side lengths of each triangle could be obtained. For example, the distance between points p_1 (x_1, y_1, z_1) and p_2 (x_2, y_2, z_2) can be calculated by Equation (3). Then, the area of each triangle was calculated through Helen's formula, as in Equation (4), and the sum of the area of all triangles was calculated, which was the surface area. The shrinkage of the potato slices during drying could be calculated by the change in the surface area at different drying time points (Equation (5)). The specific equations are as follows:

$$d_{p_1p_2} = \sqrt{(x_1-x_2)^2 + (y_1-y_2)^2 + (z_1-z_2)^2} \tag{3}$$

$$S_{ABC} = \sqrt{p(p-d_{AB})(p-d_{AC})(p-d_{BC})} \tag{4}$$

$$\text{Shrinkage} = \frac{S_0 - S_t}{S_0} \tag{5}$$

where $d_{p_1p_2}$ is the distance between the two points of p_1 and p_2; S_{ABC} is the area of the triangle ABC; and p is half of the circumference of the triangle ABC. S_0 is the surface area of the sample before drying, and S_t is the surface area of the sample during drying.

2.5.2. Height Standard Deviation

The appearance of the material changed from flat to curled during drying, which caused a change in the surface height value. The HSD could reflect the degree of dispersion of the surface height among individuals in a group. Therefore, the HSD was used to characterize the degree of curling of the material. The larger the value, the more uneven the surface of the material and the more severe the curling. The height value of the processed point cloud was extracted by the software, and the standard deviation of the height was calculated by Equation (6).

$$\text{Height standard deviation} = \sqrt{\frac{\sum_{i=1}^{n}(h_i - h_{av})^2}{n-1}} \tag{6}$$

Among them, n is the number of point clouds; h_i is the height of the i-th point, mm; and h_{av} is the average height of n points, mm.

2.6. Color Measurement

The color of fresh and dried potato slices was determined using colorimeter (SC-10; Shenzhen 3nh technology Co., Ltd., Shenzhen, China). The color was represented by coordinates L^* (lightness), a^* (redness/greenness), and b^* (yellowness/blueness). For each condition, the collection of color parameters was repeated 9 times and averaged. In addition, the total color difference (ΔE) was calculated by Equation (7).

$$\Delta E = \sqrt{(L_0^* - L^*)^2 + (a_0^* - a^*)^2 + (b_0^* - b^*)^2} \tag{7}$$

where, L_0^*, a_0^*, and b_0^* are the color parameters of the untreated dried potato slices, and L^*, a^*, and b^* are the color parameters of the pretreated dried potato slices.

2.7. Determination of Total Polyphenol Content (TPC)

Polyphenol extract was prepared by the following method: A total of 1 g of potato slice powder was extracted with 70% ethanol solvent. The potato powder and 50 mL solvent were mixed evenly at room temperature and then treated by ultrasound for 1 h at 40 °C, followed by centrifugation at 4000 rpm for 20 min to obtain the supernatant. The supernatant was the final polyphenol extract, and it was stored at 4 °C for further analysis.

The total polyphenol content (TPC) of the potato slices was determined by an improved Folin–Ciocalteu method [36]. Five hundred microliters of polyphenol extract were mixed with 1 mL Folin–Ciocalteu's reagent. After 2 min incubation at room temperature, 2 mL Na_2CO_3 (7.5%, w/v) was added and then fixed to 10 mL with distilled water. The resulting mixture was incubated for 60 min at room temperature. At the end of the incubation, the absorbance was measured at 775 nm using a UV–Vis spectrophotometer (754, Shanghai Jinghua Technology Instrument Co., Ltd., Shanghai, China). The results of the TPC were expressed as mg gallic acid equivalents (GAE) per gram of dried potato slices.

2.8. Determination of DPPH Radical Scavenging Assay

The DPPH radical scavenging assay was analyzed according to the method of Zhu et al. [37] and modified appropriately. DPPH solution (2 mL) solution was mixed with a certain volume of sample polyphenol extracts and then fixed to 5 mL with 70% ethanol solution. The reaction mixture was shaken well by a vortex blender (VORTEX-2, Shanghai Hutong Industrial Co., Ltd., Shanghai, China) and left standing for 30 min in a dark environment at room temperature. In the control group, 70% ethanol solution was used to replace the extract, and the preparation method was similar to that of the experimental group. The absorbance of the experimental group and the control group at 517 nm was measured by UV–Vis spectrophotometer (754, Shanghai Jinghua Technology Instrument Co., Ltd., Shanghai, China). The results were presented as percentage of DPPH radical scavenging activity utilizing the Equation (8).

$$\text{DPPH scavenging activity } (\%) = \frac{A_0 - A}{A_0} \times 100\% \tag{8}$$

where A_0 is the absorbance of the control group, and A is the absorbance of the sample group.

2.9. Microstructure

Microstructure images of the dried potato slices were obtained using a scanning electron microscope (SEM) (S-3400 N, Hitachi Ltd., Tokyo, Japan) according to the method described by Chu et al. [38]. Dried potato slices were cut into 5 mm × 5 mm with a blade and coated with gold in an ion sputter. The samples were observed in the high vacuum mode at an accelerating voltage of 15.0 kV. Samples were observed at a magnification of 100× and 500×.

2.10. Statistical Analysis

All statistical analyses were performed using three sets of parallel experimental data, and the experimental results were expressed as mean ± SD. Statistical analysis was performed using SPSS software (version 25.0, SPSS Inc., Chicago, IL, USA). The one-way analysis of variance and Duncan's test ($p < 0.05$) were used to determine whether there were significant differences between the groups.

3. Results and Discussion

3.1. Moisture Ratio (MR)

Figure 2 shows the MR curves and drying time of the potato slices under different pretreatments during hot-air drying. Compared with the untreated potato samples, blanching, saline immersion, and ultrasound pretreatment had obvious effects on the drying curves and drying time. The drying curve of the potato slices under different blanching times is shown in Figure 2I. The drying time was decreased by about 14.29% when the blanching time increased to 90 s. This phenomenon may be due to the fact that blanching can expel the intercellular air retention in sample tissues and weaken the resistance of cell membranes and cell walls to water diffusion through structure softening [39]. Similar results were found in studies on the drying process of apricots [40] and carrots [41].

For the saline immersion pretreatment in Figure 2II, when the salt solution concentration increased to 20%, the drying time of the potato slices decreased by about 35.71% compared with the untreated samples. The reason for this result may be that saline immersion can remove part of the free water in the material [18], which obviously led to a reduction in the drying time. In addition, it was reported that accumulation of solute (sucrose or salt) occurred in the space between the wall and plasmalemma, which plasmolyzed the cytoplasm and the vacuoles [42].

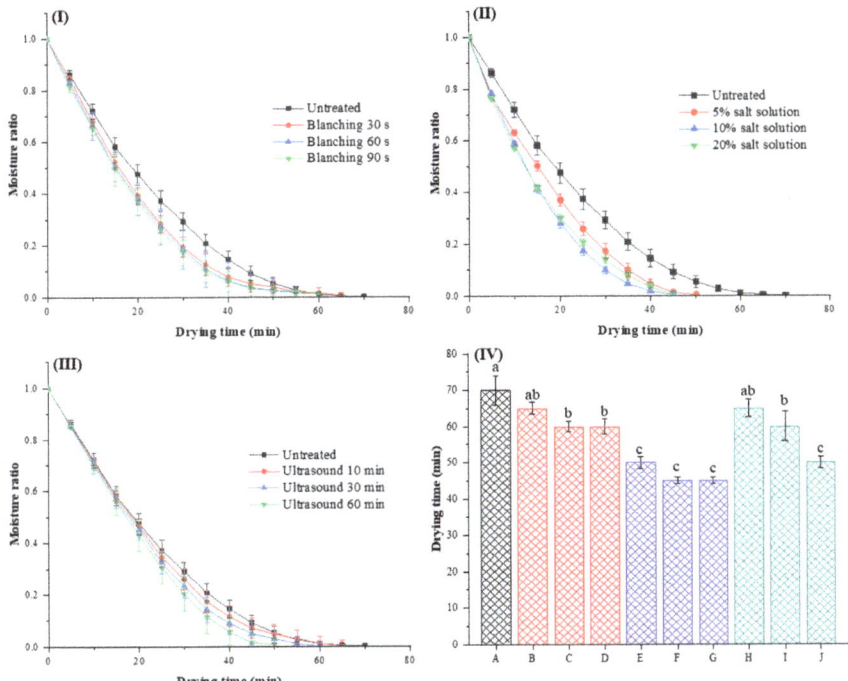

Figure 2. Drying curves and drying time of potato slices under different pretreatment conditions such as (**I**) blanching, (**II**) saline immersion, and (**III**) ultrasound pretreatment. (**IV**) The drying time for (A) untreated potato samples, (B–D) with blanching pretreatment for 30, 60, and 90 s, (E–G) with saline immersion under solution concentration of 5%, 10%, and 20%, and (H–J) with ultrasound pretreatment for 10, 30, and 60 min. Means denoted by a different lowercase letter indicate significant difference between treatments ($p < 0.05$).

The effect of ultrasound time on the drying time is shown in Figure 2III. It was found that the drying times were about 65, 60, and 50 min for the potato samples treated for 10, 30, and 60 min, respectively. This may be due to cell disruption and microscopic channels being formed after ultrasound pretreatment, which led to a reduction in the resistance against moisture migration [43].

Figure 2IV shows the drying time and variance analysis results of the potato slices under different pretreatment conditions. All three pretreatments enhanced the drying kinetics relative to the untreated samples The saline immersion pretreatment had the greatest influence on the drying time, followed by the ultrasound and blanching pretreatments. In general, the different pretreatments had different effects on the structure of the materials and further affected the process of heat and mass transfer during the drying.

3.2. Three-Dimensional Appearance Characterization

The 3D appearance images of the dried potato slices under different pretreatments are shown in Figure 3. The three images from top to bottom in each column represent the physical, 3D reconstruction, and height distribution diagrams of the potato slices. It was found that the appearance of the potato slices had significant curling, shrinkage, and browning after the drying process. Moreover, the appearance of the dried potato slices varied greatly with different pretreatments.

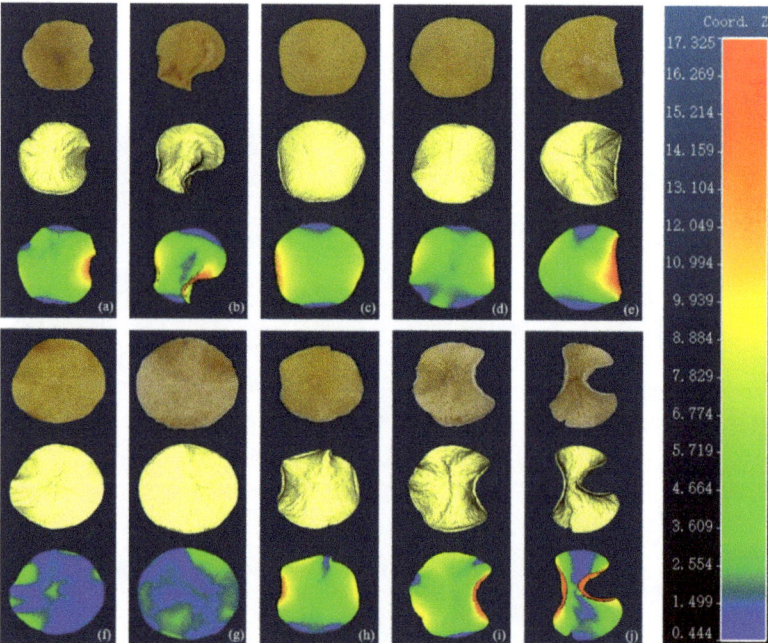

Figure 3. Three-dimensional appearance images of dried potato slices under different pretreatments. (**a**) Untreated potato samples. (**b**–**d**) Blanching pretreatment for 30, 60, and 90 s. (**e**–**g**) Saline immersion under solution concentration of 5%, 10%, and 20%. (**h**–**j**) Ultrasound pretreatment for 10, 30, and 60 min. The three images from top to bottom in each column represent the physical, three-dimensional reconstruction, and height distribution diagrams of the potato slices.

Figure 3b–d shows the appearance of the potato slices after pretreatment by blanching for 30, 60, and 90 s, respectively. When the blanching time was 30 s, the dried potato slices curled obviously. However, when the blanching time was extended to 60 s or 90 s, the potato slices became relatively flat. It has been reported that blanching can destroy the cellular structure and alter the moisture distribution of materials, which leads to a more uniform moisture distribution in materials [44]. The uniform distribution of moisture in the material could have reduced the stress caused by shrinkage in the drying process.

The appearance of the potato slices after pretreatment by saline immersion under solution concentrations of 5%, 10%, and 20% is shown in Figure 3e–g. It can be seen from the figures that, as the salt solution concentration increased to 10% and 20%, the saline immersion pretreatment obviously inhibited the shrinkage and curling of the potato slices during drying. The reason for this phenomenon may be that salt particles could fill the spaces reduced by moisture removal during the drying process. In contrast, for the samples pretreated by ultrasound pretreatment, especially for a long time (60 min), the appearance of the material was seriously curled. This may be attributed to the destruction of the material structure by the "cavitation effect" of ultrasound.

In summary, saline immersion and blanching pretreatment could effectively inhibit the shrinkage and curling of the potato slices, while ultrasound pretreatment aggravated the deformation during the drying process.

3.3. Shrinkage

The shrinkage curves of potato slices under different pretreatment conditions during drying process are shown in Figure 4I–III, and the results of the analysis of variance of the dried potato slices are shown in Figure 4IV. It can be seen that the shrinkage of the potato slices mainly took place at the early drying stage, and gradually slowed down in the later drying stage. It has been reported that the shrinkage at the initial stage of drying is approximately equal to the volume of moisture lost, while in the middle and late drying stages, with the fixation of the "skeleton", the shrinkage becomes slow [45].

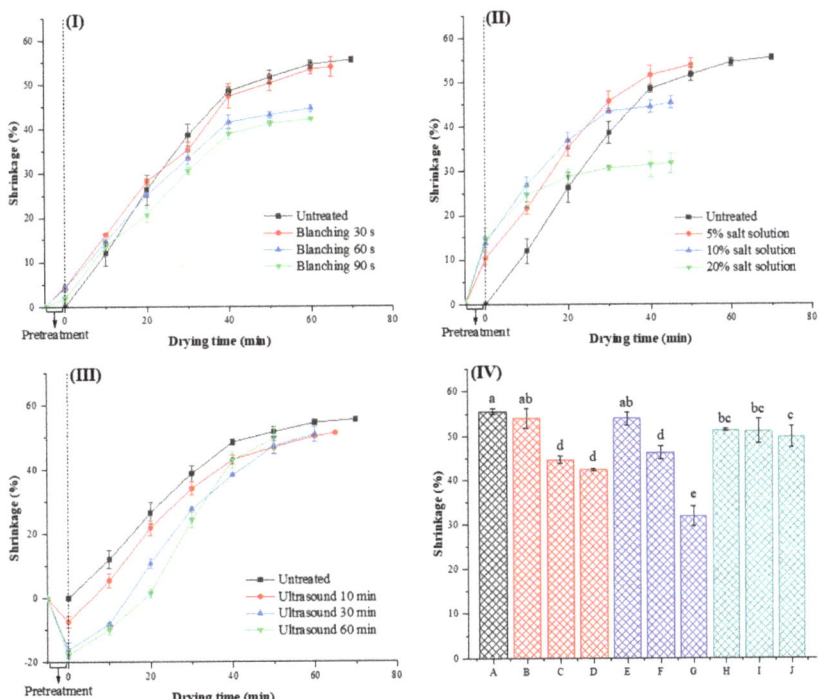

Figure 4. Shrinkage of potato slices during drying under different pretreatments, such as (**I**) blanching, (**II**) saline immersion, and (**III**) ultrasound pretreatment. (**IV**) The shrinkage for (**A**) untreated potato samples, (**B–D**) with blanching pretreatment for 30, 60, and 90 s, (**E–G**) with saline immersion under solution concentration of 5%, 10%, and 20%, and (**H–J**) with ultrasound pretreatment for 10, 30, and 60 min. Means denoted by a different lowercase letter indicate significant difference between treatments ($p < 0.05$).

As shown in Figure 4I, the blanching time had a great influence on the shrinkage of the potato slices. The shrinkage of the dried potato slices at 30, 60, and 90 s were 53.97%, 44.67%, and 42.27%, respectively, which decreased by 2.83%, 19.57%, and 23.89% compared with the untreated samples (55.54%). This was because the blanching caused the cell walls to collapse [46], which reduced the effect of surface stress. Mahiuddin et al. [47] also reported that the destruction of the cell structure has an effect on the shrinkage properties of materials.

Figure 4II indicates the shrinkage of the potato slices by saline immersion under different solution concentrations. It can be seen that the saline immersion pretreatment had a great influence on the shrinkage of the dried potato slices. The shrinkage of the potato slices decreased with the increase in the salt solution concentration. The potato slices had minimal shrinkage when the salt solution concentration reached 20%, which caused a decrease of 42.69% compared to the untreated sample. Fante et al. [48] found that an increase in sucrose solution concentration led to a decrease in the shrinkage of dried plum slices in the drying process. This may be due to the fact that salt or sucrose particles can fill the space left by the removal of moisture in the material, which would support the skeleton structure of the material to a certain extent.

From Figure 4III, it was found that the ultrasound pretreatment slightly reduced the shrinkage, but the pretreatment time had no significant effect on the shrinkage of the dried potato slices. Liu et al. [49] observed large microchannels and pores in ultrasound-pretreated samples, while the structure of the untreated material was relatively compact. In addition, ultrasound waves may have extended the intercellular spaces by the cavitation effect [50], which may have partially offset the volume reduction caused by moisture removal.

3.4. Height Standard Deviation (HSD)

The curling degree was evaluated by the HSD of the material surface. The HSD curves of the potato slices during drying under different pretreatments are shown in Figure 5. At the early stage of drying, the HSD of the material changed little or showed a downward trend, which was mainly due to the softening of the material structure by hot-air heating. The HSD increased rapidly in the middle and late drying stages, indicating that the material had an obvious curling phenomenon. The shape changes in the materials in the drying process may be due to the uneven stress caused by the shrinkage of the cells and pores [51].

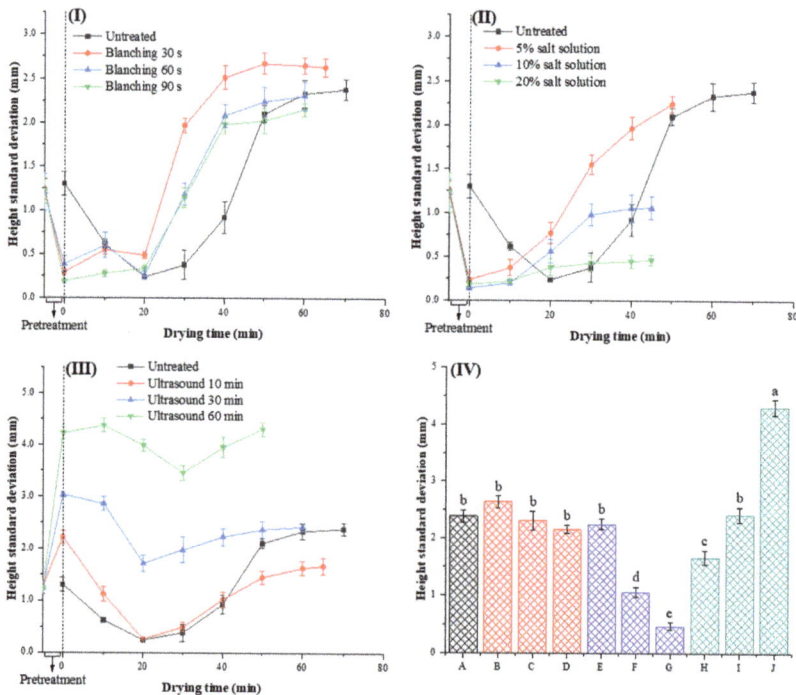

Figure 5. Height standard deviation of potato slices during drying under different pretreatments, such as (I) blanching, (II) saline immersion, and (III) ultrasound pretreatment. (IV) The height standard deviation for (A) untreated potato samples, (B–D) with blanching pretreatment for 30, 60, and 90 s, (E–G) with saline immersion under solution concentration of 5%, 10%, and 20%, and (H–J) with ultrasound pretreatment for 10, 30, and 60 min. Means denoted by a different lowercase letter indicate significant difference between treatments ($p < 0.05$).

The HSD of the dried potato slices after blanching for 30, 60, and 90 s were 2.64 mm, 2.31 mm, and 2.16 mm, respectively. However, there was no significant difference between the blanching pretreatment and the untreated samples, indicating that the blanching pretreatment could not reduce the curling phenomenon during drying. Although the structure of the material would have been damaged by the blanching process, the starch gelatinization caused by the high temperature may have played a certain role in supporting the structure.

As shown in Figure 5IV, the HSD of the dried potato slices after saline immersion pretreatment under solution concentrations of 5%, 10%, and 20% were 2.25 mm, 1.06 mm, and 0.47 mm, respectively, which decreased by 5.88%, 55.46%, and 80.25% compared with the untreated samples. The results demonstrated that saline immersion could inhibit the curling of the potato slices in the drying process, showing a relatively flat shape. This may be because osmotic ions entered the tissue and blocked the transmission of internal stress [52]. In addition, it also may have been due to the structure of "hard outside and soft inside" after processing by osmotic dehydration [53].

For the ultrasound pretreatment, the HSD after ultrasound pretreatment for 10, 30, and 60 min were 1.67 mm, 2.41 mm, and 4.30 mm, respectively. It was found that ultrasound pretreatment for 10 min could reduce the HSD of the potato slices, which indicated that a shorter time of the ultrasound pretreatment could reduce the curling degree. When the ultrasound time was extended to 60 min, the HSD (4.30 mm) increased by 80.67% compared with the untreated samples, which indicated that very serious curling of the slices occurred. This may be because the short-time ultrasound pretreatment made the potato tissue more uniform, thereby resulting in a more uniform transfer of internal stress. However, with the increase in the ultrasound time, the cavitation effect of micro-jets and micro-agitation at the bubble inter-face led to the destruction of the cell structure and formed cracks and pores [54]. The non-continuous and non-uniform structure increased the effect of stress and showed the appearance of curling from a macroscopic perspective.

3.5. Color

Color is a significant quality parameter of dried potato slices, which influences the customer's perception and purchasing power [55]. The color values of all the samples are presented in Table 1. Blanching, saline immersion, ultrasound, and drying had significant effects on the color parameters of the dried potato slices. As seen in Table 1, the L^*, a^*, and b^* values of the untreated potato slices were 72.62, 8.24, and 26.13, respectively. It was found that the untreated samples had the largest value of ΔE, which was due to browning caused by the drying process [56]. The L^* value of the potato slices pretreated with blanching was lower, which may be related to the gelatinization of starch by blanching pretreatment. Xiao et al. [57] reported that the clarity of gelatinized starch could reduce the lightness of starch products. Compared with the untreated samples, the values of a^* and b^* were significantly reduced. The value of ΔE of the dried samples after blanching pretreatment was also significantly lower than that of the untreated samples. In particular, when the blanching time was 30 s, the color change was the least, and the ΔE value was 3.10. This indicated that blanching pretreatment could better retain the original color, which may be because blanching inactivates polyphenol oxidase. It has also been reported that this phenomenon is due to the leaching of reducing sugars by blanching pretreatment, which is the substrate of the Maillard reaction [58]. Thus, this minimized the non-enzymatic browning reaction and reduce the color variation in the slices.

The effect of the saline immersion pretreatment on the color is shown in Table 1. The values of L^*, a^*, and b^* were all smaller than those of the untreated samples. With the increase in the salt concentration, the value of the sample color parameters decreased continuously, which indicated that a high concentration salt solution could achieve a better retention effect in terms of color. This may be due to the loss of polyphenol oxidase, which is due to the leakage effect of a high-concentration salt solution.

For the ultrasound pretreatment, the color parameters of the potato slices were slightly less than those of the untreated samples. With the extension of the ultrasound time, the ΔE value gradually decreased, which indicated that long-time ultrasound pretreatment was in favor of maintaining the color of the samples. This may be because the ultrasound pretreatment reduced the oxygen content of the sample and inhibited the browning reaction [38,59].

Table 1. Changes in color, total polyphenol content, and antioxidant capacity of potato slices after drying under different pretreatments.

Pretreatment Methods		L*	a*	b*	ΔE	TPC (mg/g)	DPPH Radical Scavenging Activity (%)
Untreated	-	72.67 ± 0.48 a	8.24 ± 0.09 a	26.13 ± 0.18 a	24.60 ± 0.91 a	0.31 ± 0.02 d,e	34.12 ± 1.51 c
Blanching	30 s	51.35 ± 1.13 e,f	4.44 ± 0.07 f,g	15.83 ± 0.33 e	3.45 ± 0.50 f	0.45 ± 0.05 a	56.45 ± 1.02 a
	60 s	50.50 ± 0.69 e,f	5.02 ± 0.36 e,f	17.88 ± 0.63 d	5.54 ± 0.37 e,f	0.42 ± 0.03 a,b	52.01 ± 3.94 a
	90 s	49.89 ± 1.01 f	6.10 ± 0.34 c,d	18.20 ± 0.20 d	6.17 ± 0.98 e,f	0.32 ± 0.02 c,d	38.82 ± 3.66 c
Saline immersion	5%	67.28 ± 1.44 b	7.09 ± 0.67 b	27.01 ± 2.22 a	20.82 ± 2.44 b,c	0.27 ± 0.04 e,f	26.38 ± 0.81 d
	10%	63.12 ± 1.26 c	7.10 ± 0.57 b	20.29 ± 0.44 c	13.42 ± 1.41 d	0.28 ± 0.03 d,e	25.08 ± 0.90 d
	20%	59.81 ± 0.71 d	5.31 ± 0.43 d,e	17.03 ± 0.63 d,e	8.68 ± 1.32 e	0.22 ± 0.02 g	17.15 ± 1.30 c
Ultrasound	10 min	72.23 ± 0.31 a	6.49 ± 0.22 b,c	26.01 ± 1.10 a	23.97 ± 1.48 a,b	0.40 ± 0.05 b	46.72 ± 3.13 b
	30 min	71.92 ± 0.71 a	5.87 ± 0.21 c,d	23.44 ± 1.26 c	22.34 ± 1.79 a,b,c	0.35 ± 0.04 c	45.07 ± 2.19 b
	60 min	70.86 ± 1.88 a	5.44 ± 0.39 d,e	21.30 ± 0.62 c	20.40 ± 2.08 c	0.22 ± 0.03 f,g	33.65 ± 0.98 c

Note: Data are expressed as the average ± standard deviation for three replicates. Values in the same column with different letters for each parameter are significantly different ($p < 0.05$).

3.6. Total Polyphenol Content (TPC)

The effects of the different pretreatment methods on the TPC of the dried potato slices are shown in Table 1. Compared with the untreated samples, the blanching and ultrasound pretreatment had a better retention of polyphenols, while the saline immersion pretreatment was not conducive to the retention of polyphenols.

Compared with the untreated samples, the total polyphenol content in the blanching-pretreated samples was generally increased. However, with the extension of the blanching time, the total polyphenol content gradually decreased. This indicated that short-time blanching pretreatment was beneficial to the retention of polyphenols. This may be due to the loss of polyphenol oxidase activity by blanching pretreatment, which resulted in a better retention of more polyphenols [59]. However, a prolonged blanching time made the cellular structure vulnerable to damage during drying, which led to the oxidation of polyphenols [40].

For the samples treated with saline immersion, the content of polyphenols was lower than that of the untreated samples. When the solution concentration reached 20%, the polyphenol content was the lowest. This was the loss of polyphenols due to leakage of the salt solution [60,61].

Similar to the blanching pretreatment, a shorter ultrasound treatment was more beneficial for polyphenol retention. This may be due to the fact that ultrasound pretreatment can produce stomata in plant tissues, thus improving the extraction of polyphenols during the preparation of sample [62]. However, when the ultrasound time was too long, the total phenol content decreased slightly, which was due to the loss of food ingredients caused by the enlargement of pores [63]. This was consistent with the study of polyphenol content in dried onions slices by Ren et al. [64].

3.7. DPPH Radical Scavenging Assay

The DPPH free radical activity values of the dried potato slices under different pretreatments are shown in Table 1. It was observed that the trend of DPPH was similar to that of TPC retention. The high positive correlation between phenolic compounds and antioxidant activity was also reported in another study [65]. In this study, the free radical scavenging activity of the blanched samples was the best, followed by the samples pretreated with ultrasound and saline immersion. When the blanching time was 30 s, the sample showed the highest activity (56.45%), which was similar to the results of Feng et al. [66].

3.8. Microstructure

The scanning electron microscopy (SEM) images of the dried potato slices under different pretreatments are shown in Figure 6. The microscopic results of the different pretreated samples and untreated samples differed greatly. As shown in Figure 6a, the untreated samples had both dense and porous structures, which may be caused by the non-uniform shrinkage of the material structure. From Figure 6b, we also found intact starch granules, indicating that the starch did not swell and gelatinize during the drying process.

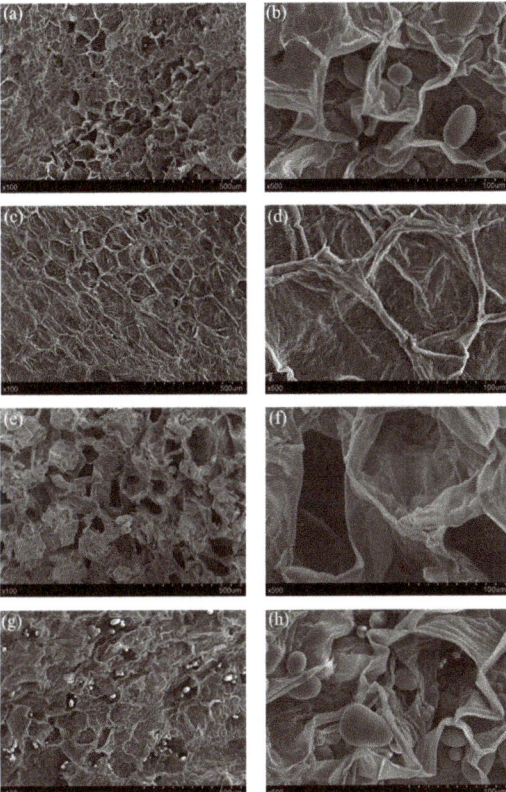

Figure 6. Microstructures of dried potato slices under different pretreatments in different magnifications. (**a**,**b**) Untreated potato samples; (**c**,**d**) blanching pretreatment for 90 s; (**e**,**f**) saline immersion under solution concentration of 20%; and (**g**,**h**) ultrasound pretreatment for 60 min.

The microstructure of the dried samples after blanching pretreatment are shown in Figure 6c,d. The tissue structure of the blanched dried potato slices was uniform and dense, and no obvious pore structure was found. This may be caused by the collapse of the cellular structure after the blanching and drying process. In addition, starch granules were not found in the micrograph field, indicating that the blanching treatment resulted in starch breakage and gelatinization [46]. This was similar to the results of a study on sweet potato bars [57].

The samples from the saline immersion pretreatment had a relatively loose and porous structure (Figure 6e,f). The cytoskeletal structure became coarse as compared to the untreated samples, and starch granules were no longer visible in the samples. This may be due to the internal modification of the starch particles by the components of osmotic solution during processing [67]. After the ultrasound pretreatment, the boundaries of the cells were fuzzy, while the starch granules could be also clearly seen (Figure 6g,h). This was because the ultrasound pretreatment caused changes in the cell structure and formed microchannels on the surface of the potato samples, and the microchannels were combined with the original pore structure, which may be due to the cavitation and sponge effects of the ultrasound waves [68]. The observation of the microstructure of the material was helpful in understanding the effects of pretreatment on the drying rate and appearance deformation.

4. Conclusions

The application of blanching, saline immersion, and ultrasound pretreatment had significant effects on the drying characteristics, 3D appearance, quality characteristics, and microstructure of the potato slices. The results showed that pretreatment significantly enhanced the drying process of the potato slices and affected the 3D appearance during drying. All the pretreatment methods reduced the shrinkage during the drying process relative to the untreated potatoes. The curling degree was quantitatively characterized by height standard deviation (HSD). The results showed that the saline immersion and blanching pretreatments inhibited the curling of the potato slices, while the ultrasound pretreatment greatly aggravated the curling.

Through the quality analysis of the dried potato slices, it was found that the color difference value, total polyphenol content, and antioxidant activity of the potato slices were significantly different under the different pretreatment conditions. The blanching pretreatment could significantly inhibit color deterioration and maintain a higher total polyphenol content and antioxidant activity. Although the blanching pretreatment could significantly improve the nutritional quality and color of the potato slices, it could not significantly reduce the curling degree. Therefore, blanching pretreatment combined with saline immersion may be an optimal alternative pretreatment method for potato slice drying.

The microstructures of the dried potato slices were observed and analyzed by SEM. The microstructures of the dried potato slices were significantly changed under the different pretreatments, which was helpful in understanding and verifying the effects of pretreatment on the drying kinetics and appearance deformation. In addition, the mechanism of the 3D appearance changes caused by pretreatment needs to be further studied. This paper can provide a certain reference for the 3D appearance change and control of agricultural products during the drying process.

Author Contributions: Conceptualization, J.-W.B. and X.-Y.T.; data curation, J.-W.B. and Y.D.; formal analysis, Y.D.; funding acquisition, J.-R.C.; investigation, J.-W.B., Y.D. and Y.-C.W.; methodology, Y.-C.W. and X.-Y.T.; project administration, X.-Y.T.; resources, L.Z.; software, Y.-C.W. and L.Z.; supervision, X.-Y.T.; validation, Y.-C.W.; visualization, Y.D. and L.Z.; writing—original draft, J.-W.B. and Y.D.; writing—review and editing, J.-W.B. and X.-Y.T. All authors have read and agreed to the published version of the manuscript.

Funding: This research was funded by the Jiangsu Key R&D Program (Modern Agriculture), Grant No: BE2019319.

Institutional Review Board Statement: Not applicable.

Informed Consent Statement: Not applicable.

Data Availability Statement: Not applicable.

Conflicts of Interest: The authors declare no conflict of interest.

References

1. Feng, X.; Hu, Q.; Zhu, A. Model and character of hot air convection drying of potato slice. *Cereals Oils* **2018**, *31*, 52–55.
2. Huang, Q.; Shu, T.; Liu, X.; Ouyang, M.; Zheng, M. Overview of the nutritional value of potato. *Mod. Food* **2018**, *16*, 58–59.
3. Wang, R.; Zhang, M.; Mujumdar, A.S. Effect of osmotic dehydration on microwave freeze-drying characteristics and quality of potato chips. *Dry. Technol.* **2010**, *28*, 798–806. [CrossRef]
4. Delaplace, P.; Brostaux, Y.; Fauconnier, M.L.; du Jardin, P. Potato (*Solanum tuberosum* L.) tuber physiological age index is a valid reference frame in postharvest ageing studies. *Postharvest Biol. Technol.* **2008**, *50*, 103–106. [CrossRef]
5. Sonnewald, S.; Sonnewald, U. Regulation of potato tuber sprouting. *Planta* **2014**, *239*, 27–38. [CrossRef]
6. Hii, C.L.; Ong, S.P.; Vap, J.Y.; Putranto, A.; Mangindaan, D. Hybrid drying of food and bioproducts: A review. *Dry. Technol.* **2021**, *39*, 1554–1579. [CrossRef]
7. Putranto, A.; Chen, X.D. Reaction engineering approach modeling of intensified drying of fruits and vegetables using microwave, ultrasonic and infrared-heating. *Dry. Technol.* **2020**, *38*, 747–757. [CrossRef]
8. Albosharib, D.; Noshad, M.; Jooyandeh, H.; Dizaji, H.Z. Effect of freezing and radiofrequency pretreatments on quality. *J. Food Process. Preserv.* **2021**, *45*, e16062. [CrossRef]
9. Kręcisz, M.; Kolniak-Ostek, J.; Stępień, B.; Łyczko, J.; Pasławska, M.; Musiałowska, J. Influence of drying methods and vacuum impregnation on selected quality factors of dried sweet potato. *Agriculture* **2021**, *11*, 858. [CrossRef]
10. Djebli, A.; Hanini, S.; Badaoui, O.; Haddad, B.; Benhamou, A. Modeling and comparative analysis of solar drying behavior of potatoes. *Renew. Energy* **2020**, *145*, 1494–1506. [CrossRef]
11. Farias, R.P.; Gomez, R.S.; Sliva, W.P.; Sliva, L.P.L.; Neto, G.L.O.; Santos, I.B.; Carmo, J.E.F.; Nascimento, J.J.S.; Lima, A.G.B. Heat and mass transfer, and volume variations in banana slices during convective hot air drying: An experimental analysis. *Agriculture* **2020**, *10*, 423. [CrossRef]
12. Deng, L.Z.; Mujumdar, A.S.; Yang, W.X.; Zhang, Q.; Zheng, Z.A.; Wu, M.; Xiao, H.W. Hot air impingement drying kinetics and quality attributes of orange peel. *J. Food Process. Preserv.* **2019**, *44*, e14294. [CrossRef]
13. Ando, Y.; Maeda, Y.; Mizutani, K.; Wakatsuki, N.; Hagiwara, S.; Nabetani, H. Impact of blanching and freeze-thaw pretreatment on drying rate of carrot roots in relation to changes in cell membrane function and cell wall structure. *LWT* **2016**, *71*, 40–46. [CrossRef]
14. Mehta, D.; Prasad, P.; Bansal, V.; Sissiqul, M.W.; Sharma, A. Effect of drying techniques and treatment with blanching on the physicochemical analysis of bitter-gourd and capsicum. *LWT* **2017**, *84*, 479–488. [CrossRef]
15. Liu, P.; Mujumdar, A.S.; Zhang, M.; Jiang, H. Comparison of Three Blanching Treatments on the Color and Anthocyanin Level of the Microwave-Assisted Spouted Bed Drying of Purple Flesh Sweet Potato. *Dry. Technol.* **2015**, *33*, 66–71. [CrossRef]
16. Gomide, A.I.; Monteiro, R.L.; Carciofi, B.A.M.; Laurindo, J.B. The Effect of Pretreatments on the Physical Properties and Starch Structure of Potato Chips Dried by Microwaves under Vacuum. *Foods* **2022**, *11*, 2259. [CrossRef]
17. Sharma, P.R.; Varma, A.J. Thermal stability of cellulose and their nanoparticles: Effect of incremental increases in carboxyl and aldehyde groups. *Carbohydr. Polym.* **2014**, *114*, 339–343. [CrossRef]
18. Zou, K.; Teng, J.; Huang, L.; Dai, X.; Wei, B. Effect of osmotic pretreatment on quality of mango chips by explosion puffing drying. *LWT Food Sci. Technol.* **2013**, *51*, 253–259. [CrossRef]
19. Dehghannya, J.; Bozorghi, S.; Heshmati, M.K. Low temperature hot air drying of potato cubes subjected to osmotic dehydration and intermittent microwave: Drying kinetics, energy consumption and product quality indexes. *Heat Mass Transf.* **2018**, *54*, 929–954. [CrossRef]
20. Chinenye, N.M.; Onyenwigwe, D.I.; Abam, F.; Lamrani, B.; Simo-Tagne, M.; Bekkioui, N.; Bennamoun, L.; Said, Z. Influence of hot water blanching and saline immersion period on the thermal effusivity and the drying kinetics of hybrid solar drying of sweet potato chips. *Sol. Energy* **2022**, *240*, 176–192. [CrossRef]
21. Pei, Y.; Li, Z.; Xu, W.; Song, C.; Li, J.; Song, F. Effects of ultrasound pretreatment followed by far-infrared drying on physicochemical properties, antioxidant activity and aroma compounds of saffron (*Crocus sativus* L.). *Food Biosci.* **2021**, *42*, 101186. [CrossRef]
22. Liu, Y.; Zeng, Y.; Hu, X.; Sun, X. Effect of ultrasonic power on water removal kinetics and moisture migration of kiwifruit slices during contact ultrasound intensified heat pump drying. *Food Bioproc. Technol.* **2020**, *13*, 430–441. [CrossRef]
23. Jarahizadeh, H.; Dinani, S.T. Influence of applied time and power of ultrasonic pretreatment on convective drying of potato slices. *Food Sci. Technol.* **2019**, *28*, 365–376. [CrossRef] [PubMed]
24. Zhang, J.; Fan, L.P. Effects of preliminary treatment by ultrasonic and convective air drying on the properties and oil absorption of potato chips. *Ultrason. Sonochem.* **2021**, *74*, 105548. [CrossRef]
25. Xu, X.; Zhang, L.; Feng, Y.; Yagoub, A.A.; Sun, Y.; Ma, H.; Zhou, C. Vacuum pulsation drying of okra (*Abelmoschus esculentus* L. Moench): Better retention of the quality characteristics by flat sweep frequency and pulsed ultrasound pretreatment. *Food Chem.* **2020**, *326*, 127026. [CrossRef] [PubMed]
26. Rashid, M.T.; Ma, H.L.; Jatoi, M.A.; Hashim, M.M.; Wali, A.; Safdar, B. Influence of Ultrasonic Pretreatment with Hot Air Drying on Nutritional Quality and Structural Related Changes in Dried Sweet Potatoes. *Int. J. Food Eng.* **2018**, *15*, 20180409. [CrossRef]
27. Bai, J.; Tian, X.; Liu, Y.; Xu, S.; Luo, H. Studies on Drying Characteristics and Shrinkage Kinetics Modelling of *Colocasia gigantea* Slices during Thin Layer Drying. *J. Chin. Inst. Food Sci. Technol.* **2018**, *18*, 124–130.
28. Khzazei, N.B.; Tavakoli, T.; Ghasemian, H.; Khoshtaghaza, M.H.; Banakar, A. Applied machine vision and artificial neural network for modeling and controlling of the grape drying process. *Comput. Electron. Agric.* **2013**, *98*, 205–213.

29. Sampson, D.J.; Chang, Y.K.; Rupasinghe, H.P.V.; Zaman, Q.U.Z. A dual-view computer-vision system for volume and image texture analysis in multiple apple slices drying. *J. Food Eng.* **2014**, *127*, 49–57. [CrossRef]
30. Cai, J.; Lu, Y.; Bai, J.; Sun, L.; Xiao, H. Three-dimensional imaging of morphological changes of potato slices during drying. *Trans. Chin. Soc. Agric. Eng.* **2019**, *35*, 278–284.
31. Wasenmüller, O.; Stricker, D. Comparison of Kinect V1 and V2 Depth Images in Terms of Accuracy and Precision. In Proceedings of the 13th Asian Conference on Computer Vision (ACCV), Taipei, Taiwan, 20–24 November 2016.
32. Esturk, O. Intermittent and Continuous Microwave-Convective Air-Drying Characteristics of Sage (*Salvia officinalis*) Leaves. *Food Bioproc. Technol.* **2012**, *5*, 1664–1673. [CrossRef]
33. Sun, L.; Zhang, P.; Zheng, X.; Cai, J.; Bai, J. Three-dimensional morphological changes of potato slices during the drying process. *Curr. Res. Food Sci.* **2021**, *4*, 910–916. [CrossRef] [PubMed]
34. Le Cozler, Y.; Allain, C.; Caillot, A.; Delouard, J.M.; Delattre, L.; Luginbuhl, T.; Faverdin, P. High-precision scanning system for complete 3D cow body shape imaging and analysis of morphological traits. *Comput. Electron. Agric.* **2019**, *157*, 447–453. [CrossRef]
35. Ruchay, A.; Kober, A.; Dorofeev, K.; Kolpakov, V.; Miroshnikov, S. Accurate body measurement of live cattle using three depth cameras and non-rigid 3-D shape recovery. *Comput. Electron. Agric.* **2020**, *179*, 105821. [CrossRef]
36. Liu, K.; Xiao, X.; Wang, J.; Chen, C.O.; Hu, H. Polyphenolic composition and antioxidant, antiproliferative, and antimicrobial activities of mushroom *Inonotus sanghuang*. *LWT Food Sci. Technol.* **2017**, *82*, 154–161. [CrossRef]
37. Zhu, K.X.; Lian, C.X.; Guo, X.N.; Wei, P.; Zhou, H.M. Antioxidant activities and total phenolic contents of various extracts from defatted wheat germ. *Food Chem.* **2011**, *126*, 1122–1126. [CrossRef]
38. Chu, Y.; Wei, S.; Ding, Z.; Mei, J.; Xie, J. Application of Ultrasound and Curing Agent during Osmotic Dehydration to Improve the Quality Properties of Freeze-Dried Yellow Peach (*Amygdalus persica*) Slices. *Agriculture* **2021**, *11*, 1069. [CrossRef]
39. Mukherjee, S.; Chattopadhyay, P.K. Whirling bed blanching of potato cubes and its effects on product quality. *J. Food Eng.* **2007**, *78*, 52–60. [CrossRef]
40. Deng, L.Z.; Pan, Z.; Mujumdar, A.S.; Zhao, J.H.; Zheng, Z.A.; Gao, Z.J.; Xiao, H.W. High-humidity hot air impingement blanching (HHAIB) enhances drying quality of apricots by inactivating the enzymes, reducing drying time and altering cellular structure. *Food Control* **2018**, *96*, 104–111. [CrossRef]
41. Wang, H.; Karim, M.A.; Vidyarthi, S.K.; Xie, L.; Liu, Z.L.; Gao, L.; Zhang, J.S.; Xiao, H.W. Vacuum-steam pulsed blanching (VSPB) softens texture and enhances drying rate of carrot by altering cellular structure, pectin polysaccharides and water state. *Innov. Food Sci. Emerg. Technol.* **2021**, *74*, 102801. [CrossRef]
42. Lagnika, C.; Jiang, N.; Song, J.; Li, D.; Liu, C.; Huang, J.; Wei, Q.; Zhang, M. Effects of pretreatments on properties of microwave-vacuum drying of sweet potato slices. *Dry. Technol.* **2019**, *37*, 1901–1914. [CrossRef]
43. Ricce, C.; Rojas, M.L.; Miano, A.C.; Siche, R.; Augusto, P.E.D. Ultrasound pre-treatment enhances the carrot drying and rehydration. *Food Res. Int.* **2016**, *89*, 701–708. [CrossRef] [PubMed]
44. Wang, J.; Mujumdar, A.S.; Deng, L.Z.; Gao, Z.J.; Xiao, H.W.; Raghavan, G.S.V. High-humidity hot air impingement blanching alters texture, cell-wall polysaccharides, water status and distribution of seedless grape. *Carbohydr. Polym.* **2018**, *194*, 9–17. [CrossRef]
45. Wang, J.; Law, C.L.; Nema, P.K.; Zhao, J.H.; Liu, Z.L.; Deng, L.Z.; Gao, Z.J.; Xiao, H.W. Pulsed vacuum drying enhances drying kinetics and quality of lemon slices. *J. Food Eng.* **2018**, *224*, 129–138. [CrossRef]
46. Li, Y.; Zhang, Y.; Liu, H.; Jin, X.; Liu, X. Impacts of different blanching pretreatments on the quality of dried potato chips and fried potato crisps undergoing heat pump drying. *Int. J. Food Eng.* **2021**, *17*, 517–527. [CrossRef]
47. Mahiuddin, M.; Rodriguez-Ramirez, J.; Khan, M.I.H.; Kumar, C.; Rahman, M.M.; Karim, M.A. Shrinkage of food materials during drying: Current status and challenges. *Compr. Rev. Food Sci. Food Saf.* **2018**, *17*, 1113–1126. [CrossRef] [PubMed]
48. Fante, C.; Correa, J.; Natividade, M.; Lima, J.; Lima, L. Drying of plums (*Prunus* sp., c.v Gulfblaze) treated with KCl in the field and subjected to pulsed vacuum osmotic dehydration. *Int. J. Food Sci. Technol.* **2011**, *46*, 1080–1085. [CrossRef]
49. Liu, Y.H.; Sun, C.Y.; Lei, Y.Q.; Yu, H.C.; Xi, H.H.; Duan, X. Contact ultrasound strengthened far-infrared radiation drying on pear slices: Effects on drying characteristics, microstructure, and quality attributes. *Dry. Technol.* **2019**, *37*, 745–758. [CrossRef]
50. Rashid, M.T.; Ma, H.; Jatoi, M.A.; Wali, A.; El-Mesery, H.S.; Ali, Z.; Sarpong, F. Effect of infrared drying with multifrequency ultrasound pretreatments on the stability of phytochemical properties, antioxidant potential, and textural quality of dried sweet potatoes. *J. Food Biochem.* **2019**, *43*, e12809. [CrossRef]
51. Aral, S.; Bese, A.V. Convective drying of hawthorn fruit (*Crataegus* spp.): Effect of experimental parameters on drying kinetics, color, shrinkage, and rehydration capacity. *Food Chem.* **2016**, *210*, 577–584. [CrossRef]
52. He, C.; Zhang, M.; Devahastin, S. Investigation on spontaneous shape change of 4D printed starch-based purees from purple sweet potatoes as induced by microwave dehydration. *ACS Appl. Mater. Int.* **2020**, *12*, 37896–37905. [CrossRef] [PubMed]
53. Barragan-Iglesias, J.; Sablani, S.S.; Mendez-Lagunas, L.L. Texture analysis of dried papaya (*Carica papaya* L., cv. Maradol) pretreated with calcium and osmotic dehydration. *Dry. Technol.* **2019**, *37*, 906–919. [CrossRef]
54. Miano, A.C.; Rojas, M.L.; Augusto, P.E.D. Structural changes caused by ultrasound pretreatment: Direct and indirect demonstration in potato cylinders. *Ultrason. Sonochem.* **2019**, *52*, 176–183. [CrossRef] [PubMed]
55. Boateng, I.D.; Yang, X.M. Process optimization of intermediate-wave infrared drying: Screening by Plackett–Burman; comparison of Box–Behnken and central composite design and evaluation: A case study. *Ind. Crop. Prod.* **2021**, *162*, 113287. [CrossRef]

56. Barani, Y.H.; Zhang, M.; Wang, B. Effect of thermal and ultrasonic pretreatment on enzyme inactivation, color, phenolics and flavonoids contents of infrared freeze-dried rose flower. *J. Food Meas. Charact.* **2021**, *15*, 995–1004. [CrossRef]
57. Xiao, H.W.; Lin, H.; Yao, X.D.; Du, Z.L.; Lou, Z.; Gao, Z.J. Effects of Different Pretreatments on Drying Kinetics and Quality of Sweet Potato Bars Undergoing Air Impingement Drying. *Int. J. Food Eng.* **2009**, *5*, 5. [CrossRef]
58. Pimpaporn, P.; Devahastin, S.; Chiewchan, N. Effects of combined pretreatments on drying kinetics and quality of potato chips undergoing low-pressure superheated steam drying. *J. Food Eng.* **2007**, *81*, 318–329. [CrossRef]
59. Chao, E.; Li, J.; Fan, L. Enhancing drying efficiency and quality of seed-used pumpkin using ultrasound, freeze-thawing and blanching pretreatments. *Food Chem.* **2022**, *384*, 132496. [CrossRef]
60. Sakooei-Vayghan, R.; Peighambardoust, S.H.; Hesari, J.; Peressini, D. Effects of osmotic dehydration (with and without sonication) and pectin based coating pretreatments on functional properties and color of hot-air dried apricot cubes. *Food Chem.* **2020**, *311*, 125978. [CrossRef]
61. Sarkar, A.; Ahmed, T.; Alam, M.; Rahman, S.; Pramanik, S.K. Influences of osmotic dehydration on drying behavior and product quality of coconut (*Cocos nucifera*). *Asian Food Sci. J.* **2020**, *15*, 21–30. [CrossRef]
62. Gamboa-Santos, J.; Soria, A.C.; Villamiel, M.; Montilla, A. Quality parameters in convective dehydrated carrots blanched by ultrasound and conventional treatment. *Food Chem.* **2013**, *141*, 616–624. [CrossRef] [PubMed]
63. Mothibe, K.J.; Zhang, M.; Nsor-atindana, J.; Wang, Y.C. Use of ultrasound pretreatment in drying of fruits: Drying rates, quality attributes, and shelf life extension. *Dry. Technol.* **2011**, *29*, 1611–1621. [CrossRef]
64. Ren, F.; Perussello, C.A.; Zhang, Z.; Kerry, J.P.; Tiwari, B.K. Impact of ultrasound and blanching on functional properties of hot-air dried and freeze dried onions. *LWT Food Sci. Technol.* **2018**, *87*, 102–111. [CrossRef]
65. Salehi, B.; Zucca, P.; Orhan, I.E.; Azzini, E.; Adetunji, C.O.; Mohammed, S.A.; Banerjee, S.K.; Sharopov, F.; Rigano, D.; Sharifi-Rad, J.; et al. Allicin and health: A comprehensive review. *Trends Food Sci. Technol.* **2019**, *86*, 502–516. [CrossRef]
66. Feng, Y.; Xu, B.; El Gasim, A.Y.A.; Ma, H.; Sun, Y.; Xu, X.; Yu, X.; Zhou, C. Role of drying techniques on physical, rehydration, flavor, bioactive compounds and antioxidant characteristics of garlic. *Food Chem.* **2021**, *343*, 128404. [CrossRef] [PubMed]
67. Ahmed, M.; Sorifa, A.M.; Eun, J.B. Effect of pretreatments and drying temperatures on sweet potato flour. *Int. J. Food Sci. Technol.* **2010**, *45*, 726–732. [CrossRef]
68. Ortuño, C.; Pérez-Munuera, I.; Puig, A.; Riera, E.; Garcia-Perez, J.V. Influence of power ultrasound application on mass transport and microstructure of orange peel during hot air drying. *Phys. Procedia* **2010**, *3*, 153–159. [CrossRef]

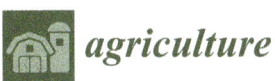

Article

Characterization of Polyphenols in a Sicilian Autochthonous White Grape Variety (PDO) for Monitoring Production Process and Shelf-Life of Wines

Mattia Rapa *, Vanessa Giannetti and Maurizio Boccacci Mariani

Department of Management, Sapienza University of Rome, 00161 Rome, Italy
* Correspondence: mattia.rapa@uniroma1.it

Abstract: Sicilian wines have shown a growing expansion in the international market, and over 60% of the production of them is focused on quality products. Grillo is a white grape variety, and it is among the best-known variety, with a cultivated area of 6300 ha and with the vocation of being particularly predisposed to aging for years or even decades. This paper aimed to perform a physiochemical (SSC and pH) and polyphenolic characterization of Grillo wines that were produced by a selected winery in the years 2011–2021 using an optimized RP-HPLC-DAD method. The polyphenols fraction was assessed by means a semiquantitative analysis on which, statistical processing was carried out. The HCA and PCA highlighted the presence of three clusters in the samples. Cluster 1 was composed of the samples from the years 2011–2014, cluster 2 composed of the samples from 2015–2017, and cluster 3 composed of the samples from 2019–2021. Using an HSD Tukey test, it was possible to point out that some compounds were makers of specific clusters and therefore, specific vintages. This preliminary study showed that polyphenols are suitable markers that can be used to identify Grillo vintages, and they should be also related to the storage conditions or different production processes.

Keywords: polyphenols; Sicily; chemometrics; Grillo; wine; grape

Citation: Rapa, M.; Giannetti, V.; Boccacci Mariani, M. Characterization of Polyphenols in a Sicilian Autochthonous White Grape Variety (PDO) for Monitoring Production Process and Shelf-Life of Wines. *Agriculture* **2022**, *12*, 1888. https://doi.org/10.3390/agriculture12111888

Academic Editor: Bengang Wu

Received: 10 October 2022
Accepted: 7 November 2022
Published: 10 November 2022

Publisher's Note: MDPI stays neutral with regard to jurisdictional claims in published maps and institutional affiliations.

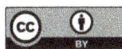

Copyright: © 2022 by the authors. Licensee MDPI, Basel, Switzerland. This article is an open access article distributed under the terms and conditions of the Creative Commons Attribution (CC BY) license (https://creativecommons.org/licenses/by/4.0/).

1. Introduction

Viticulture consists of the set of agronomic techniques that are used for the cultivation of the vine. From planting vines to their removal, viticulture embraces every aspect of the grape plant's life. The cultivation of vineyards is one of the most important and essential phases of the wine making process [1–3]. The first evidence of Sicilian viticulture seems to date back to the 2nd millennium BC. Influenced by the various dominations that have occurred on the island, Sicilian viticulture is today characterized by a complexity of native cultivars [4]. Sicily, with 17.5% of the national production, is the Italian region with the largest wine-growing area. In recent decades, Sicilian wines have experienced a growing expansion in the international market [5]. Indeed, since the early 1990s, Sicilian wine producers have understood the need to increase the quality of their production to compete with the market challenges of the global market [6]. Over 60% of the production is focused on quality wines with 24 PDO (Protected Designation of Origin) and 7 PGI (Protected Geographical Indication) certifications. Among the best-known and autochthonous ones are Nero D'Avola, Frappato, Nerello, Grillo, Catarratto, Carricante, and Marsala [6].

The wide organoleptic variety of these wines—from the more alcoholic and full-bodied ones to the fresher, elegant, and fragrant ones—is due not only to the grape variety, but to the different pedoclimatic conditions of the Sicilian Island [7]. The Mediterranean climate, in fact, is characterized by hilly and coastal areas with mild winters and low rainfall and hot summers, and sometimes it is sultry and ventilated, while the mountainous and inland areas are affected by a continental climate, which is cold and rigid, especially on the Etna and Madonie mountains, which strongly determines the daily and seasonal temperature variations [8]. The characteristics and production of the different cultivars are also influenced by the differences in the composition of the soils of the different areas [9]. For example, the lava soils of Etna are optimal for the Carricante and Nerello vines, and the calcareous and clayey soils are optimal for the Nero d'Avola vines, while those of tuff give a sugary charge and a refined aroma to the white wines, in particular to the Grillo [9].

The Grillo is a white grape variety that is famous above all for its role in the Marsala fortified wines of the island [10]. It is still widely planted in western Sicily, with there being a cultivated area of 6300 ha, despite the fall in the trend of Marsala, and it is now most commonly used in a variety of still white wines, both varietal and blended types [11]. Grillo adapts well to the hot and dry Sicilian climate and shows adequate resistance to downy mildew. Its high sugar levels and the ease with which it oxidizes make it a good option for fortification. Grillo can produce wines with an alcohol content that reaches 15/16° vol. [12]. In recent years, as the focus has shifted from quantity to quality, the Sicilian producers of it, thanks to the improvement of viticultural and vinicultural techniques, have begun to revisit the Grillo wines. This has produced Grillo wines of a great organoleptic thickness, savoury, and fragrance that are more pleasant than the rather earthy styles that were previously available. Furthermore, Grillo has the vocation of being particularly predisposed to aging for years or even decades [13].

In this regard, the present study aimed to investigate the possibility of using the total content of polyphenols as an indicator of the shelf-life of Grillo wines.

In the scientific literature, there are some studies on the subject, for example Arena et al. (2021) showed that the phenolic content in Malvasia delle Lipari wine varies over time (6 months of monitoring) and with the storage temperature (30, 35, and 45 °C), and that this aspect was not influenced by the colour of the glass bottle [14]. Diaz-Maroto et al. (2020) showed that after 12 months of bottle storage, a significant loss of the phenolic compounds was observed in all of the analyzed samples [15]. The same trend was found by Castellanos et al. (2021), but they also highlighted that after 12 months of storage, no changes in the phenolic content were reported [16]. Therefore, the studies on the subject do not show a univocal trend of the phenolic content during storage, so there is a bibliographic gap in the variation of these compounds in white wines during the aging period.

In this context, our research aimed to perform a polyphenolic characterization of the Grillo wines that were produced by a selected winery in the years 2011–2021 using an optimized RP-HPLC-DAD method. The data that were obtained were then processed by a chemometric analysis. In addition, the soluble solids content (SSC) and pH were determined due to their importance as quality indices in winemaking. The SSC are mainly organic sugars, such as glucose, sucrose, and fructose, which affect the taste and transparency of the wine. The pH was used as the measure of its acidity, which is due to the inclusion of organic acids such as lactic acid, malic acid, and others. Furthermore, the pH is an important parameter of complicated biochemical changes during fermentation and winemaking (e.g., degradation of some nutrients or formation of by-products) [17–21].

2. Materials and Methods

2.1. Reagents and Standard Solutions

All reagents used were analytical grade. The acetonitrile, methanol, and formic acid were provided by Merck (Darmstadt, Germany). The water was obtained from a Milli-Q water purification system (Millipore, Bedford, MA, USA). The standards of gallic acid (r2 = 0.9981), p-hydroxybenzoic acid (r2 = 0.9995), and ferulic acid (r2 = 0.9999) were from Sigma-Aldrich (St. Louis, MO, USA). The standard stock solutions of polyphenols were prepared in methanol and stored at 4 °C in the dark.

2.2. Sampling

A total of eighteen Grillo white wines from a Sicilian winery, called "Cantina Cellaro S.C.A.", located in Sambuca di Sicilia (Agrigento, Sicily), were analyzed. All of the samples reported that there was Grillo on the label. The samples were produced during the period of 2011–2021. For the same year of production, two bottles from different production batches were collected. No samples were included for the 2012 and 2018 vintages due to their different storage conditions. The samples were filtered through a 0.45 μm PTFE membrane filter (Merck, Darmstadt, Germany). The analyses were performed in triplicate immediately after we opened the bottle. Table 1 shows the alcohol content and the selling price of the analyzed samples.

Table 1. Sample details declared by the production company.

Production Year	Alcohol Content	Price
2011	12.5% vol	7.70 EUR
2013	13% vol	10.00 EUR
2014	13% vol	9.90 EUR
2015	13% vol	7.20 EUR
2016	13% vol	10.20 EUR
2017	12% vol	7.90 EUR
2019	12.5% vol	6.80 EUR
2020	13% vol	7.20 EUR
2021	12.5% vol	9.95 EUR

2.3. HPLC Analysis

A Waters HPLC system (600 Waters, Milford, MA, USA), which was entirely assembled with PEEK tubing, was used for the chromatographic analysis. The HPLC system was equipped with a 20 μL injection loop and coupled to a Waters Photodiode Array Detector (2998 Waters, Milford, MA, USA) set at 280 nm. A reversed-phase Kinetex C18 column (250 × 4.6 mm i.d., 5 μm pore size) (Phenomenex, Torrance, CA, USA) was used. The mobile phase consisted of a 0.5% (v/v) solution of formic acid (eluent A) and acetonitrile (eluent B). The gradient elution was as follows: 90:10% (A:B) from 0 to 2 min, 85:15% for 13 min, 50:50% for 2 min, and 10:90% for 12 min, which was followed by the cleaning and balancing of the column [22–28]. The separation was achieved after 19 min with a flow rate of 1 mL/min. Data acquisition and processing was performed using the Empower 2 software. Some polyphenols were identified by comparing their retention times with those of the pure standards, and their quantification was carried out using the external standard method.

2.4. Physiochemical Analysis

The soluble solids content (SSC) was measured using an RS PRO portable refractometer (Milan, Italy) at 20 °C. The accuracy of the refractive index was ±0.01, and the °Brix range was 0–20. The pH was measured using a pH-meter (Hanna Instruments, Woonsocket, RI, USA) with an accuracy of 0.001.

2.5. Statistical Analysis

The HSD Tukey test and chemometric data analyses (PCA and CA) were performed using the JMP software (ver. 16.2 Pro, SAS Institute, Cary, NC, USA).

3. Results and Discussions

3.1. Physiochemical Parameters

The presence of phytochemicals in the grapes (such as mineral salts, organic acids, sugars, etc.), and therefore in the wine, deriving from the metabolism of the plants, is closely related to their health properties. Furthermore, these substances are also involved in the evaluation of food quality and safety. Their level in the final product is strictly influenced by the cultivars, environmental factors, cultural practices, and genetic aspects [21]. Zietsman et al. (2015) pointed out that large differences in the SSC in the wines should reflect the variations in the annual climate conditions [29]. Rouxinol et al. (2022) reported that the SSC and pH are important quality parameters that have a great impact on the wine's quality and are usually used to select the right harvest date [17].

Table 2 shows the pH and SSC values that were measured in the analyzed samples.

Table 2. SSC and pH values for Grillo wine samples in the period of 2011–2021.

Sample Vintage	SSC (°Brix)	pH
2011	6.8 ± 0.1 [a,b]	3.36 ± 0.3 [a]
2013	7.0 ± 0.3 [a]	3.27 ± 0.1 [a,b]
2014	6.8 ± 0.1 [a,b]	3.15 ± 0.1 [d]
2015	7.1 ± 0.1 [a]	3.16 ± 0.3 [c,d]
2016	6.8 ± 0.3 [a,b]	3.21 ± 0.1 [b,c,d]
2017	6.4 ± 0.1 [a,b]	3.22 ± 0.3 [b,c]
2019	6.8 ± 0.3 [a,b]	3.17 ± 0.1 [c,d]
2020	6.9 ± 0.1 [a,b]	3.19 ± 0.3 [b,c,d]
2021	6.2 ± 0.1 [b]	3.15 ± 0.1 [c,d]

[a, b, c, d] Results not linked by the same superscript letter are statistically different from the HSD Tukey test.

As for the SSC, which is expressed in °Brix, there is not a great variability between the samples, but it is possible to highlight that the 2021 samples have a lower SSC value than the other vintages do. The only statistically significant difference was found between the 2013 and 2021 samples. The possible correlation of the evidenced difference with the climate conditions was explored. Table 3 shows the climate conditions in the years that were under review. Nevertheless, no significant difference was found with the recovered climate parameters (minimum, medium and maximum temperature, rainy days per year, and relative humidity), therefore, in this context, it is not possible to attribute the SSC difference to the climatic conditions.

Table 3. Climatic conditions in Sambuca di Sicilia, expressed as an average in the years 2013 and 2021, as provided by the producer.

Parameters	2013	2021
Minimum temperature	15.9 °C	15.8 °C
Medium temperature	19.3 °C	19.4 °C
Maximum temperature	22.2 °C	22.6 °C
Rainy days a year	133	121
Relative humidity	77.0%	77.3%

The trend of the pH values also showed a slight variation over the years, going from a maximum of 3.36 in 2011 to a minimum of 3.15 in 2021. Additionally, in this case it is not possible to highlight a significant variability between the samples.

3.2. Chromatographic Results

The polyphenol contents in the wines are related to various factors, such as the grape varieties, the winemaking process, their storage, and their shelf-life. For this purpose, in the present study, the polyphenolic fractions of 18 samples of Grillo wines, which were produced from 2011 to 2021, were investigated. Two samples were analyzed for each vintage. To avoid a bias occurring, all of the samples came from the same vine (Grillo), were produced in the same area (Sambuca di Sicilia, Ag) by the same company (Cantine Cellaro), and were stored in the same storage warehouse.

A fast and reliable chromatographic method was optimized. The separation of the polyphenolic fraction was obtained within 19 min. No extraction step was required, and the samples were only filtered before the analysis. A comparison of the chromatographic profiles of three samples (2011, 2016, and 2021) is reported in Figure 1. Sixteen peaks, each one being attributable to a specific polyphenol, were identified and are numbered (1–16) in Figure 1.

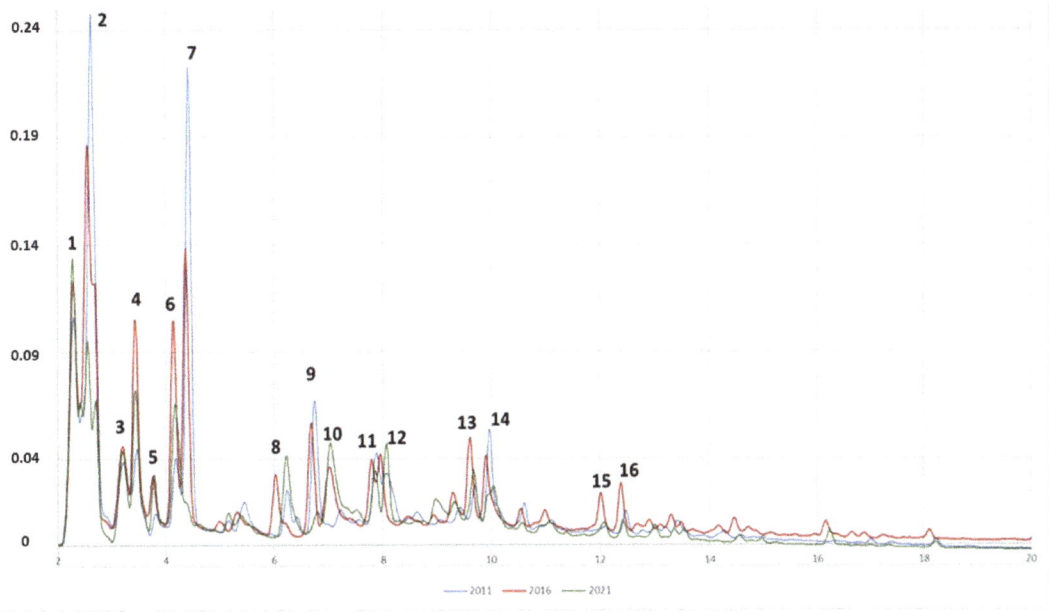

Figure 1. Chromatographic profiles of Grillo—2011 (blue), 2016 (red), and 2021 (green) wine samples.

A semi-quantitative analysis was performed using gallic acid, p-hydroxybenzoic acid, and ferulic acid as external reference standards. Gallic acid (r.t. 3.5 min) was used to quantify the compounds that were identified from peak one to peak seven (range 2–5 min). As we used a reverse phase method, these first eluted compounds are attributable to simple polyphenols. p-Hydroxybenzoic acid (r.t. 8.5 min) was used to quantify the peaks from point eight to point fourteen (range 5–11 min). The compounds that were eluted in this range could be phenolic acids or more complex polyphenols such as catechins, as can be seen from the reference literature. Ferulic acid was used to quantify peak 15 and peak 16 (range 11–19 min), which are the typical area of the anthocyanins, anthocyanidins, and stilbenes.

Table 4 shows the results of the semi-quantitative analysis, which is expressed as equivalent mg of gallic acid (GAE/L), p-hydroxybenzoic acid (PAE/L), and ferulic acid (FAE/L).

Table 4. Semi-quantitative results of the chromatographic analysis of Grillo wines, expressed as mgGAE/L (peaks 1–7), mgPAE/Kg (peaks 8–14), and mgFAE/Kg (peaks 15–16).

No. Peak	2011	2013	2014	2015	2016	2017	2019	2020	2021
1	25.30 ± 1.27	23.60 ± 8.63	31.25 ± 0.49	30.00 ± 1.41	25.90 ± 0.71	29.90 ± 0.71	19.45 ± 0.07	29.55 ± 1.91	26.50 ± 0.28
2	72.25 ± 1.91	68.70 ± 21.40	72.50 ± 0.14	79.35 ± 3.75	62.10 ± 0.99	57.85 ± 4.31	48.60 ± 0.01	18.49 ± 22.2	25.20 ± 0.14
3	11.50 ± 0.71	10.87 ± 2.86	16.35 ± 0.64	13.25 ± 0.49	12.20 ± 0.01	15.90 ± 0.42	11.30 ± 1.70	13.05 ± 0.78	9.36 ± 0.01
4	10.39 ± 0.57	10.60 ± 3.53	13.15 ± 0.35	31.70 ± 1.41	20.55 ± 0.35	26.75 ± 0.07	26.15 ± 0.21	27.45 ± 2.05	14.30 ± 0.14
5	3.32 ± 0.40	4.98 ± 1.75	5.61 ± 0.05	7.03 ± 0.35	6.89 ± 0.20	8.38 ± 0.53	8.00 ± 1.67	8.71 ± 0.53	6.02 ± 0.04
6	7.92 ± 0.03	6.77 ± 2.65	11.70 ± 0.42	14.90 ± 0.42	18.55 ± 0.071	21.30 ± 0.99	13.25 ± 1.06	9.62 ± 0.11	18.80 ± 1.27
7	41.55 ± 1.63	35.50 ± 10.90	40.80 ± 0.71	29.40 ± 2.69	27.35 ± 0.78	26.40 ± 0.99	13.00 ± 1.70	1.58 ± 0.49	0.23 ± 0.01
8	9.46 ± 0.49	7.71 ± 2.25	12.80 ± 0.42	12.05 ± 0.64	15.85 ± 0.07	16.90 ± 0.28	14.25 ± 1.63	10.52 ± 0.95	20.65 ± 0.07
9	28.20 ± 1.13	16.75 ± 5.16	27.15 ± 0.49	27.25 ± 1.06	20.80 ± 0.14	23.10 ± 1.13	12.95 ± 3.18	7.10 ± 0.25	32.55 ± 0.35
10	10.11 ± 0.26	14.20 ± 5.37	16.50 ± 0.57	19.60 ± 0.99	26.70 ± 4.10	26.25 ± 1.06	20.00 ± 5.94	39.80 ± 3.39	7.84 ± 0.27
11	18.80 ± 0.71	15.50 ± 4.53	15.55 ± 0.49	13.85 ± 1.06	14.40 ± 0.71	13.85 ± 0.78	11.10 ± 0.99	10.60 ± 0.01	12.85 ± 0.07
12	20.25 ± 0.92	11.52 ± 3.37	17.85 ± 0.64	18.30 ± 0.28	19.65 ± 0.21	20.35 ± 1.77	11.92 ± 3.37	12.78 ± 14.90	18.70 ± 3.96
13	10.85 ± 0.21	14.60 ± 4.38	15.80 ± 0.85	16.30 ± 0.71	18.85 ± 0.21	17.00 ± 0.57	8.56 ± 0.90	15.40 ± 2.12	15.00 ± 0.01
14	26.30 ± 0.99	21.10 ± 6.36	24.10 ± 1.27	24.75 ± 1.06	25.45 ± 0.21	29.30 ± 1.70	21.40 ± 6.51	7.50 ± 0.17	20.10 ± 0.28
15	1.34 ± 0.06	1.10 ± 0.38	1.22 ± 0.17	2.38 ± 0.08	2.36 ± 0.32	2.18 ± 0.36	2.05 ± 0.09	2.04 ± 0.10	0.57 ± 0.01
16	1.07 ± 0.06	2.53 ± 0.84	1.41 ± 0.13	1.80 ± 0.08	1.81 ± 0.05	1.66 ± 0.16	0.99 ± 0.02	1.76 ± 0.01	0.14 ± 0.02
Total	298.63 ± 10.80	266.05 ± 84.30	323.74 ± 5.66	341.91 ± 16.50	319.42 ± 1.26	337.08 ± 11.00	242.97 ± 22.30	215.97 ± 2.35	228.81 ± 6.21

Some differences emerged from the evaluation of the chromatographic results. For example, in regard to the area of the simple polyphenols, peak two and peak seven showed a similar trend. Their values decreased over time (2011–2017), passing from a value of 75.25 mgGAE/L in peak two in the 2011 sample to 18.45 mgGAE/L in 2020; while for peak seven, this was from 41.55 mgGAE/L in 2011 to 0.23 mg GAE/L in 2021. An opposite trend occurred for peaks four and five, and in fact, their content tended to increase during the shelf-life (peak four: 10.40 mgGAE/L in 2011 and 27.45 mgGAE/L in 2020; peak five: 3.32 mgGAE/L in 2011 and 8.71 mgGAE/L in 2020). Peak six showed an even different trend, its content increased from 7.92 mgGAE/L in 2011 to 21.3 mgGAE/L in 2017, and then, it decreased to 9.62 mgGAE/L in 2020. For the remaining peaks, only peak eight—in the phenolic acids zone—showed a particular trend. Its content, in fact, decreased from 18.8 mgPAE/L in 2011 to 10.6 mgPAE/L in 2020.

Due to the variability of the values that were obtained in the wine of the same cultivar but from subsequent vintages and the different trends that were manifested by each single compound, it was not possible to give a univocal interpretation of the results. To this end, a statistical processing was carried out after the preliminary evaluation.

3.3. Chemometric Analysis

As previously reported, the physiochemical and chromatographic results showed some differentiations between the samples, however, they were not significant to reach an effective conclusion. Therefore, several chemometric tools were applied to the data matrix to improve the characterization and to highlight the possible categorizations. The first chemometric application was the Hierarchical Cluster Analysis (HCA). Figure 2 shows the resulting constellation diagram of the observed clusters. The samples appear to be classified into three main clusters which are distributed by their years of production. In fact, one cluster includes samples of the years 2011, 2013, and 2014, and the second one contains samples of the years 2015, 2016, and 2017, while the third one contains samples of the years 2019, 2020, and 2021. The only deviation was found for a sample that was produced in 2013 which differs from the composition trend of the other samples that were produced in the period of 2011–2014. This sample, in fact, showed a total content of polyphenols that was lower than that of the samples that were produced in a similar vintages, and it was included in the cluster of samples that were produced in the period of 2019–2021, which were characterized instead by a lower level of these compounds. The deviation of the 2013 sample which is highlighted by the HCA results could be related to inadequate storage conditions that influenced the polyphenol content.

The clustering analysis revealed that the dataset consisting of the physiochemical and polyphenol analysis results is suitable for a sample classification.

After the clustering analysis, a Principal Component Analysis (PCA) was performed to highlight the natural grouping of the samples. The autoscaling pre-treatment was performed on the dataset to exclude the variance that is related to the different units of measurement. The unsupervised PCA scores and loadings are plotted in Figure 3. The first two PCs explain 54.1% of the total variability. The PCA plots confirm the groupings that were noted earlier in the HCA. In fact, the samples from 2011 to 2014 are located in the lower right area, the samples from 2015 to 2017 are in the upper right area, while the samples from 2019 to 2021 are all in the left area of the score plot. Additionally, in this case, one sample belonging to the 2013 vintage was located in a different area from that of the 2011–2014 ones.

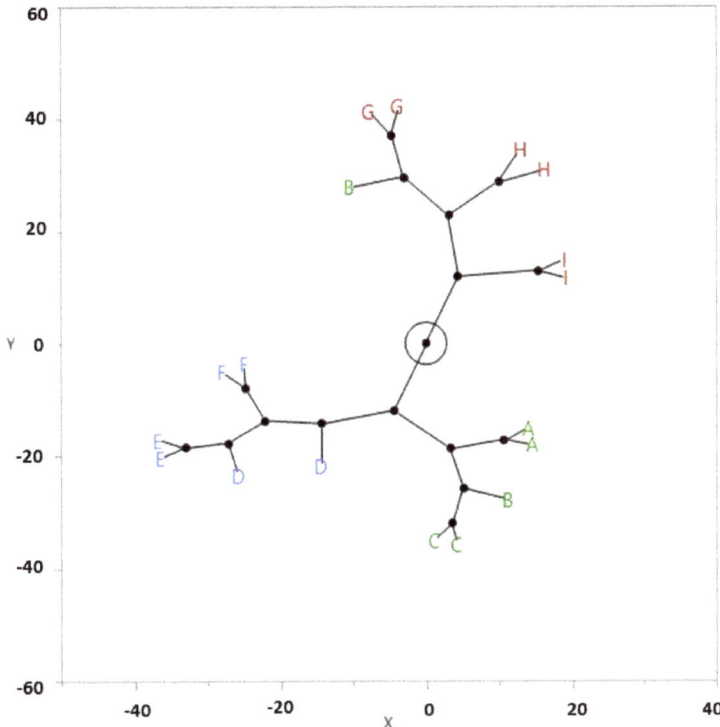

Figure 2. Constellation diagram from HCA on physiochemical and chromatographic results. Green: 2011–2014, Blue: 2015–2017, Red: 2019–2021. A: 2011, B: 2013, C: 2014, D: 2015, E: 2016, F: 2017, G: 2019, H: 2020, I: 2021.

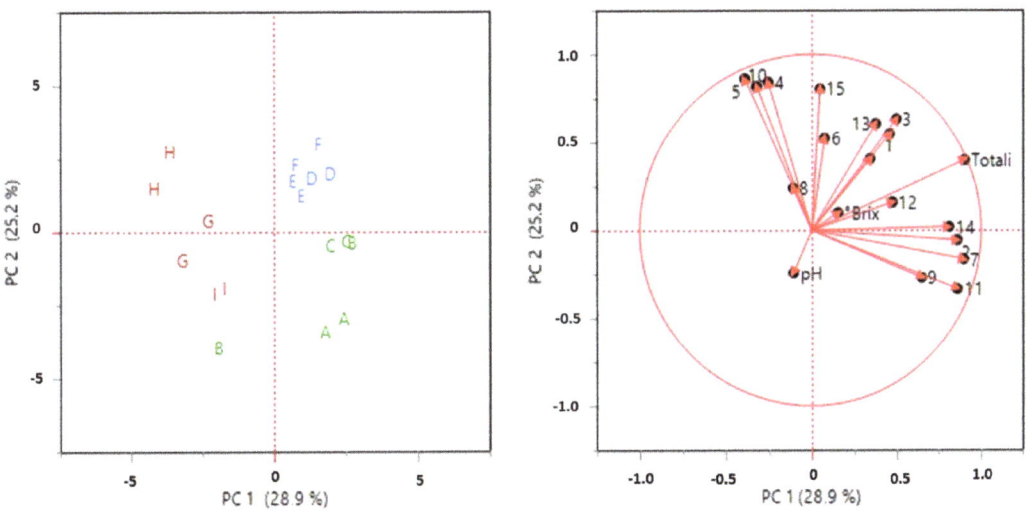

Figure 3. Score and loading plots by PCA on physiochemical and chromatographic results. Green: 2011–2014, Blue: 2015–2017, Red: 2019–2021. A: 2011, B: 2013, C: 2014, D: 2015, E: 2016, F: 2017, G: 2019, H: 2020, I: 2021.

It can be noted that on PC1, it is possible to distinguish the 2019–2021 samples from the others, and the variable that most influenced this grouping were the compounds related to peaks 14, 2, and 7, while with PC2, it is possible to the separate the samples from 2011–2014 and from 2015–2017, and the compounds no. 15 and no. 6 affected this partition.

From the HCA and PCA, it was found that the samples could be grouped into three clusters without any supervision. The three highlighted clusters are characterized by the samples from the same production years, i.e., cluster 1: 2011–2014, cluster 2: 2015–2017, and cluster 3: 2019–2021. Based on these results, the mean and standard deviation of the physiochemical and polyphenol content were calculated according to the three clusters (Table 5).

Table 5. Mean and standard deviation of the physiochemical and polyphenol content according to the three clusters, expressed as mgGAE/L (peak 1–7), mgPAE/L (peak 8–14), and mgFAE/L (peak 15–16).

Variables	2011–2014	2015–2017	2019–2021
Peak 1	26.70 ± 5.31 [a]	28.60 ± 2.23 [a]	25.20 ± 4.71 [a]
Peak 2	71.20 ± 9.78 [a]	66.40 ± 10.5 [a]	30.80 ± 17.30 [b]
Peak 3	12.90 ± 3.00 [a]	13.80 ± 1.73 [a]	11.20 ± 1.85 [a]
Peak 4	11.40 ± 2.11 [b]	26.30 ± 5.04 [a]	22.60 ± 6.55 [a]
Peak 5	4.64 ± 1.33 [b]	7.44 ± 0.80 [a]	7.58 ± 1.47 [a]
Peak 6	8.80 ± 2.60 [b]	18.30 ± 2.91 [a]	13.90 ± 4.20 [a]
Peak 7	39.30 ± 5.75 [a]	27.70 ± 1.91 [b]	4.94 ± 6.32 [c]
Peak 8	9.99 ± 2.54 [a]	14.90 ± 2.30 [a,b]	15.10 ± 4.66 [b]
Peak 9	24.00 ± 6.14 [a]	23.70 ± 3.01 [a]	17.50 ± 12.00 [a]
Peak 10	13.60 ± 3.77 [a]	24.20 ± 4.05 [a]	22.50 ± 14.70 [a]
Peak 11	16.60 ± 2.67 [a]	14.00 ± 0.726 [a,b]	11.50 ± 1.15 [b]
Peak 12	16.50 ± 4.33 [a]	19.40 ± 1.23 [a]	14.50 ± 7.78 [a]
Peak 13	13.80 ± 3.05 [a,b]	17.40 ± 1.25 [a]	13.00 ± 3.59 [b]
Peak 14	23.80 ± 3.75 [a,b]	26.50 ± 2.37 [a]	16.30 ± 7.46 [b]
Peak 15	1.22 ± 0.219 [b]	2.31 ± 0.24 [a]	1.55 ± 0.77 [b]
Peak 16	1.67 ± 0.783 [a]	1.76 ± 0.11 [a]	0.96 ± 0.72 [a]
Total	296.00 ± 46.10 [a]	333.00 ± 13.80 [a]	229.00 ± 15.90 [b]
SSC (°Brix)	6.87 ± 0.10 [a]	6.77 ± 0.31 [a]	6.63 ± 0.33 [a]
pH	3.26 ± 0.09 [a]	2.70 ± 1.24 [a]	3.17 ± 0.01 [a]

[a, b, c] Values in the same row not linked by the same superscript letters are significantly different from the HSD Tukey test.

An HSD Tukey test was performed to highlight the significant differences between the variables in the three clusters. It can be seen that the quantity of compound no. 2, which is attributable to a simple polyphenol, is significantly lower in the 2019–2021 samples than they is in the 2011–2014 and 2015–2017 ones. The compounds that are related to the phenolic acids, i.e., compounds no. 4, no. 5, and no. 6, showed a significantly lower concentration in the samples from the period of 2011–2013. Compound no. 7 could be considered as a possible shelf-life marker; in fact, its concentration significantly decreases from cluster 1 (2011–2014) to cluster 3 (2019–2021).

As for the complex polyphenols, such as the flavonoids and stilbenes, only compound no. 15 showed a significantly higher content in the 2015–2017 samples. These compounds give the wine the typical red-brown colour, so their content in white wine is not relevant.

In general, there is also a significant decrease in the polyphenols content. Therefore, the total amount of polyphenols is significantly lower in the 2019–2021 samples.

Following an interview with the winery that supplied the samples, it emerged that in 2015, there was a change in the production process, i.e., during the bleaching phases, and together with bentonite, the use of active carbon was started. In 2019, however, bentonite was totally replaced by active carbon.

These changes in the production process took place precisely in the years that divided the clusters, 2015 and 2019, so the different polyphenol content could also be correlated to these variations.

4. Conclusions

This study aimed to perform a physiochemical (SSC and pH) and polyphenolic characterization of the Grillo wines that were produced by a selected winery in the years 2011–2021 using an optimized RP-HPLC-DAD method.

For the physiochemical parameters, the only statistically significant difference was found for the SSC between the 2013 and 2021 samples. The SSC content should be related to different climatic conditions, but it is not attributable to them in this case.

The polyphenolic fraction was evaluated by a semi-quantitative analysis using gallic acid (r.t. 2–5 min), p-hydroxybenzoic acid (r.t. 5–11 min), and ferulic acid (range 11–19 min) as the external reference standards. These standards were used to quantify the simple polyphenols, phenolic acids, or more complex polyphenols, and anthocyanins, anthocyanidins, and stilbenes, respectively. Due to the variability of the values that were obtained in the wine of the same cultivar but from subsequent vintages, different trends manifested in each single compound, and it was not possible to give a univocal interpretation of the results. To this end, a statistical processing was carried out after the preliminary evaluation.

The HCA and PCA highlighted the presence of three clusters of samples. One cluster includes the samples from the years 2011, 2013, and 2014, the second contains the samples from the years 2015, 2016, and 2017, while the third one the samples from 2019, 2020, and 2021. The means and standard deviation were recalculated based on this clustering, and the HSD Tukey test was applied to show the significant differences. It was possible to highlight how some compounds (no. 2, no. 4, no. 5, no. 6, no. 7, and no. 15) were markers of specific clusters and therefore, of specific vintages. Overall, the 2011–2014 and 2015–2017 vintages were richer in polyphenols (296.00 ± 46.10 mg/L and 333.00 ± 13.80 mg/L, respectively) when they were compared to the 2019–2021 ones (229.00 ± 15.90 mg/L).

This preliminary study showed that polyphenols are suitable markers that can be used to identify Grillo vintages. However, it is not possible to attribute the difference in the polyphenol content to a single event. This evidence, in fact, should be related to the real differences in the polyphenol content in the grapes or to the different opening times of the bottles.

Another variable to take into consideration, as indicated by the company, are the changes in the production process that took place in the years which divided the clusters, in 2015 and in 2019, so the different polyphenol content could also be correlated to these variations.

Author Contributions: Conceptualization, M.R., V.G. and M.B.M.; methodology M.R., V.G. and M.B.M.; software, M.R., V.G. and M.B.M.; validation, M.R., V.G. and M.B.M.; formal analysis, M.R., V.G. and M.B.M.; investigation, M.R., V.G. and M.B.M.; resources, M.R., V.G. and M.B.M.; data curation, M.R., V.G. and M.B.M.; writing—original draft preparation, M.R., V.G. and M.B.M.; writing—review and editing, M.R., V.G. and M.B.M.; visualization, M.R., V.G. and M.B.M.; supervision, M.R., V.G. and M.B.M.; project administration, M.R., V.G. and M.B.M.; funding acquisition, M.R., V.G. and M.B.M. All authors have read and agreed to the published version of the manuscript.

Funding: This research was funded by the Sapienza University of Rome, SEED PNR funds.

Acknowledgments: The authors warmly thank the company Cantina Cellaro S.C.A. for sample procurement and for sharing the information.

Conflicts of Interest: The authors declare no conflict of interest.

References

1. Carrasco, D.; Zhou-Tsang, A.; Rodriguez-Izquierdo, A.; Ocete, R.; Revilla, M.A.; Arroyo-García, R. Coastal Wild Grapevine Accession (*Vitis vinifera* L. Ssp. Sylvestris) Shows Distinct Late and Early Transcriptome Changes under Salt Stress in Comparison to Commercial Rootstock Richter 110. *Plants* **2022**, *11*, 2688. [CrossRef] [PubMed]
2. Alkan, A.; Abdullah, M.Ü.; Abdullah, H.O.; Assaf, M.; Zhou, H. A Smart Agricultural Application: Automated Detection of Diseases in Vine Leaves Using Hybrid Deep Learning. *Turk. J. Agric. For.* **2021**, *45*, 717–729. [CrossRef]
3. Benjak, A.; Ercisli, S.; Vokurka, A.; Maletić, E.; Pejić, I. Erratum: Genetic Relationships among Grapevine Cultivars Native to Croatia, Greece and Turkey. *Vitis J. Grapevine Res.* **2005**, *44*, 73–77.
4. Nesto, B.; di Savino, F. *The World of Sicilian Wine*; University of California Press: Berkeley, CA, USA, 2019.
5. Tudisca, S.; di Trapani, A.M.; Donia, E.; Sgroi, F.; Testa, R. Entrepreneurial Strategies of Etna Wine Farms. *Int. J. Entrep. Small Bus.* **2014**, *21*, 155. [CrossRef]
6. Bellia, C.; Pilato, M. Competitiveness of Wine Business within Green Economy: Sicilian Case. *Qual—Access Success* **2014**, *15*, 74–78.
7. Lanfranchi, M.; Schimmenti, E.; Campolo, M.G.; Giannetto, C. The Willingness to Pay of Sicilian Consumers for a Wine Obtained with Sustainable Production Method: An Estimate through an Ordered Probit Sample-Selection Model. *Wine Econ. Policy* **2019**, *8*, 203–215. [CrossRef]
8. Crescimanno, M.; Ficani, G.B.; Guccione, G. The Production and Marketing of Organic Wine in Sicily. *Br. Food J.* **2002**, *104*, 274–286. [CrossRef]
9. Borsellino, V.; Varia, F.; Zinnanti, C.; Schimmenti, E. The Sicilian Cooperative System of Wine Production: The Strategic Choices and Performance Analyses of a Case Study. *Int. J. Wine Bus. Res.* **2020**, *32*, 391–421. [CrossRef]
10. Fracassetti, D.; Stuknytė, M.; la Rosa, C.; Gabrielli, M.; de Noni, I.; Tirelli, A. Thiol Precursors in Catarratto Bianco Comune and Grillo Grapes and Effect of Clarification Conditions on the Release of Varietal Thiols in Wine. *Aust. J. Grape Wine Res.* **2018**, *24*, 125–133. [CrossRef]
11. Corona, O.; Bambina, P.; de Filippi, D.; Cinquanta, L. Influence of Pre-Fermentative Addition of Aqueous Solution Tannins Extracted from Oak Wood (*Quercus petraea*) on the Composition of Grillo Wines. *Eur. Food Res. Technol.* **2021**, *247*, 1595–1608. [CrossRef]
12. Nerva, L.; Moffa, L.; Giudice, G.; Giorgianni, A.; Tomasi, D.; Chitarra, W. Microscale Analysis of Soil Characteristics and Microbiomes Reveals Potential Impacts on Plants and Fruit: Vineyard as a Model Case Study. *Plant Soil* **2021**, *462*, 525–541. [CrossRef]
13. Alfonzo, A.; Francesca, N.; Mercurio, V.; Prestianni, R.; Settanni, L.; Spanò, G.; Naselli, V.; Moschetti, G. Use of Grape Racemes from Grillo Cultivar to Increase the Acidity Level of Sparkling Base Wines Produced with Different Saccharomyces Cerevisiae Strains. *Yeast* **2020**, *37*, 475–486. [CrossRef]
14. Arena, E.; Rizzo, V.; Licciardello, F.; Fallico, B.; Muratore, G. Effects of Light Exposure, Bottle Colour and Storage Temperature on the Quality of Malvasia Delle Lipari Sweet Wine. *Foods* **2021**, *10*, 1881. [CrossRef]
15. Díaz-Maroto, M.C.; Viñas, M.L.; Marchante, L.; Alañón, M.E.; Díaz-Maroto, I.J.; Pérez-Coello, M.S. Evaluation of the Storage Conditions and Type of Cork Stopper on the Quality of Bottled White Wines. *Molecules* **2021**, *26*, 232. [CrossRef]
16. Castellanos, E.R.; Jofre, V.P.; Fanzone, M.L.; Assof, M.V.; Catania, A.A.; Diaz-Sambueza, A.M.; Heredia, F.J.; Mercado, L.A. Effect of Different Closure Types and Storage Temperatures on the Color and Sensory Characteristics Development of Argentinian Torrontes Riojano White Wines Aged in Bottles. *Food Control* **2021**, *130*, 108343. [CrossRef]
17. Rouxinol, M.I.; Martins, M.R.; Murta, G.C.; Barroso, J.M.; Rato, A.E. Quality Assessment of Red Wine Grapes through NIR Spectroscopy. *Agronomy* **2022**, *12*, 637. [CrossRef]
18. Benelli, A.; Cevoli, C.; Ragni, L.; Fabbri, A. In-Field and Non-Destructive Monitoring of Grapes Maturity by Hyperspectral Imaging. *Biosyst. Eng.* **2021**, *207*, 59–67. [CrossRef]
19. Zhang, X.; Zhang, T.G.; Mu, W.S.; Fu, Z.T.; Zhang, X.S. Prediction of Soluble Solids Content for Wine Grapes During Maturing Based on Visible and Near-Infrared Spectroscopy. *Guang Pu Xue Yu Guang Pu Fen Xi Spectrosc. Spectr. Anal.* **2021**, *41*, 229–235. [CrossRef]
20. Ye, M.; Yue, T.; Yuan, Y.; Li, Z. Application of FT-NIR Spectroscopy to Apple Wine for Rapid Simultaneous Determination of Soluble Solids Content, PH, Total Acidity, and Total Ester Content. *Food Bioproc. Tech.* **2014**, *7*, 3055–3062. [CrossRef]
21. Rapa, M.; Ciano, S.; Gobbi, L.; Ruggieri, R.; Vinci, G. Quality and Safety Evaluation of New Tomato Cultivars. *Ital. J. Food Sci.* **2021**, *33*, 35–45. [CrossRef]
22. Buiarelli, F.; Bernardini, F.; di Filippo, P.; Riccardi, C.; Pomata, D.; Simonetti, G.; Risoluti, R. Extraction, Purification, and Determination by HPLC of Quercetin in Some Italian Wines. *Food Anal. Methods* **2018**, *11*, 3558–3562. [CrossRef]
23. Porgali, E.; Büyüktuncel, E. Determination of Phenolic Composition and Antioxidant Capacity of Native Red Wines by High Performance Liquid Chromatography and Spectrophotometric Methods. *Food Res. Int.* **2012**, *45*, 145–154. [CrossRef]
24. Kharadze, M.; Japaridze, I.; Kalandia, A.; Vanidze, M. Anthocyanins and Antioxidant Activity of Red Wines Made from Endemic Grape Varieties. *Ann. Agrar. Sci.* **2018**, *16*, 181–184. [CrossRef]
25. Tuberoso, C.I.G.; Serreli, G.; Congiu, F.; Montoro, P.; Fenu, M.A. Characterization, Phenolic Profile, Nitrogen Compounds and Antioxidant Activity of Carignano Wines. *J. Food Compos. Anal.* **2017**, *58*, 60–68. [CrossRef]

26. Ragusa, A.; Centonze, C.; Grasso, M.E.; Latronico, M.F.; Mastrangelo, P.F.; Sparascio, F.; Maffia, M. HPLC Analysis of Phenols in Negroamaro and Primitivo Red Wines from Salento. *Foods* **2019**, *8*, 45. [CrossRef]
27. Bai, S.; Cui, C.; Liu, J.; Li, P.; Li, Q.; Bi, K. Quantification of Polyphenol Composition and Multiple Statistical Analyses of Biological Activity in Portuguese Red Wines. *Eur. Food Res. Technol.* **2018**, *244*, 2007–2017. [CrossRef]
28. Pajović Šćepanović, R.; Wendelin, S.; Raičević, D.; Eder, R. Characterization of the Phenolic Profile of Commercial Montenegrin Red and White Wines. *Eur. Food Res. Technol.* **2019**, *245*, 2233–2245. [CrossRef]
29. Zietsman, A.J.J.; Moore, J.P.; Fangel, J.U.; Willats, W.G.T.; Trygg, J.; Vivier, M.A. Following the Compositional Changes of Fresh Grape Skin Cell Walls during the Fermentation Process in the Presence and Absence of Maceration Enzymes. *J. Agric. Food Chem.* **2015**, *63*, 2798–2810. [CrossRef]

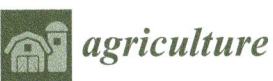

Article

Characterisation of Pasting, Structural and Volatile Properties of Potato Flour

Haining Zhuang [1,2], Shiyi Liu [1], Kexin Wang [1], Rui Zhong [1], Joshua Harington Aheto [1], Junwen Bai [1] and Xiaoyu Tian [1,*]

[1] School of Food and Biological Engineering, Jiangsu University, Zhenjiang 212013, China
[2] School of Health and Social Care, Shanghai Urban Construction Vocational College, Shanghai 201415, China
* Correspondence: tianxiaoyucau@163.com; Tel.: +86-139-5294-2608

Abstract: Potato flour is an important raw material for potato staple food products; nevertheless, the quality and flavor vary significantly due to process changes. In this study, the physicochemical features of fresh and five different dehydration temperature potato samples, including the degree of starch gelatinization (DG), pasting, structure properties and volatile components, were compared to investigate the effect of hot air drying (HAD) on potato flour. The results showed that the degree of pasting, viscosity and volatile aroma components changed significantly with differences in drying temperature. With the increase in drying temperature, the gelatinization degree and peak viscosity of potato powder increased or decreased, the breakdown viscosity of HAD-50 was higher, the setback viscosity of HAD-90 was higher, while the crystallization zone of HAD-90 was destroyed due to the high temperature. The flavor components of potato flour are increased during processing due to lipid oxidation, Maillard reaction and thermal degradation. The level of aldehydes,3,5-Octadien-2-one and E,E)-3,5-Octadien-2-one gradually reduced as the processing temperature increased, while the content of furans grew and then decreased, nonanal and 2-Penty-l-Furan increased. Overall, lower HAD temperatures are beneficial for the quality and flavor of potato flour. The information presented here will be useful for the further development of potato flour products.

Keywords: potato flour; gelatinization; viscosity; X-ray diffraction; volatile aroma components

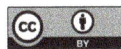

1. Introduction

Potato, a highly nutritious agricultural commodity with a rich source of high-quality protein, starch, basic vitamins, minerals and trace elements, is widely used as a food and industrial crop [1]. With a yearly output of more than 370 million tons, potato is among the most important crops, making it the third largest after wheat and rice in total output [2]. Considering the important role of potato as a vital food-security crop, there has been a concerted policy from the Chinese Government that potatoes be promoted as the fourth major staple food in China, next to wheat, rice and corn [3]. Potato flour is an indispensable intermediate raw material in processed potato food; the potato is processed into whole flour and then added to the staple food in a certain proportion (processed into a new, staple potato food product), which is conducive to improving the nutritional value of traditional staple foods, to meet the current demand for nutritious staple foods [4]. However, the research and development of nutritional potato staple food products is confronted with lots of constraints. For instance, the dehydration of fresh potatoes can affect the profile of endogenous compositions, such as moisture, pasting properties and volatile and non-volatile precursors of potatoes, which can significantly affect the quality of the end products [5]. In order to improve the quality of potato flour, it is essential to reduce the drying time by using modern drying technologies to replace traditional natural drying methods [6–8].

Free starch content, microstructure, pasting characteristics and color are often used to characterize the quality of potato flour [9]. To address the problems of high pasting and processing performance limitations of traditional whole potato flour, it is necessary to seek some new processing processes to obtain potato flour with lower pasting [10]. In addition, starch crystallinity is an important parameter that characterizes the crystalline nature of starch granules, and its size directly affects the application performance of raw potato powder products [11].

Different processing conditions have been noted to have a great effect on the qualities and volatile compositions of processed potatoes. For example, Yang used SPME GC-MS to identify key volatile compound differences between fresh potato puree and potato puree stored at 4 °C for 1 day and identified more than 30 compounds in both types of puree at varied concentrations [12]. Processing with a microwave oven, which is considered a quick cooking method, has been reported by Jansky to produce the least flavor compounds in potatoes [13]. Such chemical reactions during processing also lead to the development of a blend of volatile and non-volatile chemical compounds that can make food tastier or create desirable or unwanted flavors [14]

Many techniques and methods are available for identifying and quantifying volatile compounds in potatoes, including simultaneous distillation and extraction [15], solvent-assisted flavor evaporation [16], dynamic headspace extraction [17] and solid-phase microextraction (SPME), have been investigated [18]. Others include gas chromatography-mass spectrometry (GC-MS) [19] and gas chromatography-olfactometry (GC-O) [20], whereby volatile compounds are separated by GC, and the human nose is used as a "sniffing port" to describe the various aromas as they exit the GC column. A portion can also be diverted for simultaneous identification by MS (GC-MS-O). Relatively, more research has been performed on the identification of volatiles and reaction products in raw and cooked potatoes, but few on dehydrated potatoes. Therefore, much remains to be learned about the dynamic flavor traits of potatoes and the key components that contribute to them.

Nowadays, most studies focus on the characteristics of potato starch [21], a small number of scholars have begun to pay attention to the properties of potato flour and potato flour added to steamed wheat bread, including rheological and texture properties, viscoelasticity and volatile aroma components [5], but little information is available on the potato flour's properties. Therefore, the aim of the current work is to investigate the influence of the processing temperature on the pasting properties and flavor of potato flour. In this regard, we aim to monitor the viscosity, X-ray diffraction and the profiling of volatile compositions of raw and dehydrated potato flour by means of a rapid visco analyzer, X-ray diffractometer and headspace solid-phase microextraction coupled with gas chromatography-mass spectrometry (HS-SPME GC-MS).

2. Materials and Methods

2.1. Raw Material and Processing Procedures

Fresh potato tubers of the *Longshu 10* variety were purchased from Gansu province, the main potato-producing area in northwest China. To ensure the uniformity of physical characteristics of the experimental materials, the samples were carefully selected for size uniformity, no rot, no bad odor, no sprouts, no pests or diseases infections and no mechanical damage or greening.

Potato tubers were washed to remove residual sediment and other impurities prior to peeling. Upon peeling, the potato tubers were sliced into uniformly thick (1 mm) slices. In order to prevent the browning of potatoes during processing, a phenomenon that reduces the color attributes of potato flour, slices were treated with color protectant by dipping into 2 g/L citric acid solution and maintained for 10 min. The potato slices were then put on a sieve to drain the color fixative and then thin-layer hot air drying (HAD). The dryer, which was engineered and built at Jiangsu University prior to the commencement of the experiment, is equipped with a temperature adjustment ranging from 0 to 99.9 °C. The drying temperatures used for this experiment were set at 50 (HAD-50), 60 (HAD-60), 70 (HAD-70), 80 (HAD-80) and 90 °C (HAD-90), and HAD-0 means raw potato materials that are not dried. Once the dryer had reached a steady state for the set points (at least

30 min), the single slices were uniformly distributed on a perforated sieve tray. Sample weight was recorded every 20 min until the moisture content was less than 8% or a constant value was achieved. The dried slices were ground, screened through a 120 mesh sieve and packed in low-density polyethylene bags.

2.2. Degree of Gelatinization

The degree of starch gelatinization (DG) was determined according to the Chemical Industry Standards of the People's Republic of China (HG/T 3932-2007). The DG value of potato starch was determined by means of enzymatic hydrolysis. Gelatinized starch is hydrolyzed to glucose by glucose amylase and can be determined by titration of iodine-thiosulphate [22]. The principle is: the glucose is oxidized by iodine in an alkaline solution to gluconic acid, and the excess acidified iodine is then titrated with sodium thiosulfate.

2.3. Rapid Visco Analyzer (RVA) Pasting Properties

Pasting properties were analyzed using a Brabender Amylograph (Brabender-803201, Micro Visco-Amyl-Graph, Germany), which was carried out according to Xu [23]. Each sample was suspended with deionized water (6% (w/w, dry basis) in an RVA aluminum can, and a heating and cooling program was used where the initial equilibrium temperature was 40 °C, heating from 40 to 95 °C, holding at 95 °C for 5 min, cooling from 95 to 50 °C and holding at 50 °C for 10 min with a heating/cooling rate of 7.5 °C/min while stirring at 250 rpm. The peak, breakdown, hot paste, cold paste, setback viscosities, peak time and pasting temperature, were recorded.

2.4. X-ray Diffraction Analysis

The crystalline structure of the sample powder (200 mesh) was investigated using a Bruker D8-Advance X-ray powder diffractometer (Bruker, Germany), according to the method of Yang [10]. The diffractograms were collected under the conditions of 40 kV, 30 mA, with a scanning angle (2θ) set from 5 to 45°, with a 0.02° step interval, at a scanning rate of 1°/min and Cu Kα radiation source (λ = 0.154 nm). The data were analyzed by Jade 5.0 software (Materials Data Inc., Livermore, CA, USA).

2.5. HS-SPME Sampling

An SPME extraction fiber (50/30 μm) coated with divinylbenzene/carboxen/polydimethylsiloxane (Supelco, Inc., Bellefonte, PA, USA) was used for headspace analyses of potato sample volatiles. This fiber is commonly used for flavor analysis and is especially useful for pyrazines [24,25]. The SPME fiber was aged in the GC inlet port at 270 °C for 1 h to ensure the removal of residual gas. Then, 2 g of potato flour sample was weighed and placed in a 20 mL glass sample vial to make way for the extraction of volatile components.

The sealed vial was placed in a 50 °C constant temperature water bath with thermal equilibrium for 10 min. The SPME extraction head was inserted into the headspace of the sample through the cap, and the fiber was exposed for 30 min. After the extraction, the SPME fiber head was removed from the headspace bottle, inserted into the GC inlet and was thermally desorbed for 5 min and transferred to the GC system.

2.6. Identification of Volatile Compounds Based on GC–MS Analysis

GC condition: Compounds were separated on a DB-Wax column (30 m × 0.25 mm inside diameter, 0.25 μm film thickness, Agilent Technologies). The injection was performed in the splitless mode, and the injector temperature was 250 °C. Helium (99.999%) was used as the carrier gas with a constant flow rate starting at 1.0 mL/min. The oven temperature was programmed as follows: 40 °C for 1 min, 5 °C/min to 100 °C, 3 °C/min to 130 °C, 10 °C/min to a final temperature of 220 °C, with a final holding time of 3 min.

MS condition: The detector adopted an electron impact ion source with the ionizing potential of 70 eV set at 230 °C. The quadrupole temperature was set to 150 °C, and the transfer line temperature was kept at 250 °C. Total ion chromatograms were acquired by scanning from 30 to 450 u.

The GC-MS experimental data were processed by Jade 6.0 software (Materials Data Inc., Livermore, CA, USA). Volatile components of the potato flour samples were identified by comparison of the mass spectra in the commercial computer library as NIST (107k compounds) and Wiley (320k compounds, version 6.0), and only volatiles with matching degrees of more than 800 was recorded.

2.7. Statistical Analysis

The experiments were performed in triplicate, and the values are represented as mean ± standard deviation, using one-way ANOVA in SPSS 21.0 (SPSS Inc., Chicago, IL, USA), and comparisons were made using Duncan's multiple-range test at a significant level of $p < 0.05$. A clustered heat map of the volatile compounds obtained following GC-MS analysis was created using the Heat Map Dendrogram App in OriginLab 2021(Northampton, MA, USA).

3. Results and Discussion

3.1. The Effect of Drying Temperature on Gelatinization Degree

Figure 1 shows the DG (%) of potato flour processed at different drying temperatures. In general, the DG (%) of raw potato was around 15%, and the pasting degree of cooked powder was almost 95% or higher. It could be said, as shown in Figure 1, that the potato flour has not yet gelatinized (a value of 15.79–22.10%) when the temperature was below 50 °C, and a slight gelatinization began to occur at 60 °C, but at 70 °C, almost half of the starch in the potato flour has been gelatinized (the value is 48.72%). The results were consistent with the DG (%) of low gelatinization potato four (hot air drying at 65°C) by Zhang [26]. The DG (%) was already very high when the drying temperature reached 80 and 90 °C, approaching full gelatinization (the value is 86.51–90.57%). Different hot air temperatures change the temperature, moisture and particle structure of potato starch, resulting in different DGs of the product starch. According to the observation of the microstructure of starch granules [6], it was found that a high temperature would destroy the structure of starch granules, which may be due to serious gelation.

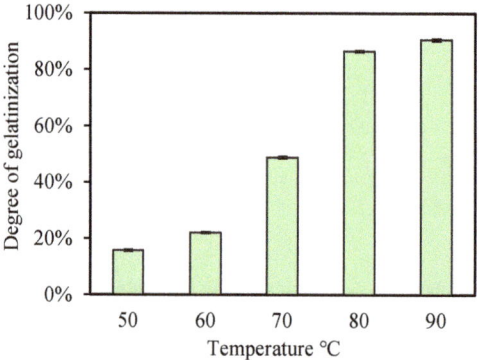

Figure 1. Degree of gelatinization at different drying temperatures.

3.2. XRD Analysis

The various temperature treatments applied in this study exerted a significant impact on the functional properties of the starch in the potato flour. Figure 2 shows the X-ray diffraction patterns of the diverse potato starches. The X-ray diffraction patterns revealed the typical B-type diffractions characteristic of potato starch with a doublet peak at 15° and a very strong reflection at $2\theta = 17$ and $22°$ [27]. There were also some minor reflections at $2\theta = 20$, 24 and 35°.

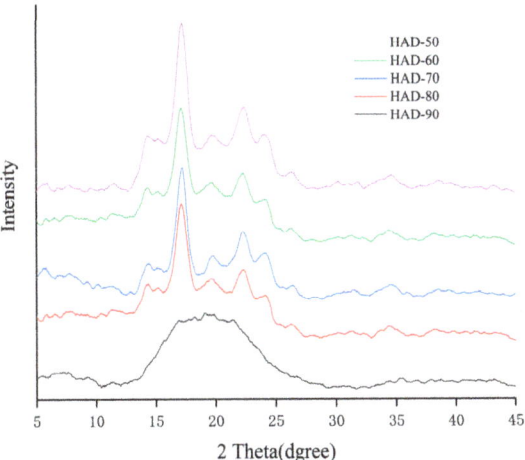

Figure 2. Structural characteristics of the potato flour. X-ray diffractograms showing the effects of drying conditioning of samples in X-ray diffraction.

The intensity of peaks for treated samples HAD-50, HAD-60, HAD-70 and HAD-80 were on par or very similar, implying that the molecular arrangement of the starch under these treatment conditions was not adversely affected, the crystalline shape of starch was not altered and the diffraction intensity of HAD-50 was the highest. On the contrary, after high-temperature dehydration processing, the crystal diffraction peak of HAD-90 completely disappeared, and the diffraction curve showed a typical amorphous structure diffraction curve, indicating that the crystalline structure of starch granules had been destroyed by heating and shear force.

3.3. Pasting Properties

Starch's pasting behavior is a mixture of complex processes that occur after gelatinization, including starch granules transitioning from swelling to rupturing, amylose leaching and high-energy gel development [28,29]. Figure 3 presents the pasting properties of potato starch under different temperature regimes. As shown in Figure 3, the peak viscosity and valley viscosity of HAD-50 and HAD-60 were higher, whereas those for HAD-90 and HAD-80 were lower, which may be attributed to the following potential explanations. The HAD-90 samples may have undergone varying degrees of heat treatment during the production process, and some of the starch has undergone gelatinization and aging, causing the starch crystals to be partially damaged; the aged starch after gelatinization cannot be re-gelatinized at high temperatures, which also results in a decrease in the starch gelation temperature [30]. Secondly, because low-temperature drying can significantly reduce the loss of heat-sensitive nutrients and prevent starch crystals from being destroyed, it is clear that HAD-50 and HAD-60 are difficult to gelatinize, while the gelatinization temperature of HAD-90 was low [31].

According to the characteristic value of the gelatinization characteristic curve, the breakdown viscosity of HAD-50 is large, which indicates that the viscosity stability is not good, and the setback viscosity of HAD-90 is large, which indicates that the gel ability formed after cooling is poor and easily subject to aging.

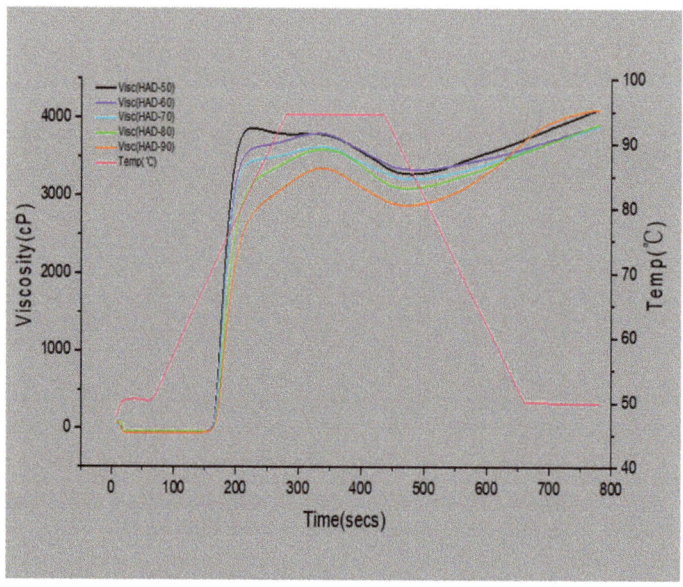

Figure 3. Pasting curves of potato flour dried at 50, 60, 70, 80 and 90 °C.

In addition, in potato flour, a certain proportion of protein on the surface of starch granules can also inhibit the swelling of starch granules, according to Bharti [32] and Regina [33], which can also effectively reduce the gelatinization degree of HAD-50 and HAD-60. However, with the increase in HAD temperature, protein bond breakage may occur, resulting in the rapid transition of starch particles from expansion to decomposition. This claim is based on the fact that proteins are denatured during cooking, making them inactive [34,35].

Researchers have recently reported on the impact of various processing techniques on the quality of whole potato powder. The findings demonstrate that low-temperature hot-air drying and freeze-drying improve various aspects of potato powder [26,36]. However, there is no further study on the effect of different hot-air drying temperatures, which is supplemented by the results of this study. According to our findings, potato flour produced by low-temperature HAD had better processing characteristics, including low levels of gelatinization, internal starch particles that were completely intact and good gel stability, which was consistent with the findings of Zhang [26] and Shen [37].

3.4. Identification of Volatile Compounds in Different Potato Samples

The volatile compounds in raw and processed potato samples were extracted at different temperatures by HS-SPME and then analyzed by GC-MS. A total of 52 compounds were tentatively identified using the NIST and Wiley MS Library Database (Table 1). These included 9 alcohols, 12 hydrocarbons, 15 aldehydes, 7 ketones, 2 furans and 7 additional compounds. Hexanal, a major constituent of processed potato (above 30% of the total area), was not found in the raw samples.

Table 1. Volatiles and their relative content (%) in raw and dehydrated potatoes at different drying temperatures.

No.	Compounds	Retention Time (min)	The Relative Peak Area (%)					
			HAD-0	HAD-50	HAD-60	HAD-70	HAD-80	HAD-90
	Alcohol							
1	Ethyl alcohol	10.16	ND	1.63 ± 0.10	2.48 ± 0.09	1.74 ± 0.06	3.98 ± 0.14	2.75 ± 0.11
2	1-Pentanol	20.52	ND	1.66 ± 0.12	1.3 ± 0.07	2.17 ± 0.09	ND	1.09 ± 0.15
3	1-Octen-3-ol	26.93	9.56 ± 0.11	1.92 ± 0.04	1.8 ± 0.09	2.21 ± 0.08	ND	2.18 ± 0.07
4	1-Methoxy-2-propanol	15.52	ND	ND	2.69 ± 0.10	ND	2.82 ± 0.12	2.48 ± 0.05
5	2-Ethyl-1-hexanol	28.37	ND	ND	1.16 ± 0.11	1.73 ± 0.06	1.71 ± 0.13	1.14 ± 0.05
6	1-Pentanol	15.9	6.3 ± 0.08	ND	ND	ND	ND	ND
7	Benzyl alcohol	25.71	2.58 ± 0.10	ND	ND	ND	ND	ND
8	3-Methyl-1-butanol	8.39	2.55 ± 0.07	ND	ND	ND	ND	ND
9	1-Penten-3-ol	14.08	2.32 ± 0.06	ND	ND	ND	ND	ND
	Hydrocarbon							
10	Hexane	5.72	1.14 ± 0.07	ND	0.7 ± 0.04	1.12 ± 0.04	1.6 ± 0.03	ND
11	Methylene Chloride	9.88	ND	1.77 ± 0.07	1.75 ± 0.06	ND	1.56 ± 0.09	0.96 ± 0.08
12	Octamethyl-cyclotetrasiloxane	11.08	0.71 ± 0.05	1.69 ± 0.12	ND	0.97 ± 0.06	1.24 ± 0.07	1.02 ± 0.05
13	Decamethyl-cyclopentasiloxane	16.1	ND	0.83 ± 0.08	0.7 ± 0.03	1.78 ± 0.09	0.62 ± 0.03	0.85 ± 0.05
14	Dodecane	18.43	ND	1.89 ± 0.06	2.06 ± 0.05	2.39 ± 0.09	2.99 ± 0.10	3.02 ± 0.07
15	Tridecane	21.16	ND	ND	ND	ND	2.7 ± 0.09	ND
16	Tetradecane	24.9	ND	ND	1.8 ± 0.03	1.75 ± 0.11	2.63 ± 0.04	1.88 ± 0.03
17	Trichloromethane	11.88	ND	ND	ND	ND	ND	0.87 ± 0.04
18	3-Methyl-tridecane	22.64	ND	ND	ND	ND	1.38 ± 0.06	ND
19	Hexamethyl-cyclotrisiloxane	7.71	ND	ND	ND	ND	1.61 ± 0.05	ND
20	cis-1-Ethyl-2-Methyl-cyclopentane	18.62	5.5 ± 0.03	ND	ND	ND	ND	ND
21	3-ethyl-2-methyl-1,3-hexadiene	19.08	1.03 ± 0.10	ND	ND	ND	ND	ND
	Aldehydes							
22	Pentanal	11.31	ND	2.38 ± 0.08	1.79 ± 0.08	1.74 ± 0.08	1.05 ± 0.09	1.32 ± 0.05
23	Hexanal	14.62	ND	51.73 ± 1.23	43.99 ± 0.77	37.7 ± 0.92	31.26 ± 0.95	28.63 ± 1.16
24	(Z)-2-Heptenal	23.24	ND	1.1 ± 0.06	1.12 ± 0.26	1.78 ± 0.06	1.32 ± 0.08	2.08 ± 0.04
25	Nonanal	25.43	ND	2.58 ± 0.08	5.84 ± 0.05	6.58 ± 0.17	7.13 ± 0.19	7.32 ± 0.47
26	Decanal	28.27	ND	2.65 ± 0.06	3.53 ± 0.05	1.53 ± 0.07	5.26 ± 0.08	ND
27	Octanal	22.16	0.31 ± 0.04	ND	ND	ND	ND	2.56 ± 0.12
28	Heptanal	18.24	ND	2.18 ± 0.03	2.42 ± 0.04	2.38 ± 0.04	2.35 ± 0.10	ND
29	Benzaldehyde	29.07	ND	2.54 ± 0.08	2.38 ± 0.05	2.49 ± 0.08	2.7 ± 0.06	2.73 ± 0.05
30	(E)- 2-Octenal	26.62	1.22 ± 0.06	ND	ND	1.67 ± 0.19	ND	ND
31	2-Dodecenal	29.82	ND	ND	ND	1.95 ± 0.07	ND	ND
32	4-Ethyl-Benzaldehyde	33.62	ND	ND	ND	ND	ND	0.85 ± 0.05
33	2-Methy-l-Butanal	8.32	6.36 ± 0.10	ND	ND	ND	ND	ND
34	Benzeneacetaldehyde	22.77	4.65 ± 0.11	ND	ND	ND	ND	ND
35	3-Methy-l-Butanal	8.39	2.84 ± 0.57	ND	ND	ND	ND	ND
36	2-Methyl-Propanal	6.48	2.7 ± 0.10	ND	ND	ND	ND	ND
	Ketone							
37	Acetone	7.62	ND	1.24 ± 0.06	1.63 ± 0.06	2.41 ± 0.13	2.7 ± 0.11	5.84 ± 0.14
38	6-Methyl-5-Hepten-2-one	23.01	ND	1.78 ± 0.09	2.89 ± 0.11	2.14 ± 0.06	3.22 ± 0.09	2.41 ± 0.03
39	3-Octen-2-one	25.97	ND	4.62 ± 0.17	4.4 ± 0.12	3.82 ± 0.14	3.74 ± 0.17	3.18 ± 0.11
40	3,5-Octadien-2-one	28.84	ND	7.64 ± 0.15	6.85 ± 0.10	5.71 ± 0.16	5.2 ± 0.10	4.75 ± 0.14
41	(E,E)-3,5-Octadien-2-one	29.96	ND	4.12 ± 0.01	3.57 ± 0.15	2.71 ± 0.07	1.98 ± 0.10	1.73 ± 0.18
42	1-Penten-3-one	10.76	7.66 ± 0.10	ND	ND	ND	ND	ND
43	2,3-Octanedione	16.96	0.82 ± 0.06	ND	ND	ND	ND	ND
	Furan							
44	2-Ethy-l-Furan	10.08	ND	ND	ND	3.21 ± 0.09	3.7 ± 0.06	3.88 ± 0.11
45	2-Penty-l-Furan	18.96	ND	1.66 ± 0.60	3.31 ± 0.08	8.29 ± 0.13	3.2 ± 0.16	6.0 ± 0.16
	Additional volatiles							
46	Toluene	12.62	0.44 ± 0.09	ND	ND	ND	1.29 ± 0.02	1.42 ± 0.14
47	15-Crown-5	35.67	ND	ND	ND	ND	0.89 ± 0.07	ND
48	1-Methyl-naphthalene	25.99	ND	ND	ND	ND	0.87 ± 0.06	0.87 ± 0.08
49	Triethylamine	7.18	ND	ND	ND	ND	ND	1.93 ± 0.04
50	Acetic acid	27.33	ND	ND	ND	ND	ND	3.87 ± 0.10
51	1,3-dichloro-Benzene	19.43	1.14 ± 0.07	ND	ND	ND	ND	ND
52	2-Methyl-7-phenylindole	24.07	0.88 ± 0.03	ND	ND	ND	ND	ND

Note: The relative peak area (%) of each compound was mean value ± SD. Abbreviations: ND, not found.

Based on the GC-MS results in Table 1, a stacking histogram was created and displayed in Figure 4. As shown in Figure 4, the volatile flavor components of raw potato samples differed significantly from those of dehydrated potatoes, while in dehydrated potato samples, some substances tended to change regularly with the drying temperature course.

The content of aldehydes gradually decreased with increasing processing temperature, while furans first rose and then decreased, with the highest content in the HAD-70 samples. Alcohols and ketones were not linearly correlated to the grades but were obviously rich in HAD-0, and hydrocarbons were rich in HAD-50 and HAD-60 samples.

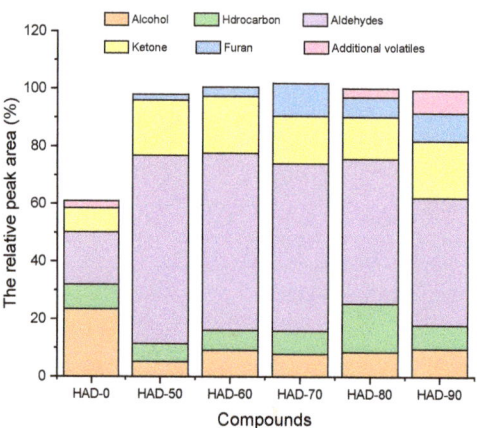

Figure 4. Comparison of the types and contents of volatile substances in different processed samples.

3.4.1. Volatile Composition of Raw Potato Samples

In total, there were 20 volatile compounds identified in the raw potato samples prior to processing; they include: five alcohols, four hydrocarbons, six aldehydes, two ketones and three additional compounds. Alcohols have been considered the main odorants of raw potato aroma, higher concentrations of which were detected in varieties of potatoes such as Longshu 11, Atlantic and Shepody [38]. Among the alcoholic compounds identified, 1-octen-3-ol, which is a degradation product of hydroperoxide in linoleic acid, was predominant. 3-Methyl- 1-butanol was also present, which is common in plant materials resulting from enzymatic deamination and the decarboxylation of amino acids [39]. It was reported that most unsaturated aldehydes have a pleasant odor; for instance, 3-methyl-butyraldehyde has a pleasant fruit aroma [40], and 2-methyl-butyraldehyde has a sweet and fruity flavor [41]. Chloride is present in fresh potatoes at room temperature and reacts with starch to produce ethers [42]. Methoxyphenyl-oxime, which is a kind of nitrogen-containing compound with a musty taste and meaty flavor, was also detected in the raw potato.

3.4.2. Volatile Composition of Dehydrated Potato Samples

The results of this study, as presented in Table 1, revealed that the types and concentrations of volatile compounds in potato flour changed at varying processing temperatures. From Table 1, the samples treated at 80 and 90 °C had the highest concentrations of volatile compounds with three and five alcohols, nine and six hydrocarbons, seven aldehydes, five ketones, two furans and three and four additional non-identified compounds, respectively. The rest of the samples yielded 20, 23 and 25 kinds of main volatiles at the processing temperature of 50, 60 and 70 °C, respectively.

Aldehydes, alcohols and furans are key components of dehydrated potato aromas. For instance, hexanal is the basic product of linoleic acid oxidation [43], playing a major role in the formation of the characteristic flavors of potato flour. Among the aldehydes detected in the present work, hexanal recorded the highest relative contents at all levels of processing (Table 1). According to Pérez [44], Linoleic acid containing double bonds easily oxidizes in the air to produce peroxide and aldehydes. They also serve as a precursor to many other aldehydes and alcohols, including (E)-2-heptenal and nonanal. Regarding the characteristic aromas of the various aldehydes detected in this study, hexanal has a nutty and roasted odor, and benzaldehyde has a roasted peanut or almond aroma and fruity flavor. Nonanal is known to have a strong aroma of sweet orange and can be similar to fried peanuts, decanal has a sweet floral aroma, while heptaldehyde has a strong smell of grease [45], and phenylacetaldehyde has a rich aroma of Oriental hairpin. 1-amyl alcohol and 2-ethyl-1-hexanol, known to originate from linoleic acid oxidation, have a mushroom aroma, while 2-undecanone is considered to be the main compound responsible for the fruity aroma.

3.4.3. The Effect of Drying Temperature on Volatile Compounds during Processing

The relative peak area matrix of the GC-MS results for volatile potato components at different temperatures as also analyzed by heat map clustering analysis, as shown in Figure 5. The results show that the distance between 50 and 60 °C is the closest, and the component similarity is higher, then the distance increases at 70, 80 and 90 °C. The difference between all dried materials and fresh materials was the most significant. This can correspond to the result of gelatinization of Figure 5, because at low temperatures, the gelatinization degree of potato is lower, and the flavor component is close, but after high-temperature processing, the potato is basically gelatinized and the flavor substances produced have changed greatly.

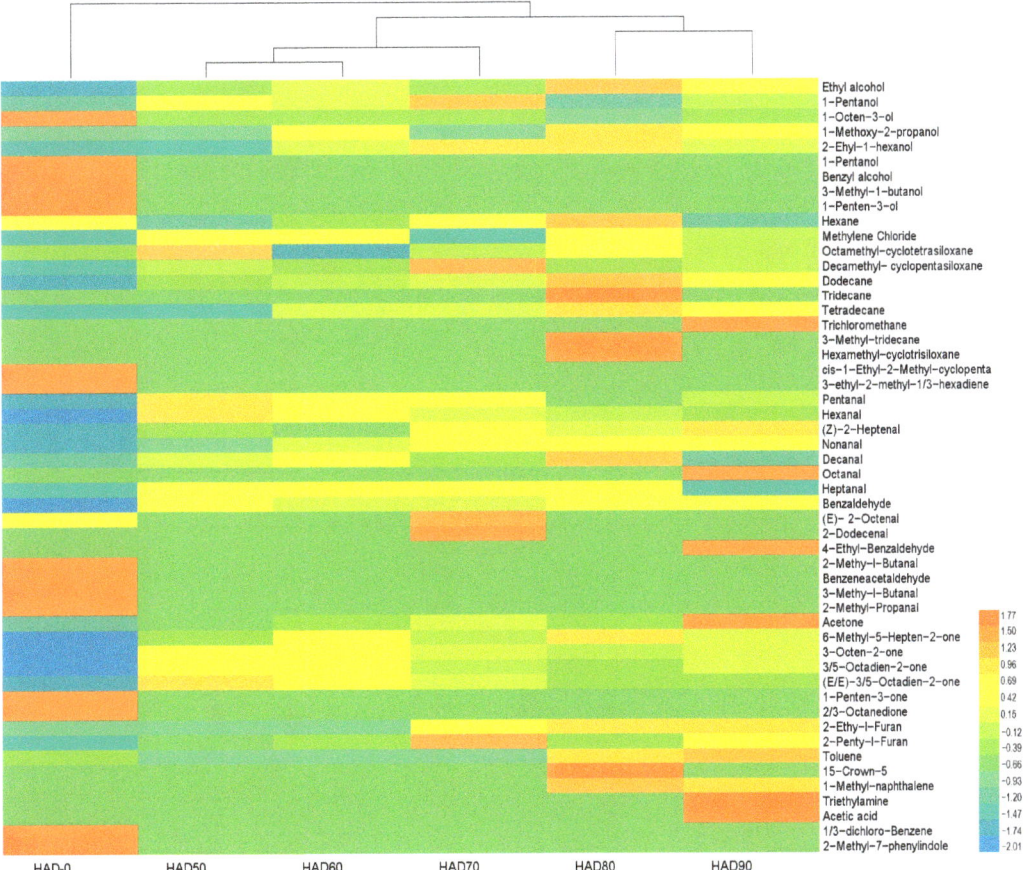

Figure 5. Heatmap of volatile matter in different processed samples.

High concentrations of 1-octen-3-ol in raw tubers, which decreased significantly in dehydrated potatoes from 9.55% to 1.72%, and 1-penten-3-one, 1-pentanol were found only in raw samples. This may be from sample tissue degradation as a result of cutting or because the compounds were generated through lipid oxidation and lipoxygenase-initiated reaction. Several new volatile components were generated as a result of Maillard reaction and lipid oxidation during dehydration processing.

This exhibited an obvious difference in the variety of aldehyde compounds between raw and processed samples. Hexanal was found only in the processed potato, of which the concentration reached 51.73% with a 50 °C drying process. The formation of hexanal, reported in previous potato studies, depends on the time and opportunity for lipoxygenase to be in contact with the substrate [18]. It has been observed that high lipoxygenase activity at a lower temperature (50 °C) with a longer dehydration period results in a relatively high aldehyde content. On the contrary, higher temperatures lead to the rapid dehydration of potato slices and also to a reduction in lipoxygenase activity and oxidation of linoleic acid, which reduces the concentration of aldehydes.

The total amount of lipid degradation products formed by different processing methods are quite different. Oruna-Concha reported that different cooking methods (boiling, conventional baking and microwave baking) resulted in a unique profile of flavor compounds and a relatively high concentration of lipid oxidation products in boiled tubers [18]. More opportunities were provided for the interaction of lipoxygenase with the substrate during the slicing and boiling, while gradual heating of the tuber provides more time for oxidizing reaction. The flavor compounds of boiled potatoes are mainly caused by lipid degradation and Maillard reaction and/or sugar degradation, while those in roasted potatoes are formed by thermal degradation. Another oxidative product contributing to the flavor of the boiled potato is c4-heptanal, which produces a soil aroma at low concentrations [46], while high concentrations cause a stale flavor of potato tubers [47].

The concentration of aromatic compounds and furan in processed potatoes was higher. Benzaldehyde is an aromatic aldehyde with a pleasant aroma resulting from the enzyme breakdown of the diglucoside amygdalin [48]. Furans are formed during heating by Maillard sugar-amine reactions and thermal degradation of sugars, such as fructose and glucose [49]. The furans detected in the present work were 2-ethy-l-furan and 2-Penty-l-Furan. 2-ethy-l-furan was formed in potatoes processed at a higher temperature (above 70 °C). They have a very strong meat flavor and a low aroma threshold; in almost all food, 2-pentylfuran has a ham flavor, making a special contribution to the flavor of cooked potato [50].

According to Figure 6, new volatile compounds produced formed via several chemical reactions that occurred during drying, and the relative content changed according to the temperature. The concentration of hexanal dropped dramatically from 51.73% to 28.63%, 3,5-Octadien-2-one and E,E)-3,5-Octadien-2-one also decreased from 7.64% and 4.12% to 4.75% and 1.73%, respectively. Significant increases in Maillard reactions and thermal degradation as a result of lipid oxidation were noted for two volatiles: nonanal and 2-Penty-l-Furan. Some bad flavors were produced, while some of the aromas were lost. It has been reported that the temperature of the gelatinization of potato starch is approximately 57–69 °C [51]; hence, a processing temperature higher than 70 °C will result in starch gelatinization, which is unfavorable for the preparation of raw potato flour. It is, therefore, important to note that high temperatures reduce the processing properties of staple foods, such as water absorption, kneading properties, gluten-like strength, viscosity, amylase activity and regenerative properties. Therefore, 60 °C is a moderate HAD temperature, which is beneficial to the formation of comprehensive properties of potato powder.

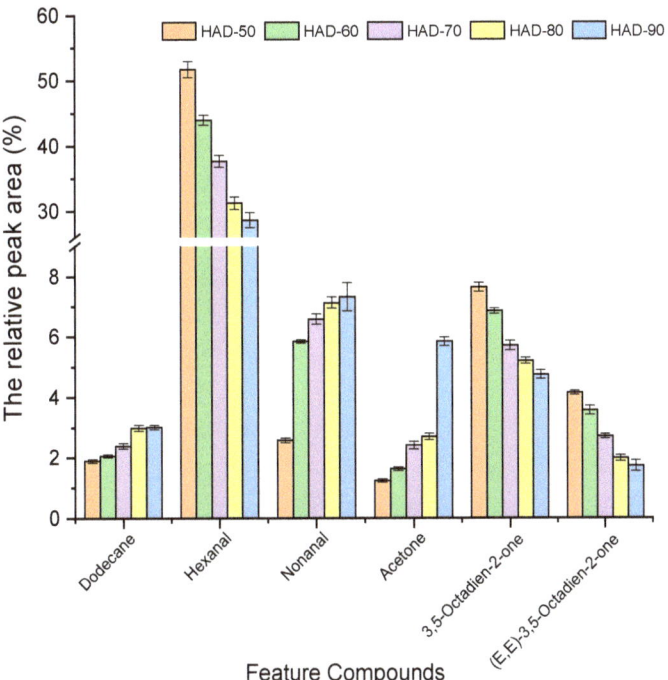

Figure 6. Changing trend of feature volatile component contents in different processed samples.

4. Conclusions

Potato is an important raw food material, but the limited storage and transportation of fresh potato lead to fewer types of processed products, while after drying and milling, potato can retain most of the nutrients, is easy to use, has stable storage and can provide special tastes and aromas. Compared with potato starch, potato flour has more comprehensive nutrition and superior processing performance and is an important raw material for staple potato food products. The variation in physicochemical properties, including viscosity, X-ray diffraction and volatile compositions, of HAD potato flour were observed using enzyme hydrolysis, rapid visco analyzer, X-ray diffractometer and headspace solid-phase microextraction coupled with gas chromatography-mass spectrometry (HS-SPME GC-MS). The results indicate that HAD temperature is an important index affecting the quality of potato powder. Higher temperatures lead to an increase in DG value, a decrease in peak viscosity, poor gel ability and aging, the destruction of the crystal structure and the loss of bad flavor and key flavors of potato powder. However, low-temperature HAD for a long time will also reduce the viscosity stability; HAD-60 has more comprehensive nutrition and flavor and better processability. The results provide more detailed data for the raw material processing technology of staple potato foods and can effectively guide the process optimization and quality classification of potato flour. However, there are other ways to process potato flour, such as infrared drying, microwave drying, etc. The influence of different drying methods needs to be further analyzed in future research.

Author Contributions: Methodology, J.B.; software, R.Z.; validation, J.H.A.; formal analysis, S.L.; investigation, K.W.; resources, J.B.; data curation, X.T.; writing—original draft preparation, X.T.; writing—review and editing, J.B.; visualization, H.Z.; supervision, J.B.; project administration, H.Z.; funding acquisition, H.Z. All authors have read and agreed to the published version of the manuscript.

Funding: This research was funded by Shanghai Municipal Human Resources and Social Security Bureau, Shanghai Pujiang Program, grant number 2021PJD021; Shanghai Urban Construction Vocational College, Key Scientific Research Project of Shanghai Urban Construction Vocational College, grant number cjky202209; Ministry of Science and Technology of China, National Key Research and Development Plan, grant number 2016YFD0401302.

Institutional Review Board Statement: Not applicable.

Informed Consent Statement: Not applicable.

Data Availability Statement: Not applicable.

Conflicts of Interest: The authors declare no conflict of interest.

References

1. Dreyer, H. Towards Sustainable Potato Production: Partnering to Support Family Farmers in Africa. *Potato Res.* **2017**, *60*, 237–238. [CrossRef]
2. Zhang, H.; Fen, X.; Yu, W.; HU, H.; Dai, X. Progress of potato staple food research and industry development in China. *J. Integr. Agric.* **2017**, *16*, 2924–2932. [CrossRef]
3. Huang, G. China to grow and eat more potatoes. *Front. Ecol. Environ.* **2015**, *13*, 68. [CrossRef]
4. Liu, X.; Mu, T.; Sun, H.; Zhang, M.; Chen, J. Influence of potato flour on dough rheological properties and quality of steamed bread. *J. Integr. Agr.* **2016**, *15*, 2666–2676. [CrossRef]
5. Zeng, F.; Liu, H.; Yu, H.; Cheng, J.; Gao, G.; Shang, Y. Effect of potato flour on the rheological properties of dough and the volatile aroma components of bread. *Am. J. Potato Res.* **2018**, *96*, 69–78. [CrossRef]
6. Raigond, P.; Singh, B.; Gupta, V.K.; Singh, B. Potato flavour: Profiling of umami 5′-nucleotides from indian potato cultivars. *Indian J. Plant Physiol.* **2014**, *19*, 338–344. [CrossRef]
7. Bai, J.; Cai, J.; Tian, X. Crust Formation and Microstructural Changes of Gingko Biloba Seeds During Drying. *Food Bioprocess Technol.* **2019**, *12*, 1041–1051. [CrossRef]
8. Wang, H.; Zhang, M.; Adhikari, B. Drying of shiitake mushroom by combining freeze-drying and mid-infrared radiation. *Food Bioprod. Process.* **2015**, *94*, 507–517. [CrossRef]
9. Krystyjan, M.; Gumul, D.; Areczuk, A.; Khachatryan, G. Comparison of physico-chemical parameters and rheological properties of starch isolated from coloured potatoes (*Solanum tuberosum* L.) and yellow potatoes. *Food Hydrocoll.* **2022**, *131*, 107829. [CrossRef]
10. Yang, S.; Dhital, S.; Zhang, M.; Wang, J.; Chen, Z. Structural, gelatinization, and rheological properties of heat-moisture treated potato starch with added salt and its application in potato starch noodles. *Food Hydrocoll.* **2022**, *131*, 107802. [CrossRef]
11. Warren, F.J.; Gidley, M.J.; Flanagan, B.M. Infrared Spectroscopy as a Tool to Characterise Starch Ordered Structure—A Joint FTIR–ATR, NMR, XRD and DSC Study. *Carbohydr. Polym.* **2016**, *139*, 35–42. [CrossRef] [PubMed]
12. Zhao, Y.; Wang, X.; Liao, W.; Xu, D.; Liu, G. Study on nutritional quality and volatile aroma compounds of the stir-fried shredded potatoes. *Am. J. Potato Res.* **2022**, *99*, 191–205. [CrossRef]
13. Jansky, S.H. Potato flavor. *Am. J. Potato Res.* **2010**, *87*, 209–217. [CrossRef]
14. Diez-Simon, C.; Mumm, R.; Hall, R.D. Mass spectrometry-based metabolomics of volatiles as a new tool for understanding aroma and flavour chemistry in processed food products. *Metabolomics* **2019**, *15*, 41. [CrossRef] [PubMed]
15. Oruna-Concha, M.; Duckham, S.; Ames, J.M. Comparison of volatile compounds isolated from the skin and flesh of four potato cultivars after baking. *J. Agric. Food Chem.* **2001**, *49*, 2414–2421. [CrossRef] [PubMed]
16. Engel, W.; Bahr, W.; Schieberle, P. Solvent assisted flavour evaporation—A new and versatile technique for the careful and direct isolation of aroma compounds from complex food matrices. *Eur. Food Res. Technol.* **1999**, *209*, 237–241. [CrossRef]
17. Oruna-Concha, M.; Bakker, J.; Ames, J.M. Comparison of the volatile components of two cultivars of potato cooked by boiling, conventional baking and microwave baking. *J. Sci. Food Agr.* **2002**, *82*, 1080–1087. [CrossRef]
18. Xu, D.; Chen, C.; Zhou, F.; Liu, C.; Tian, M.; Zeng, X.; Jiang, A. Vacuum packaging and ascorbic acid synergistically maintain the quality and flavor of fresh-cut potatoes. *LWT-Food Sci. Technol.* **2022**, *163*, 113356. [CrossRef]
19. Hou, F.; Mu, T.; Ma, M.; Blecker, C. Optimization of processing technology using response surface methodology and physico-chemical properties of roasted sweet potato. *Food Chem.* **2019**, *278*, 136–143. [CrossRef]
20. Majcher, M.; Jelen, H.H. Comparison of suitability of SPME, SAFE and SDE methods for isolation of flavor compounds from extruded potato snacks. *J. Food Compos. Anal.* **2009**, *22*, 606–612. [CrossRef]
21. Sarker, M.Z.I.; Yamauchi, H.; Kim, S.J.; Matsumura-Endo, C.; Takigawa, S.; Hashimoto, N. A farinograph study on dough characteristics of mixtures of wheat flour and potato starches from different cultivars. *Food Sci. Technol. Res.* **2008**, *14*, 211–216. [CrossRef]
22. Zhang, W.; Shan, C.; Jiang, H.; Liu, Y.; Zhang, J. Enzymatic Hydrolysis Treatment for Determination of Polysacchrides in Chinese Yam. *Food Sci.* **2009**, *20*, 385–387, (In Chinese with English abstract).
23. Xu, B.; Zhou, S.L.; Miao, W.J.; Dong, Y. Microstructure and pasting characteristics of wheat germ treated by microwave radiation. *Trans. Chin. Soc. Agric. Mach.* **2012**, *43*, 151–157, (In Chinese with English abstract).
24. Bail, S.; Stuebiger, G.; Unterweger, H.; Buchbauer, G.; Krist, S. Characterization of volatile compounds and triacylglycerol profiles of nut oils using SPME-GC-MS and MALDI-TOF-MS. *Eur. J. Lipid Sci. Technol.* **2009**, *111*, 170–182. [CrossRef]

25. Beltran, A.; Ramos, M.; Grane, N.; Martin, M.L.; Garrigos, M.C. Monitoring the oxidation of almond oils by HS-SPME-GC-MS and ATR-FTIR: Application of volatile compounds determination to cultivar authenticity. *Food Chem.* **2011**, *126*, 603–609. [CrossRef]
26. Zhang, K.; Tian, Y.; Liu, C.; Xue, W. Effects of temperature and shear on the structural, thermal and pasting properties of different potato flour. *BMC Chem.* **2020**, *14*, 20. [CrossRef]
27. Hu, H.; Li, S.; Pan, D.; Wang, K.; Qiu, M.; Qiu, Z.; Liu, X.; Zhang, J. The Variation of Rice Quality and Relevant Starch Structure during Long-Term Storage. *Agriculture* **2022**, *12*, 1211. [CrossRef]
28. Schirmer, M.; Jekle, M.; Becker, T. Starch gelatinization and its complexity for analysis. *Starch-Stärke* **2015**, *67*, 30–41. [CrossRef]
29. Zhu, L.; Zhang, Y.; Wu, G.; Qi, X.; Dag, D.; Kong, F.; Zhang, H. Characteristics of pasting properties and morphology changes of rice starch and flour under different heating modes. *Int. J. Biol. Macromol.* **2020**, *149*, 246–255. [CrossRef]
30. Ahmed, M.; Akter, M.S.; Lee, J.C.; Eun, J.B. Encapsulation by spray drying of bioactive components, physicochemical and morphological properties from purple sweet potato. *LWT-Food Sci. Technol.* **2010**, *43*, 1307–1312. [CrossRef]
31. Tian, J.; Zhang, Y. Progress on the effects of pretreatment and drying on quality of potato flour. *Sci. Technol. Food Ind.* **2018**, *39*, 347–351, (In Chinese with English abstract).
32. Bharti, I.; Singh, S.; Saxena, D.C. Exploring the influence of heat moisture treatment on physicochemical, pasting, structural and morphological properties of mango kernel starches from Indian cultivars. *LWT-Food Sci. Technol.* **2019**, *110*, 197–206. [CrossRef]
33. Regina, A.; Kosar, H.B.; Ling, S.; Li, Z.; Rahman, S.; Morell, M. Control of starch branching in barley defined through differential RNAi suppression of starch branching enzyme IIa and IIb. *J. Exp. Bot.* **2010**, *61*, 1469–1482. [CrossRef] [PubMed]
34. Corzo-Ríos, L.J.; Sánchez-Chino, X.M.; Cardador-Martínez, A.; Martínez-Herrera, J.; Jiménez-Martínez, C. Effect of cooking on nutritional and non-nutritional compounds in two species of Phaseolus (*P. vulgaris* and *P. coccineus*) cultivated in Mexico. *Int. J. Gastron. Food Sci.* **2020**, *20*, 100206. [CrossRef]
35. Divekar, M.T.; Karunakaran, C.; Lahlali, R.; Kumar, S.; Chelladurai, V.; Liu, X.; Borondics, F.; Shanmugasundaram, S.; Jayas, D.S. Effect of microwave treatment on the cooking and macronutrient qualities of pulses. *Int. J. Food Prop.* **2017**, *20*, 409–422. [CrossRef]
36. Yadav, A.R.; Guha, M.; Tharanathan, R.N.; Ramteke, R.S. Changes in characteristics of sweet potato flour prepared by different drying techniques. *LWT-Food Sci. Technol.* **2006**, *29*, 20–26. [CrossRef]
37. Shen, C.; Wang, L.; Wang, R.; Luo, X.; Li, Y.; Chen, Z. Influence of drying techniques on the physicochemical properties of potato flours. *Food Ferment Ind.* **2016**, *42*, 117–121. [CrossRef]
38. Wu, Y.; Zhou, J.; Ming, T.; Tang, S.; Bu, H.; Chen, Y.; Jiang, J.; Tian, W.; Su, X. Analysis of volatile components of potato from different habitats by electronic nose and GC-MS. *Food Sci.* **2016**, *37*, 130–136, (In Chinese with English abstract).
39. Tieman, D.; Taylor, M.; Schauer, N.; Fernie, A.R.; Hanson, A.D.; Klee, H.J. Tomato aromatic amino acid decarboxylases participate in synthesis of the flavor volatiles 2-phenylethanol and 2-phenylacetaldehyde. *Proc. National. Acad. Sci. USA* **2006**, *103*, 8287–8292. [CrossRef]
40. Akyol, H.; Riciputi, Y.; Capanoglu, E.; Caboni, M.F.; Verardo, V. Phenolic Compounds in the Potato and Its Byproducts: An Overview. *Int. J. Mol. Sci.* **2016**, *17*, 835. [CrossRef]
41. Tang, Q.; Liu, X.; Chi, J.; Chen, Z.; Li, S.; Yang, C. Effects of different drying methods on quality and volatile components of *Pleurotus eryngii*. *Food Sci.* **2016**, *37*, 25–30, (In Chinese with English abstract).
42. Xu, L.; Yang, L.; Zhang, B. A Study on Starch Etherification with 2-Chloroethanol. *Mat. Rev.* **2007**, *21*, 152–154. (In Chinese with English abstract)
43. Kotsiou, K.; Tasioula-Margari, M. Changes occurring in the volatile composition of Greek virgin olive oils during storage: Oil variety influences stability. *Eur. J. Lipid Sci. Technol.* **2015**, *17*, 514–522. [CrossRef]
44. Li, K.; Yin, Y.; Wang, Q.; Lin, T.; Guo, H. Correlation analysis of volatile flavor components and metabolites among potato varieties. *Sci. Agric. Sin.* **2021**, *54*, 792–803, (In Chinese with English abstract).
45. Iglesias, J.; Medina, I.; Bianchi, F.; Careri, M.; Mangia, A.; Musci, M. Study of the volatile compounds useful for the characterisation of fresh and frozen-thawed cultured gilthead sea bream fish by solid-phase microextraction gas chromatography-mass spectrometry. *Food Chem.* **2009**, *115*, 1473–1478. [CrossRef]
46. Josephson, D.B.; Lindsay, R.C. C4-heptenal: An influential volatile compound in boiled potato flavor. *J. Food Sci.* **1987**, *52*, 328–331. [CrossRef]
47. Pérez, A.G.; Sanz, C.; Olías, R.; Olías, J.M. Lipoxygenase and hydroperoxide lyase activities in ripening strawberry fruits. *J. Agr. Food Chem.* **1999**, *47*, 249–253. [CrossRef]
48. Sanchez-Perez, R.; Jorgensen, K.; Olsen, C.E.; Dicenta, F.; Moller, B.L. Bitterness in almonds. *Plant Physiol.* **2008**, *146*, 1040–1052. [CrossRef]
49. Vazquez-Araujo, L.; Enguix, L.; Verdu, A.; Garcia-Garcia, E.; Carbonell-Barrachina, A.A. Investigation of aromatic compounds in toasted almonds used for the manufacture of turron. *Eur. Food Res. Technol.* **2008**, *227*, 243–254. [CrossRef]
50. Qiao, L.; Wang, H.; Shao, J.; Lu, L.; Tian, J.; Liu, X. A novel mitigator of enzymatic browning-hawthorn leaf extract and its application in the preservation of fresh-cut potatoes. *Food Qual. Saf.* **2021**, *5*, fyab015. [CrossRef]
51. Xu, Z.; Xu, Q.; Wang, S.; Wang, Z.; Zhao, D. Comparison of microstructure and thermodynamic properties of starch from different varieties of potato. *Sci. Technol. Food Ind.* **2014**, *38*, 132–136. (In Chinese with English abstract)

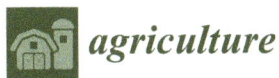

Opinion

Efficacy of Gas-Containing Conditioning Technology on Sterilization and Preservation of Cooked Foods

Dan Li [1,†], Dong Liang [2,†], Zhonghua Li [1], Yang Liu [1], Zhonghua Guo [3], Zhicai Wu [3], Chunping Cao [3], Chunhong Zhang [1,*] and Cunkun Chen [4,*]

1. Navy Special Medical Center, Naval Medical University, Shanghai 200433, China
2. Translational Medicine Research Center, Naval Medical University, Shanghai 200433, China
3. Sichuan Meining Food, Suining 629000, China
4. National Engineering Technology Research Center for Preservation of Agriculture Products, Key Laboratory of Storage of Agricultural Products, Ministry of Agriculture and Rural Affairs, Tianjin Key Laboratory of Postharvest Physiology and Storage of Agricultural Products, Tianjin 300384, China
* Correspondence: z-chunhong@163.com (C.Z.); chencunkun@126.com (C.C.)
† These authors have contributed equally to this work.

Abstract: Gas-containing conditioning technology (GCT) employs mild sterilization methods to preserve the original qualities and nutrients of foods and is particularly suitable for processing various cooked foods or food ingredients. In this study, five kinds of dishes from daily life were processed with GCT. Thermal penetration detection technology was utilized to monitor the internal temperature of food and ambient temperature in real-time, and the optimal scheduled processes of each food were summarized. Additionally, foods were processed after GCT, and the total number of bacteria (<10^2 cfu/g) and coliform colonies (<50 MPN/100 g) were significantly reduced. Moreover, to detect the preservation effect of GCT, the processed foods were stored at 37 °C for 14 days, and the total number of colonies remained low (<10 cfu/g). These results revealed the multistage mild sterilization process, confirmed the excellent sterilization and preservation effects of GCT, and provided important experimental data for further applications of GCT in special environment foods.

Keywords: gas-containing conditioning technology; mild sterilization; scheduled process; preservation

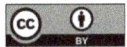

1. Introduction

With the development of social living standards, customers have paid increasing attention to the nutrition and taste of food, resulting in the increasingly strict demand for fresh food preservation. Given the limited, traditional conditions on food processing and preservation, food acceptability is rather poor, with the original odor, flavor, texture and nutrition largely affected [1]. To solve these problems, the international society has newly developed a kind of gas-containing conditioning technology (GCT) for food processing and preservation [2].

GCT indicates a technology applicable to the processing of various convenience foods or semi-finished products preserved at room temperature. It was developed to overcome the shortcomings of traditional sterilization methods, such as vacuum packaging and dry heat sterilization [3]. With this new technology, the original color, flavor, taste, form, and nutrients of cooked foods can be perfectly preserved by using mild sterilization methods, including raw material sterilization treatment, nitrogen-filled packaging, and multi-stage heating without any preservative additives [4,5]. GCT is particularly suitable for processing various cooked foods or food ingredients, such as meat, eggs, vegetables, fruits, and staple foods. The preservation effect can be rather impressive, especially for soft foods and foods for which deoxidizers cannot be used [6]. This technology can be widely applied to traditional food industry processing for further developing new food varieties, expanding the application scope of food processing, and exploiting a new food market [6–8]. Since food products can be stored, transported, and sold at room temperature, the cost of distribution is dramatically reduced [6].

At present, special environment foods mainly consist of canned foods and dried foods, and the canned foods had become the most commonly used food because of the rich nutrition and ready-to-eat feature, which fully satisfy modern emergency needs [9]. However, for persons working in special environments for a long time, the present flavor and taste of canned foods (high salt, high sugar) are not suitable for long-term large consumption. Therefore, developing high-quality, instant food with low salt and few additives as the major daily component of finished foods can be considered an imperative research direction [10,11].

GCT adopts a multi-stage mild sterilization technique, which allows it to preserve food nutrition and original qualities [12]. The biggest difference between the food processed with GCT and traditional dry heat sterilization is the taste after sterilization. One of the main causes is that the latter is subjected excessively to high temperature and pressure [1]. In the processing of food with GCT, the pretreatment of food ingredients should be combined with flavoring and steaming, while the bacterial reduction treatment should be performed simultaneously. Sterilization treatment should be complementary to multi-stage temperature rising, and the optimal sterilization conditions should be set according to the different food materials [13]. Generally, sterilization at a low F-value (generally below 4) can meet commercial sterility requirements, contributing to limiting the temperature and time of food being heated to a minimum, maximizing the changes in the physical properties of the food, and maintaining the original color, aroma, and intact taste of the food [1]. Moreover, GCT uses flexible packaging to substitute traditional tinplate packaging. The former not only improves the acceptability of food but also reaches the same storage period and shelf life of tin cans. Additionally, applications of the flexible packaging technology has largely resolve problems of difficult opening and disposal of waste. Hence, the nitrogen-filled method can be employed to process dry food so as to avoid fat oxidation and extend shelf life. Collectively, these advantages of GCT provide technical support for the safety and nutrition of foods in special environments.

Most of the advanced technology of food sterilization and preservation in the world is based on GCT. A research group headed by Xiong Shanbai, a professor in Food Science and Technology at Huazhong Agricultural University, systematically studied the law of microbial growth and quality. Based on the study of microbial changes and quality during the processing and storage of surimi products, ice temperature preservation and air-controlled preservation technology were combined to establish the related quality evaluation index system and HACCP quality control system for surimi products. Compared with traditional freezing preservation technology, ice temperature and gas-controlled preservation technology can extend the shelf life of food products by 3–4 times. The new method not only extends the shelf life of processed products but also contributes to the better appearance, color, and taste of the processed products. Moreover, a targeted-sterilization technology for the preparation of dishes has been developed in France. The ingredients of the dish are mixed in specific bags and sterilized under vacuum conditions with low-temperature conditioning, which can prevent the negative effects of repeated heat sterilization on the quality of the finished product. The packaging of special collective rations for US ships has been largely improved based on the UGR~H system in the US. The general specifications are for flexible bags, and the bagged rations can be heated directly and have a shelf life up to 18 months. In addition, Chinese chestnuts are characterized by a sweet taste and high quality. Thus, they are well-known around the world and are very popular among Japanese consumers. For the last 200 years, chestnuts from Hebei and other regions have been exported to Japan through the ports of Tianjin. For this reason, the name "Tianjin chestnuts" was formed. At present, "Tianjin Sweet Chestnut" has become a generic term for chestnuts in Japan, and the new chestnuts in small packages containing gas are natural in flavor, preservative-free, long in shelf life, and easy-to-use. They are also a favorite food among consumers in the Chinese mainland, Hong Kong, and Taiwan.

China is currently adapting to building a well-off society in an all-around way, and the food security level and die-tary needs transitioned from simple physiological satisfaction to the pursuit of physiological and psycho-logical satisfaction. Moreover, psychological needs in special environments should be concerned and satisfied.

In the present study, five kinds of food products, including fish fillet in chili sauce, preserved vegetables and pork, fried mixed vegetables, roast pork with bamboo shoots, and stewed bamboo were processed with GCT and evaluated for sterilization and preservation effects. This study will provide experimental support for the widespread application of GCT.

2. Materials and Methods

2.1. Raw Materials, Acceptance, and Bagging

We used bamboo shoots, carrots, kelp, pork, grass carp, dried plum vegetables, vegetable oil, edible salt, white granulated sugar, yellow rice wine, green onion, ginger, star anise, sodium glutamate, soy sauce, monosodium glutamate, and other raw and auxiliary materials. All raw materials and additives were obtained from the qualified suppliers of the company, inspected according to the company's Procurement and Acceptance Standards for Raw and Auxiliary Materials, and stored and used only after passing inspection.

We weighed the ingredients accurately, and tipped them into bags with food bagger. The discharge port of the food bagger should be cleaned regularly so as not to influence the sealing effect. Also notice that the air of bags should be exhausted before seal, then inject nitrogen, and finally heat sealing. Sealing widths were $\geq$8 mm; thermal bonding strengths were $\geq$40 N/15 mm; bag mouths were tight and smooth after sealing. After sealing, the mouth of bags is tight and smooth, and keep the vacuum inside bags. During the production process, visual inspection was conducted every 5 min, and sealing strengths were tested and recorded every 2 h.

2.2. Product Sterilization, Cleaning and Drying

A water bath spray sterilization pot was used. The products were not stacked in multiple, overlapping layers in the sterilization cage to avoid incomplete sterilization. The sterilization process was divided into three stages, and the main parameters (time, temperature, and pressure) of each stage are as follows: stage 1 (100 °C, 10 min, 0.12 Mpa), stage 2 (110 °C, 30 min, 0.15 Mpa) and stage 3 (121 °C, 25 min, 0.18 Mpa).

The sterilized products were transferred to the automatic cleaning and drying production line for cleaning and drying. The dried products were placed in clean turnover boxes or cartons. If the undried products were found, they were dried again. The products should not be over pressed during the packing process

2.3. Product Inspection

The insulation time was 10 d, the insulation temperature was controlled at 37 $\pm$ 2 °C, and records were made. After heat preservation, the samples were tested for quality (color, taste, tissue morphology, taste, and odor), and PH values were detected. We performed microbiological tests and recorded when the PH dropped. We conducted X-ray foreign body detection using a machine on the packaged products one by one to eliminate the products with problems and ensure that the canned products after testing were qualified products. After heat preservation and qualified inspection, the products were packed as required. The entire process was performed exactly as required by the HACCP system.

2.4. Thermal Penetration Detection

Through Sichuan Meining Food Co., Ltd., the horizontal static all-water sterilization pot (Weifang, China, R2020-0111) was used to sterilize five kinds of canned food (fish fillet in chili sauce, preserved vegetables and pork, fried mixed vegetables, roast pork with bamboo shoots, and stewed bamboo), and the wireless temperature verification system (Esbjerg, Denmark, TrackSense Pro) was used to detect the temperature [14]. The net weight of the tested food was 1000 g/bag. The thermal processing of the products was divided into several stages, such as water injection, temperature rise, constant temperature, and cooling. The sterilization process was realized by the automatic control program operation of the sterilization pot. The temperature verification system was used, in which 2 probes (LC11 and LC12) were used to test the ambient temperature in the sterilization pot and the remaining 10 probes were inserted into the centers of the products and placed at the cold point of the sterilization pot to test the center temperature of the products. The above tests were carried out according to the relevant provisions of industry standard SN/T 0400.13-2014 for thermodynamic sterilization.

2.5. Total Colony Determination

The aerobic plate and coliforms count were measured according to the methods of GB 4789.2-2022 Determination of Total Colonies in Food Microbiology Test of National Food Safety Standard and GB 4789.3-2016 Coliform Count in Food Microbiology Test of National Food Safety Standard, respectively. The 25 g sample was weighed and put into 225 mL of sterile normal saline, and the homogenizer was beat twice/s for 1–2 min and then diluted 10-fold to an appropriate dilution. Two petri dishes were made for each dilution and then cultured at 37 °C for 48 h to calculate the total number of aerobic plate and coliforms.

3. Results and Discussion

3.1. Thermal Penetration Detection of Foods

In this study, heat penetration tests were carried out on five kinds of food (1000 g each) in Sichuan Meining Food Co., Ltd., including fish fillet in chili sauce, preserved vegetables and pork, fried mixed vegetables, roast pork with bamboo shoots, and stewed bamboo. According to the detection results, the environmental temperature in the sterilization pot experienced three constant temperature stages [6]: Since the sterilization pot began to time the temperature rise, after 4–6 min in the first phase of constant temperature, all sites reached 103 °C and maintained that for 12 min; after 2 min of heating, the pot entered the second stage of constant temperature, and all points reached above 110.0 °C and maintained that for 31 min; and after 3 min of heating, the three stages of constant temperature were entered, and all points reached above 121.0 °C and maintained that for 20–30 min (Figure 1). Under the above hot working conditions, the F0 value (Standard sterilization time) of the product was less than 10 after the stages of water injection, heating, and cooling. According to the above data and combined with Ball's formula method, we summarized the optimal scheduled processes (Tables S1–S5) to be used as the reference basis for enterprises to set the critical limit values of thermal processing.

3.2. Detection of GCT Sterilization Effect

Five kinds of food were processed with GCT. Table 1 shows the changes of the total number of bacteria and coliform bacteria in the products before and after GCT processing. Before food processing, the total number of bacteria was greater than 10^4 cfu/g, and the coliform colonies were greater than 100 MPN/100 g. After processing, the total number of bacteria ($<10^2$ cfu/g) and coliform colonies (<50 MPN/100 g) were significantly reduced, which fully reached the standard of the total number of food colonies. These results indicate that GCT had an obvious bactericidal effect and could effectively prevent food nutrition destruction and food contamination [13,15].

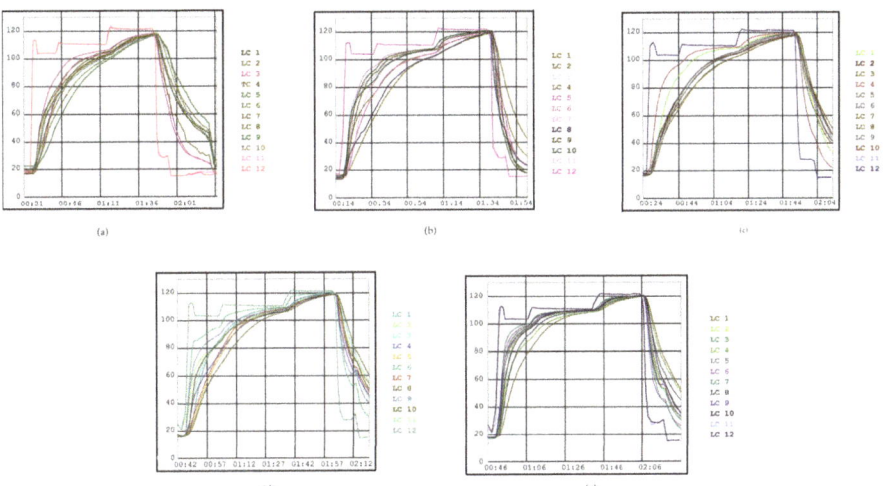

Figure 1. Heat penetration curves of 1 kg/bag of (**a**) fish fillet in chili sauce, (**b**) preserved vegetables and pork, (**c**) fried mixed vegetables, (**d**) roast pork with bamboo shoots, and (**e**) stewed bamboo products in sterilization workshop.

Table 1. Changes in the amount of food bacteria before and after GCT.

Foods	Before GCT		After GCT	
	Total Bacterial Count cfu/g	Coliforms MPN/100 g	Total Bacterial Count cfu/g	Coliforms MPN/100 g
Fish fillet in chili sauce	6.8×10^6	190	$<10^2$	<42
Preserved vegetables and pork	5.3×10^5	170	$<10^2$	<335
Roast pork with bamboo shoots	5.8×10^5	160	$<10^2$	<30
Fried mixed vegetables	4.7×10^5	120	$<10^2$	<30
Stewed bamboo	8.0×10^4	100	$<10^2$	<30

3.3. Detection of GCT Preservation Effect

In order to further test the fresh-keeping ability of GCT, the food was stored at 37 °C for 14 days to detect the viable bacterial count. The results show that the viable bacterial count of each food was less than 10 cfu/g, the F-values were lower than 2, and no potential pathogens, such as *Escherichia coli*, *Staphylococcus aureus*, *Salmonella* and *Clostridium botulinum*, were detected (Table 2). These results suggest that GCT can effectively inhibit the growth of microorganisms and well-control the number of microorganisms during food storage at room temperature.

Table 2. F-values and amounts of bacteria amount in processed foods.

Samples	Weight g	F-Value	Kept at 37 °C for 14 d	
			Viable Count	Facultative Anaerobic Bacteria
Fish fillet in chili sauce	200	1.92	<10	Negative
Preserved vegetables and pork	250	1.83	<10	Negative
Roast pork with bamboo shoots	250	1.70	<10	Negative
Fried mixed vegetables	150	0.91	<10	Negative
Stewed bamboo	150	0.84	<10	Negative

4. Conclusions

In this study, five kinds of dishes (fish fillet in chili sauce, preserved vegetables and pork, fried mixed vegetables, roast pork with bamboo shoots, and stewed bamboo) in daily life were processed with GCT, and the optimal scheduled processes were summarized. Additionally, excellent sterilization and preservation effects of GCT were confirmed by calculating the total number of viable bacteria. The present study provides important experimental data for further applications of GCT in special environment foods.

GCT is a revolutionary technology, completely different from existing preservation methods. It can successfully seal cooked dishes inside a package filled with inert gas, which can perform continuous seasoning and sterilizing for the food. After that, it can be circulated, stored, transported, and sold at room temperature without changing the tastes, colors, and flavors of the ingredients. GCT provides a potential strategy for Chinese cooking to enter an era of standardization, of large-scale and automatic production, and provides new impetus for the development of food deep processing technology [8,13].

Supplementary Materials: The following supporting information can be downloaded at: https://www.mdpi.com/article/10.3390/agriculture12122010/s1, Table S1–S5: Scheduled process of Fish fillet in chili sauce (Table S1), Preserved vegetables & Pork (Table S2), Roast pork with bamboo shoots (Table S3), Fried mixed vegetables (Table S4), and Stewed bamboo (Table S5).

Author Contributions: Conceptualization, D.L. (Dan Li), D.L. (Dong Liang), C.Z., and C.C. (Cunkun Chen); methodology, D.L. (Dan Li) and D.L. (Dong Liang); investigation, D.L. (Dan Li), Z.L., Y.L., Z.G., Z.W., and C.C. (Chunping Cao); resources, D.L. (Dan Li); data curation, D.L. (Dan Li); writing—original draft preparation, D.L. (Dan Li) and D.L. (Dong Liang); writing—review and editing, D.L. (Dong Liang); visualization, D.L. (Dan Li) and D.L. (Dong Liang); supervision, C.Z. and C.C. (Cunkun Chen); pro-ject administration, D.L. (Dan Li), C.Z., and C.C. (Cunkun Chen); funding acquisition, D.L. (Dan Li), C.Z., and C.C. (Cunkun Chen). All authors have read and agreed to the published version of the manuscript.

Funding: This work was funded by Key Laboratory of Storage of Agricultural Products, Ministry of Agriculture and Rural Affairs (kf2022002), Research Projects of National Priority (14A644), Departmental scientific Research Project (20M0603), and 2021 Excellent Construction Project (21TPQN0601).

Institutional Review Board Statement: Not applicable.

Data Availability Statement: Most of the data are available in the tables and figures of the manuscript. If scholars need more specific data, they can send an email to the corresponding author or the first author.

Conflicts of Interest: The authors declare no conflict of interest.

References

1. Guan, Y.Q.; He, M.X. Gas-containing conditioning technology. *Meat Ind.* **2010**, *5*, 8–10.
2. Zhang, H. New gas-containing conditioning technology of processing and preservatio. *Sci. Technol. Food Ind.* **1999**, *20*.
3. Lu, J. Brief analysis of new gas-conditioning conditioning technology. *Cereals Oils Process.* **2002**, *7*, 37–39.
4. Hu, J.Q. *Food Apparatus and Equipment*; China Light Industry Press Ltd.: Beijing, China, 2006; ISBN 7-5019-2436-8.
5. Create fresh, delicious and healthy for life—The application of the new gas-containing conditioning cooking and preservation technology in food processing. *Grain Oil Process. Food Mach.* **2002**, *6*, 25–26.
6. Li, Z.H.; Wang, X.H. Application of new gas-containing conditioning food processing technology in ship food for long voyage. *J. Navy Med.* **2007**, *4*, 330–332.
7. Wang, F. Japan has presented gas-containing conditioning food soft bags. *China New Packag.* **2005**, *1*, 82–83.
8. Zhang, H. New technical gas cooking system. *China Food Ind.* **1998**, *2*, 38–40.
9. Zhang, X.J.; Qian, P.; Yu, J.Y. Effect of new gas cooking sterilization technology on the quality of military soft can. Docking of science and Technology and Industry. In Proceedings of the 10th Annual Meeting of Chinese Society of Food Science and Technology and the Seventh China-US High-level Forum on Food Industry, Nanjing, China, 29 October 2009.
10. Naval Logistics Department Munitions Material Oil Department. *The Latest Development of Foreign Naval Food Support*; China Ocean Press: Beijing, China, 2007; ISBN 7-5027-6736-3.
11. Qian, S. *China Promotes the 21st Century Food Technology*; Packaging; e RAND Corporation: Santa Monica, CA, USA, 2000; Volume 1.

12. Zhang, H. Application of new gas-containing food processing technology in health food safety. In Proceedings of the 4th China International Health Festival Food Nutrition and Safety High-level Forum, Beijing, China, 1 October 2001.
13. Pan, T.T.; Su, G.S.; Zeng, G.X. Study on the production technology of fresh water product of the new gas-containing cooking. *Food Res. Dev.* **2007**, *9*, 97–101.
14. Huang, X.Y.; Han, Y.H. A test method for heat distribution and heat penetration test. *Pharm. Today* **2012**, *22*.
15. Zhang, H. Quality and application prospect of new gas-containing food. *Guangzhou Food Sci. Technol.* **1998**, *14*, 3–8. [CrossRef]

MDPI
St. Alban-Anlage 66
4052 Basel
Switzerland
Tel. +41 61 683 77 34
Fax +41 61 302 89 18
www.mdpi.com

Agriculture Editorial Office
E-mail: agriculture@mdpi.com
www.mdpi.com/journal/agriculture

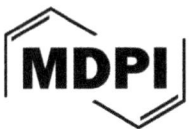

www.ingramcontent.com/pod-product-compliance
Lightning Source LLC
LaVergne TN
LVHW070627100526
838202LV00012B/745